T0344306

Integrating AI in IoT Analytics on the Cloud for Healthcare Applications

D. Jeya Mala
School of CS&IT, Jain University, Bangalore, India

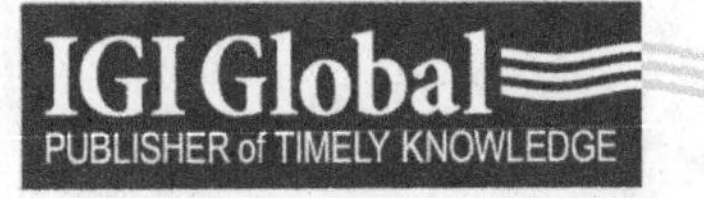

A volume in the Advances in Computational Intelligence and Robotics (ACIR) Book Series

Published in the United States of America by
IGI Global
Engineering Science Reference (an imprint of IGI Global)
701 E. Chocolate Avenue
Hershey PA, USA 17033
Tel: 717-533-8845
Fax: 717-533-8661
E-mail: cust@igi-global.com
Web site: http://www.igi-global.com

Copyright © 2022 by IGI Global. All rights reserved. No part of this publication may be reproduced, stored or distributed in any form or by any means, electronic or mechanical, including photocopying, without written permission from the publisher. Product or company names used in this set are for identification purposes only. Inclusion of the names of the products or companies does not indicate a claim of ownership by IGI Global of the trademark or registered trademark.

Library of Congress Cataloging-in-Publication Data

Names: Jeya Mala, D., 1974- editor.
Title: Integrating AI in IoT analytics on the cloud for healthcare applications / D. Jeya Mala, editor.
Description: Hershey, PA : Engineering Science Reference, [2022] | Includes bibliographical references and index. | Summary: "The objectives of the book are to apply AI in edge analytics for healthcare applications and to analyze the impact of tools, techniques and security solutions in Edge Analytics for Healthcare"-- Provided by publisher.
Identifiers: LCCN 2021035500 (print) | LCCN 2021035501 (ebook) | ISBN 9781799891321 (hardcover) | ISBN 9781799891338 (paperback) | ISBN 9781799891345 (ebook)
Subjects: LCSH: Medical informatics--Technological innovations. | Artificial intelligence--Medical applications. | Data mining.
Classification: LCC R858.A3 I58 2022 (print) | LCC R858.A3 (ebook) | DDC 610.285--dc23
LC record available at https://lccn.loc.gov/2021035500
LC ebook record available at https://lccn.loc.gov/2021035501

This book is published in the IGI Global book series Advances in Computational Intelligence and Robotics (ACIR) (ISSN: 2327-0411; eISSN: 2327-042X)

British Cataloguing in Publication Data
A Cataloguing in Publication record for this book is available from the British Library.

All work contributed to this book is new, previously-unpublished material. The views expressed in this book are those of the authors, but not necessarily of the publisher.

For electronic access to this publication, please contact: eresources@igi-global.com.

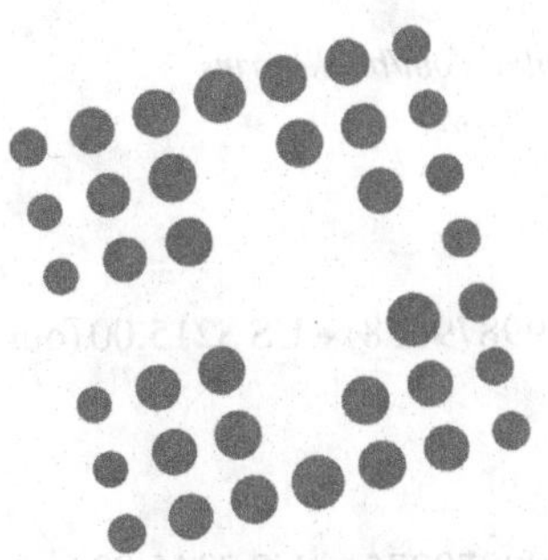

Advances in Computational Intelligence and Robotics (ACIR) Book Series

Ivan Giannoccaro
University of Salento,Italy

ISSN:2327-0411
EISSN:2327-042X

Mission

While intelligence is traditionally a term applied to humans and human cognition, technology has progressed in such a way to allow for the development of intelligent systems able to simulate many human traits. With this new era of simulated and artificial intelligence, much research is needed in order to continue to advance the field and also to evaluate the ethical and societal concerns of the existence of artificial life and machine learning.

The **Advances in Computational Intelligence and Robotics (ACIR) Book Series** encourages scholarly discourse on all topics pertaining to evolutionary computing, artificial life, computational intelligence, machine learning, and robotics. ACIR presents the latest research being conducted on diverse topics in intelligence technologies with the goal of advancing knowledge and applications in this rapidly evolving field.

Coverage

- Fuzzy Systems
- Artificial Intelligence
- Synthetic Emotions
- Computational Logic
- Computer Vision
- Robotics
- Cyborgs
- Algorithmic Learning
- Automated Reasoning
- Neural Networks

IGI Global is currently accepting manuscripts for publication within this series. To submit a proposal for a volume in this series, please contact our Acquisition Editors at Acquisitions@igi-global.com or visit: http://www.igi-global.com/publish/.

The Advances in Computational Intelligence and Robotics (ACIR) Book Series (ISSN 2327-0411) is published by IGI Global, 701 E. Chocolate Avenue, Hershey, PA 17033-1240, USA, www.igi-global.com. This series is composed of titles available for purchase individually; each title is edited to be contextually exclusive from any other title within the series. For pricing and ordering information please visit http://www.igi-global.com/book-series/advances-computational-intelligence-robotics/73674. Postmaster: Send all address changes to above address.
Copyright © 2022 IGI Global. All rights, including translation in other languages reserved by the publisher. No part of this series may be reproduced or used in any form or by any means – graphics, electronic, or mechanical, including photocopying, recording, taping, or information and retrieval systems – without written permission from the publisher, except for non commercial, educational use, including classroom teaching purposes. The views expressed in this series are those of the authors, but not necessarily of IGI Global.

Titles in this Series

For a list of additional titles in this series, please visit: www.igi-global.com/book-series

Socrates Digital™ for Learning and Problem Solving
Mark Salisbury (University of St. Thomas, USA)
Engineering Science Reference • copyright 2022 • 383pp • H/C (ISBN: 9781799879558) • US $215.00 (our price)

Regulatory Aspects of Artificial Intelligence on Blockchain
Pardis Moslemzadeh Tehrani (University of Malaya, Malaysia)
Engineering Science Reference • copyright 2022 • 273pp • H/C (ISBN: 9781799879275) • US $245.00 (our price)

Genetic Algorithms and Applications for Stock Trading Optimization
Vivek Kapoor (Devi Ahilya University, Indore, India) and Shubhamoy Dey (Indian Institute of Management, Indore, India)
Engineering Science Reference • copyright 2021 • 262pp • H/C (ISBN: 9781799841050) • US $225.00 (our price)

Handbook of Research on Innovations and Applications of AI, IoT, and Cognitive Technologies
Jingyuan Zhao (University of Toronto, Canada) and V. Vinoth Kumar (MVJ College of Engineering, India)
Engineering Science Reference • copyright 2021 • 570pp • H/C (ISBN: 9781799868705) • US $325.00 (our price)

Decision Support Systems and Industrial IoT in Smart Grid, Factories, and Cities
Ismail Butun (Chalmers University of Technology, Sweden & Konya Food and Agriculture University, Turkey & Royal University of Technology, Sweden)
Engineering Science Reference • copyright 2021 • 285pp • H/C (ISBN: 9781799874683) • US $245.00 (our price)

Deep Natural Language Processing and AI Applications for Industry 5.0
Poonam Tanwar (Manav Rachna International Institute of Research and Studies, India) Arti Saxena (Manav Rachna International Institute of Research and Studies, India) and C. Priya (Vels Institute of Science, Technology, and Advanced Studies, India)
Engineering Science Reference • copyright 2021 • 240pp • H/C (ISBN: 9781799877288) • US $245.00 (our price)

AI Tools and Electronic Virtual Assistants for Improved Business Performance
Christian Graham (University of Maine, USA)
Business Science Reference • copyright 2021 • 300pp • H/C (ISBN: 9781799838418) • US $245.00 (our price)

Transforming the Internet of Things for Next-Generation Smart Systems
Bhavya Alankar (Jamia Hamdard, India) Harleen Kaur (Hamdard University, India) and Ritu Chauhan (Amity University, India)

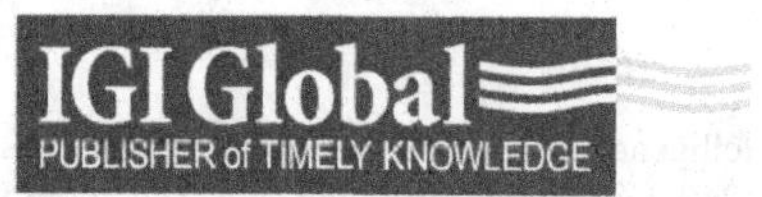

701 East Chocolate Avenue, Hershey, PA 17033, USA
Tel: 717-533-8845 x100 • Fax: 717-533-8661
E-Mail: cust@igi-global.com • www.igi-global.com

Editorial Advisory Board

T. Anathkumar, IFET College of Engineering, India
Micheal Arock, National Institute of Technology, Trichy, India
C. Deisy, Thiagarajar College of Engineering, India
Anto Cordelia Tanislaus Antony Dhanapal, Universiti Tunku Abdul Rahman (Perak Campus), Kampar, Malaysia
S. Geetha, Vellore Institute of Technology, Chennai, India
Ricordo Gonclaves, UNINOVA, Portugal
K.Gopalakrishnan, New Horizon College of Engineering, India
Brij Gupta, National Institute of Technology, Krukshetra, India
C. P. Indhumathy, Anna University (BIT Campus), Trichy, India
Sarika Jain, National Institute of Technology, Krukshetra, India
Vishal Jain, BVICAM, India
P. Mary Jeyanthi, Jaipuria Institute of Management, India
M.N.Nachappa, Jain University, Bangalore, India
Sara Paiva, Instituto Politécnico de Viana do Castelo, Portugal
George Dharma Prakash Raj, Bharathidasan University, India
B. Ramadevi, KITSW, India
Anil Kumar Singh, M. J. P. Rohilkhand University, India
Ranjotha Kumari Swain, Rourkela Institute of Management Studies, India
S. Vidya, Fatima College, Madurai, India

Table of Contents

Chapter 5
Relevance of Artificial Intelligence in Modern Healthcare 67
Dhanabalan Thangam, Acharya Institute of Graduate Studies, India
Anil B. Malali, Acharya Institute of Graduate Studies, India
Gopalakrishanan Subramaniyan, Acharya Institute of Graduate Studies, India
Sudha Mariappan, Acharya Institute of Graduate Studies, India
Sumathy Mohan, Bharathiar University, India
Jin Yong Park, Konkuk University, South Korea

Chapter 6
Secured Healthcare Data Analytics on the Cloud Using Blockchain-Based Techniques 89
Subashini B., Department of Computer Science, Thiagarajar College, Madurai, India

Chapter 7
IoT Security Issues, Challenges, Threats, and Solutions in Healthcare Applications 104
Sudhakar Hallur, KLS Gogte Institute of Technlogy, India
Roopa Kulkarni, Dayanand Sagar Academy of Technology and Management, India
Prashant Patavardhan, RV Institute of Technology and Management, Bengaluru, India
Vishweshkumar Aithal, KLS Gogte Institute of Technology, India

Chapter 8
Edge Analytics With Machine Learning Technique for Medical IoT Applications 131
Jeya Mala D., Jain University, Bangalore, India
Pradeep Reynold A., GEMS Polytechnic College, India

Chapter 9
AI-Based IoT Analytics on the Cloud for Diabetic Data Management System 143
S. V. K. R. Rajeswari, SRM Institute of Science and Technology, India
Vijayakumar Ponnusamy, SRM Institute of Science and Technology, India

Chapter 10
Edge Computing for Secured IoT Analytics on the Cloud 162
S. Meenakshi Sundaram, GSSS Institute of Engineering and Technology for Women, India
Tejaswini R. Murgod, GSSS Institute of Engineering and Technology for Women, India

Chapter 11
Automated Early Prediction of Anomalies Due to Diabetes Using Fundus Images 176
Sharmila Devi Sivakumar, Loyola ICAM College of Engineering and Technology, India
Vaishnavi Seenuvasan, Loyola ICAM College of Engineering and Technology, India
Gunasri B., Loyola ICAM College of Engineering and Technology, India
Balaji Srinivasan, Loyola ICAM College of Engineering and Technology, India

Chapter 12
Internet of Things-Empowered Next-Generation Healthcare Systems 201
J. Manga, Sathyabama Institute of Science and Technology, India
V. J. K. Kishor Sonti, Sathyabama Institute of Science and Technology, India

Detailed Table of Contents

Preface xv

Acknowledgment xxiii

Chapter 1
Virtual Digital Twins: A Renaissance in Precision Nutrition Approach 1
Anto Cordelia Tanislaus Antony Dhanapal, Universiti Tunku Abdul Rahman, Malaysia
Sylvia Subapriya M., Avinashilingam Institute for Home Science and Higher Education for Women, India
Kavitha Subramaniam, Universiti Tunku Abdul Rahman, Malaysia
Mahenderan Appukutty, Universiti Teknologi MARA, Malaysia

Healthy ageing and disease prevention depends on nutritional and lifestyle changes. Available evidence accentuates the influence of genetic, metabolic, and host gut microbiota characteristics on how individuals respond to each nutrient leading the way for the stratification of dietary guidelines. In recent days, state-of-the-art changes are pursued in therapeutic nutrition services integrating information and communication technologies (ICT) such as big data analytics, artificial intelligence (AI), and deep learning. Furthermore, we live in the 'omics' era, where individuals' dietary needs can be tailored according to their gene pattern. Digital twin typifies virtual representation that provides real-time digital technology counterpart of a physical process or object. This chapter discusses how to converge genetic information with other biochemical parameters to conceptualize a digital replica of oneself that may well be a reference tool to guide personalized nutrition.

Chapter 2
Smart Medical Kit in Chronic Kidney Disease Management 24
Pitchumani Angayarkanni Sekaran, Sri Ramachandra Institute of Higher Education and Research, India

Internet of things (IoT)-enabled devices perform remote monitoring of patients and keep them healthy. They also facilitate physicians to provide high-quality care to their patients with accurate data. Chronic disease involves a wide range of health issues like diabetics, asthma, heart disease, kidney disease, and other disorders. To avoid disease progression, the IoT-based smart medical kit helps in episodic patient monitoring, continuous patient monitoring in acute conditions, and patient alarm monitoring. The chapter focuses on the deployment of interconnected devices (sensors, actuators, monitors, detectors, and camera systems) to collect data from heterogeneous systems. The output is connected to a think speak dashboard for monitoring the variation over the period. The smart kit provides more accurate and reliable recommendations to assist patients in controlling their chronic disease and assists in remote monitoring of a patient's health conditions.

As there are several data sets available, this chapter gives insight on which regions of India have been heavily impacted during the first wave of COVID-19 and the classification of patient status using an ML-based data analytics algorithm. The chapter provides a greater insight on the background work and the reports generated based on the analytical results gathered from the data set. In this pandemic situation, such reports will be a great benefit to assess the history of occurrence and the current status of the COVID-19 situation in India.

In low and middle-income countries, people die as a result of unhygienic water quality each year. The proposed method monitors stagnant water quality. Improving sanitation facilities by prior detection of contamination depends on both knowledge and resources (both microbiological and personnel). The proposed method uses Node MCU as core controller and various sensors to monitor the water quality. The micro controller will access the data from different sensors and then processes the data. Once the data is collected, the data is fed into machine learning models, and it is trained using machine learning algorithms (classification - SVM) or neural networks (ANN). Productive decision can be made out of the results from the model. Model will be trained using the parameters such as temperature, dissolved oxygen (D.O.), pH, biochemical oxygen demand (B.O.D), Nitrate-N and Nitrite-N, and fecal coliform. The outcome of the proposed work gives a complete report about contamination in the stagnant water and gives early alert to municipalities for preventing water-borne diseases.

Artificial intelligence (AI) and machine learning (ML) are playing a major role in addressing and understanding better the COVID-19 crisis in recent days. These technologies are simulating human intelligence into the machines and consume large amounts of data for identifying and understanding the patterns and insights quickly than a human and preparing us with new kinds of technologies for preventing and fighting with COVID-19 and other pandemics. It helps a lot to notice the people who got infected by the virus and to forecast the infection rate in the upcoming days with the earlier data. Healthcare and medical sectors are in requirement of advanced technologies for taking accurate decision to manage this

the IoT devices and to be sent to the cloud for further processing and decision making. In life-critical applications such as healthcare, the time taken to send the data to the cloud and then getting back the processed data to take decisions will not be acceptable. Hence, in these kinds of MIoT applications, it is essential to have analytics to be done on the edge in order to avoid such delays. Hence, this chapter is providing an abstract view on the application of machine learning in MIoT so that the data analytics provides fruitful results to the stakeholders.

Chapter 9
AI-Based IoT Analytics on the Cloud for Diabetic Data Management System.................................. 143
S. V. K. R. Rajeswari, SRM Institute of Science and Technology, India
Vijayakumar Ponnusamy, SRM Institute of Science and Technology, India

It is very evident by looking at the current technological advancements that the interrelation and association of artificial intelligence (AI) and IoT in the Cloud have transformed the way healthcare has been working. AI and Cloud-empowered IoT boosts operational efficiency enhanced risk management. This combination creates products and services by enhancing the existing products while increasing scalability. To reduce costs, data analytics on the Cloud is much preferred in the current formation of technologies. This chapter focuses on the integration of different AI techniques in Cloud datasets for IoT data analytics. Analyzing, predicting, and making decisions by comparing the current data with historical data. The theory of AI-based IoT analytics will be much investigated with a healthcare application. Different approaches to implementing data analytics on the Cloud for a diabetic management system will be explored (human body). Finally, future trends and possible areas of research are also discussed.

Chapter 10
Edge Computing for Secured IoT Analytics on the Cloud.. 162
S. Meenakshi Sundaram, GSSS Institute of Engineering and Technology for Women, India
Tejaswini R. Murgod, GSSS Institute of Engineering and Technology for Women, India

This chapter provides an insight into building healthcare applications that are deployed in the cloud storage using edge computing and IoT data analytics approaches. Data is collected from environments both within or external to the hospital. The devices that are connected enable the healthcare providers to monitor patients at large distances, manage chronic disease, and manage medication dosages. The data from these devices can be added to clinical research to gain an insight into the participant's experiences. Artificial intelligence techniques like machine learning or deep learning can be employed at the edge of the networks for IoT analytics of multiple data streams in online mode. The industrial edge computing is growing rapidly from 7% in 2019 to being expected to reach approximately 16% by 2025. The total market for intelligent industrial edge computing that includes hardware, software, services has reached \$11.6B in 2019 and is expected to increase to \$30.8B by 2025.

Chapter 11
Automated Early Prediction of Anomalies Due to Diabetes Using Fundus Images.......................... 176
Sharmila Devi Sivakumar, Loyola ICAM College of Engineering and Technology, India
Vaishnavi Seenuvasan, Loyola ICAM College of Engineering and Technology, India
Gunasri B., Loyola ICAM College of Engineering and Technology, India
Balaji Srinivasan, Loyola ICAM College of Engineering and Technology, India

Diabetes is one of the common diseases in the world that cannot be permanently cured, but with proper medication one can lead a long and healthy life by curbing extreme complications. The skills and equipment required to identify the conditions take a longer time to provide an accurate result and are not an affordable means for all the income groups. In order to overcome this issue, an ML model is created and deployed in an application so it will be used by many in predicting the presence of the disease. The chapter focuses on detecting the presence of two major anomalies, namely diabetic retinopathy (DR) and glaucoma, which were caused due to diabetes. All the dataset used for the project is gathered from Kaggle and Messidor. Around six machine learning algorithms that fall under supervised learning techniques are executed. Among the many models, the random forest model has a high accuracy of 73% for DR prediction. Simultaneously, glaucoma detection is performed using different algorithms showing that Naive Bayes has the highest accuracy of 98%.

Chapter 12
Internet of Things-Empowered Next-Generation Healthcare Systems... 201
J. Manga, Sathyabama Institute of Science and Technology, India
V. J. K. Kishor Sonti, Sathyabama Institute of Science and Technology, India

Internet of things is seen in many fields like civil engineering, consumer goods, oil and gas fields, smart cities, agriculture, etc. Apart from these, it is applicable to the medical field to detect and treat many kinds of diseases and can find the different health parameters quickly. It became important in the health sector to mitigate the challenges of health problems. Internet of things (IoT) is an amalgamation of pervasive computing, intelligent processing, and real-time response systems. Mechanics, devices, sensors make this machine-to-machine communication a feasible solution to dynamic requirements of tech-aspiring world. This chapter highlights the possibilities of further empowerment of healthcare systems using IoT or in other words IoMT (internet of medical things). Nanotechnology-driven IoT development or internet of nano things (IoNT) has become an added advantage in healthcare applications. So, IoNT with IoMT is another exciting research prospect of the near future. This chapter introduces a technique used in healthcare applications, PUF (physical unclonable function), and it is technique for solving many problems related to privacy and security. Security of data transmission, issues pertinent to reliability, and inter-operability are inherently affecting the progress of IoT-based healthcare systems. This chapter of focuses upon these issues and feasible solutions viewed from the dimension of technology-driven healthcare costs in the modern world and economic implications. The treatment used in this chapter will be more interesting for the casual readers. The analysis of IoMT implications in the near future will be helpful to the ardent learners. The research dimensions of IoT-empowered healthcare systems will add value to the thought process of young researchers.

Chapter 13
Information Science in the Analytics of Healthcare Data 219
Sofia Jonathan G., Lady Doak College, Madurai, India

Information science is an interdisciplinary field that deals with the effective collection, storage, retrieval, and use of information for better decision making through related technologies. Today, healthcare organizations are looking for more efficient and sophisticated means of collecting, managing, analyzing data, and delivering medical information to physicians, clinicians, and nurses. The role of information science in the healthcare domain is to improve the quality of patient care, reduce operational cost, and make the entire internal management process well organized for better decision making. Through the application of technology, data analytics and information science practitioners help drive data-informed healthcare decisions. Hence, this chapter covers the techniques that are useful for data analytics and information management in healthcare such as data mining, machine learning, cloud computing, and data visualization.

Chapter 14
Smart Healthcare IoT Applications Using AI 238
Hema D., Lady Doak College, Madurai, India

Globally, healthcare professionals strive to diagnose, monitor, and save human lives. An application that advances the medical field to the next level is the need of the hour. Smart healthcare systems using IoT help in the process of monitoring human health by minimizing human intervention. Taking care and monitoring of human health has a significant contribution in declining the mortality rate as well. IoT in healthcare has aided smarter communications and prompt treatment to save lives. Patient data are sensed by sensors/microcontrollers, sent over the internet, stored in the cloud, and received by healthcare professionals during emergencies. Applications of such smart healthcare using IoT are blood glucose meters, medical vehicles, sphygmomanometer, pulse oximeter, Holter monitor, etc. This chapter elucidates several smart healthcare IoT applications using artificial intelligence and cloud computing technology. The chapter also elaborates the importance and functions of various cloud and AI components in designing a smart healthcare application.

Chapter 15
Futuristic Research Perspectives of IoT Platforms 258
Dhaya R., King Khalid University, Saudi Arabia
Kanthavel R., King Khalid University, Saudi Arabia

Future IoT innovation patterns will assist offices with getting the greatest proficiency and efficiency out of their hardware and assembling parts. IoT is an essential element of digital transformation enterprises in business and industrial sections. Service suppliers and utilities have also been taking on IoT to get pioneering services to keep competitive. Services with security, power management, asset presentation, healthcare effectiveness, and threat and agreement management must be resolved properly in order to enhance the IoT effectively and efficiently. As new tech turns up, hackers prepare to capture the benefits of its potential flaws, and this is precisely why enhancing the precautions of associated strategy is the top IoT technology development. Objectives of this chapter are to analyze and access the future of IoT in healthcare, security, education, and agriculture. This chapter will focus on edge computing, a hybrid approach to process the data that allows connected devices to distribute, compute, examine, and maintain data locally.

Compilation of References 276

About the Contributors 304

Index 310

Preface

As the need for Healthcare Analytics has become the most important part in healthcare industry; several books have provided details about it. This book provides high important research aspects and mechanisms on: how IoT analytics can be combined with AI and ML algorithms, techniques and tools used in healthcare data analytics and so on.

Nowadays, "Data Analytics" is the buzzword that rules the businesses in order to get higher profit in their existing products and predictions on how to improve their business to compete the future market.

However, apart from business analytics, nowadays Healthcare analytics becomes the most crucial area of research as it deals with human life. Due to the current pandemic situations, the researchers are highly focusing on data analytics to predict the impact of some diseases like Corona – Covid 19, analysis on drug discoveries, root cause for certain diseases by analyzing the historical data etc. In these situations, the data patterns need to be analyzed with higher degree of accuracy in order to minimize the uncertainty.

Hence, the term "Data Analytics" not only benefits the business world to improve their profit, it extends its hands to the analytics of healthcare data to provide important predictions and to generate meaningful reports. As the data associated with healthcare domain is voluminous in nature, the analytics needs to be done in higher end platforms rather than the traditional way of data analytics.

Prior to Data Analytics, 'Data analysis' has ruled the World. It has the ability to spot patterns in a set and make predictions about past events' accounts for a large part of its value. 'Data Mining' is the term used to describe the act of finding patterns in data sets in order to better understand trends. Despite the many advantages that data analysis and big data provide, much of its potential is untapped because employees lack quick and reliable access to the information.

In healthcare, especially the diseases have countless variants and the impact of different types of drugs, the regions which are highly affected by a particular disease, periodic occurrences of some of the diseases etc., have played a key role in deciding a novel technical platform to do this data analytics.

In this scenario, the need for cloud computing in data analytics has became the nurturing trend to make data analytics in a faster and efficient manner. As the use of Cloud computing is now ruling the World by its tremendous advantages, naturally the healthcare analytics has also used this as the paradigm shift to provide effective outcomes from it. The consolidation of both analytics and cloud help to store, interpret, and process the big data associated with the healthcare domain to better meet the demands expected from them.

Cloud computing is the term coined around a set of hardware and software that can be accessed through any web browser remotely. Cloud computing is the most important and emerging field in computer science that helps to do analytics in streamlining the business intelligence process. It helps in business decision making by gathering data, integrate them based on the pattern and then processing them using some analytical algorithms.

There are several cloud tools and platforms available for cloud analytics in order to provide relevant reports from huge data generated in a problem domain. Cloud analytics can give an efficient approach to data processing, by providing an organization's decision-makers to quickly access critical business data. This includes having access to various sorts of data as well as data from various sources. Anyone can quickly examine, test, and review data to uncover key insights that help a company to grow.

A cloud-based analytics platform can offer a centralized and secure data access point. A cloud analytics platform also improves data governance by providing more precise access controls to those who have access to what data, as well as auditing capabilities to see who has viewed what data.

Cloud computing offers various types of services such as SaaS, PaaS, IaaS etc. to make the software, platform and infrastructure to be available to anyone on need basis. This ultimately helps reduce the need for dedicated infrastructure setup for an organization.

Data science work is typically comprised of the tasks of working with unstructured data, implementing machine learning (ML) concepts and techniques, and generating insights. Machine learning is a critical element of the process, but training ML models is often a time-consuming process that requires a lot of resources. In the past, gaining access to ML resources was difficult and expensive. Today, many cloud computing vendors offer resources for data science in the cloud.

The crux of machine learning is the application of advanced technology to improve healthcare. Some artificial intelligence applications, such as speech recognition in voice assistants, and personalized online shopping experiences that make use of learning associations, may be familiar to many people. Electronically-stored medical imaging data is plentiful today, and Deep Learning algorithms can be provided with these kinds of datasets, to detect and discover patterns and anomalies.

Different types of data collected from the health care domains such as clinical data, sensor data, Omics data etc., are generally in the raw format and cannot be used as such for getting any insights on these meta-data. For instance, the sensor data is directly collected from the sensors of wearable devices, monitoring devices etc. and Omics data includes genome and proteome data etc. In order to process this meta-data, the Machine Learning algorithms came as a real boon to get relevant insights and to provide analytical reports.

To avoid having medicine or injection shortages in the event of an emergency, pharmaceutical logistics models in particular hospitals can be used to forecast the local demand for the product Especially during the pandemic situation of Covid-19, where there was a huge shortage of vaccines has lead to several chaos in many places of India. In these kind of situations, predictive analytics shall help in properly planning and identifying the worst affected areas and prioritize them to give vaccines.

Target Audience of this book include researchers all over the world working in healthcare domain, data analytics, IoT and AI/ML. Also, this book can be prescribed as a reference book for graduate students to understand the different ways of applying AI/ML, IoT and cloud analytics to the healthcare data to derive useful outcomes. Apart from that, the medical practitioners can also use this book as a baseline to understand the application of AI/ML in healthcare analytics.

In this book, a total of 29 chapter proposals have been received and based on the initial review, 19 chapter proposals have been accepted. Out of the full chapter submissions, only 15 chapters have been accepted after review for final publication in the book. The acceptance percentage rate is 51% which definitely ensures the quality of the book.

DESCRIPTION OF THE CHAPTERS

Chapter 1: Virtual Digital Twins – A Renaissance in Precision Nutrition Approach.

This chapter provides details on Healthy ageing and disease prevention which depends on nutritional and lifestyle changes. Available evidence accentuates the influence of genetic, metabolic and host gut microbiota characteristics on how individual's respond to each nutrient leading way for the stratification of dietary guidelines. In recent days, state-of-the art changes are pursued in therapeutic nutrition services integrating Information and Communication Technology (ICT) such as big data analytics, artificial intelligence (AI) and deep learning. Furthermore, we live in 'omics' era, where individuals' dietary needs can be tailored according to their dietary needs and gene pattern. Digital Twin typifies virtual representation that provides real-time digital technology counterpart of a physical process or object. This chapter discusses about how to converge genetic information other biochemical parameters to conceptualize a digital replica of oneself that may well be a reference tool to guide personalized nutrition.

Chapter 2: Smart Medical Kit in Chronic Kidney Disease Management

This chapter focuses on an Internet of Things (IoT) enabled devices to perform remote monitoring of patients and keep them healthy. It also facilitates physicians to provide high-quality care to their patients with accurate data. Chronic disease involves a wide range of health issues like diabetics, asthma, heart disease, kidney disease, and other disorders. To avoid disease progression, the IoT-based smart medical kit helps in episodic patient monitoring, continuous patient monitoring in acute conditions, and patient alarm monitoring. The chapter focuses on the deployment of interconnected devices (sensors, actuators, monitors, detectors, and camera systems) to collect data from heterogeneous systems The output is connected to a Think speak dashboard for monitoring the variation over the period. The smart kit provides more accurate and reliable recommendations to assist patients in controlling their chronic disease and assists in remote monitoring of a patient's health conditions.

Chapter 3: Application of Machine Learning in Data Analytics on COVID-19 First Wave in India: COVID-19 First Wave Analytics on the Cloud

This chapter deals with Covid-19 first wave analytics. As Covid-19 has impacted the entire world to suffer to the level higher than imagination, it is highly essential to compare the current situation and the first wave's impact in India. As there are several data sets available, this chapter gives an insight on which regions are heavily impacted during the first wave and the classification of patients' status using an ML-based Data analytics algorithm. The chapter provides a greater insight on the background work and the reports generated based on the analytical results gathered from the data set. In this pandemic situation, such kinds of reports will be a great benefit to assess the history of occurrence and the current status of the Covid-19 situation in India.

Chapter 4: An IoT-Based Sanitation Monitoring System Using Machine Learning for Stagnant Water to Prevent Water-Borne Diseases

This chapter gives details on how IoT based sanitation system helps in developing and under developed countries. In low and middle-income countries, over 8,20,000 people die as a result of unhygienic water quality each year. The proposed method monitors stagnant water quality and to improve sanitation facilities by prior detection of contamination depends on both knowledge and resources (both microbiological and personnel). The proposed method uses Node MCU as core controller and various sensors to monitor the water quality. The Micro controller will access the data from different sensors and then processes the data. Once the data is collected, the data is fed into Machine Learning model and it is trained using machine learning algorithms (classification - SVM) or Neural networks (ANN). Productive decision can be made out of the results from the model. Model will be trained using the parameters such as Temperature, Dissolved Oxygen(D.O.), pH, Biochemical Oxygen Demand(B.O.D), Nitrate-N and Nitrite-N and Fecal Coliform. The outcome of the proposed work gives the complete report about the contaminations in the stagnant water and gives early alert to municipal for preventing water-borne diseases.

Chapter 5: Relevance of Artificial Intelligence in Modern Healthcare

This chapter focuses on how AI/ML is used in modern healthcare. Artificial intelligence (AI) and Machine Learning (ML) are playing a major role in addressing and understanding better the Covid-19 crisis in recent days. These technologies are simulating human intelligence into the machines and consume large amounts of data for identifying and understanding the patterns and insights quickly than a human and preparing us with new kinds of technologies for preventing and fighting with Covid-19 and other pandemics. It helps a lot to notice the people who got infected by the virus and to forecast the infection rate in the upcoming days with the earlier data. Healthcare and medical sectors are in requirement of advanced technologies for taking accurate decision to manage this virus spread. AI-enabled technologies are working in a talented way to do things intelligently like human intelligence. Thus the AI-enabled technologies are employed for attaining accurate health results by examining, forecasting, and checking present infected and possibly future cases.

Chapter 6: Secured Healthcare Data Analytics on the Cloud Using Blockchain-Based Technique

In this chapter how blockchain based technique is applied in secured heathcare analytics. Blockchain and the Internet of Things (IoT) are progressive technologies that are changing the world with additional special care within the health care system. In health care, IOT is a remote patient monitoring system that allows IOT devices to collect patient information such as remote monitoring, test results, pharmacy details and medical insurance details etc., and allow doctors to provide excellent care. In order to facilitate data sharing among different hospitals and other organizations, it is necessary to secure data with caution. Block chain is a decentralized, distributed and an immutable digital ledger that records, healthcare transactions using peer-to-peer technology in an extremely secure manner. It uses the cloud environment to store the huge amount of data on health care. The data generated from IOT devices uses Blockchain technology to share medical information being analyzed by health care professionals in different hospitals in a secure manner. The objective is to benefit patient monitoring remotely and overcome the problem of information blocking.

Chapter 7: IoT Security Issues, Challenges, Threats, and Solutions in Healthcare Applications

This chapter discusses about the issues and challenges with threats and solutions in healthcare applications. Majority of the applications now go wireless, involving IoT as a technology to communicate to their respective destination about the status . IoT is considered as a future of Internet. The Internet of Things integration and efficient communication of the patient health monitoring parameters is the need of the hour in this pandemic. This chapter discusses the three-layer architecture involving hardware communication protocols supporting a layer of healthcare services and applications. Also, the data-guarantee, security and integrity issues, threats risks and solutions involving deployment of efficient privacy, control, integration methods to confront various prominent and erroneous data manipulation techniques, malicious and a series of cyber-attacks are proposed. The deployment of various efficient privacy and security protocols in IoT networks is of extreme need to ensure the confidentiality, access-control, authentication and integrity of the health data transferred. Also, to guarantee the availability of the services to the user at any point of time.

Chapter 8: Edge Analytics With Machine Learning Technique for Medical IoT Applications

This chapter focuses on how edge analytics is coupled with ML technique for MIoT applications, Edge analytics are tools and algorithms that are deployed in the internal storage of IoT devices or IoT gateways that collect, process, and analyze the data locally rather than transmitting it to the cloud for analysis. Edge Analytics is applied in a wide range of applications in which immediate decision making is required. In the case of general IoT data analytics on the cloud, the data need to be collected from the IoT devices and to be sent to the cloud for further processing and decision making. In life critical applications such as Healthcare, the time taken to send the data to the cloud and then getting back the processed data to take decisions will not be acceptable. Hence, in these kind of MIoT applications, it is essential to have analytics to be done on the edge in order to avoid such delays. Hence, this chapter is providing an abstract view on the application of Machine Learning in MIoT so that, the data analytics provides fruitful results to the stakeholders.

Chapter 9: AI-Based IoT Analytics on the Cloud for Diabetic Data Management System

This chapter has provided insights on the application of AI based IoT analytics for diabetic data management system. It is very evident by looking at the current technological advancements that the interrelation and association of Artificial Intelligence (AI) and IoT in the Cloud have transformed the way healthcare has been working.AI and cloud empowered IoT boosts operational efficiency enhanced risk management. This combination creates products and services by enhancing the existing products while increasing scalability. To reduce costs, data analytics on the cloud is much preferred in the current formation of technologies. This chapter focuses on the integration of different AI techniques in cloud datasets for IoT data analytics. Analyzing, predicting and making decisions by comparing the current data with historical data . The theory of AI-based IoT analytics will be much investigated with a healthcare application. Different approaches to implementing data analytics on the cloud for a diabetic management system will be explored (human body). Finally, future trends and possible areas of research are also discussed.

Chapter 10: Edge Computing for Secured IoT Analytics on the Cloud

This chapter provides an insight into building health care applications that are deployed in the cloud storage using edge computing and IoT data analytics approaches. Data is collected from environments both within or external to the hospital. The devices that are connected enable the healthcare providers to monitor patients at large distances, manage chronic disease, and manage medication dosages. The data from these devices can be added to clinical research to gain an insight into the participant's experiences. Artificial Intelligence techniques like machine learning or deep learning can be employed at the edge of the networks for IoT analytics of multiple data streams in online mode. The Industrial edge computing is growing rapidly from 7% in 2019 to expected reach approximately to 16% by 2025. The total market for intelligent industrial edge computing that includes hardware, software, services has reached $11.6B in 2019 and is expected to increase to $30.8B by 2025.

Chapter 11: Automated Early Prediction of Anomalies Due to Diabetes Using Fundus Images

Diabetes is one of the common diseases in the world that cannot be permanently cured, but with proper medication one can lead a long and healthy life by curbing extreme complications. The skills and equipment required to identify the conditions take a longer time to provide an accurate result and are not an affordable means for all the income groups. In order to overcome this issue an ML model is created and deployed in an application so it will be used by many in predicting the presence of the disease. Our paper focuses on detecting the presence of two major anomalies namely, Diabetic Retinopathy (DR) and Glaucoma which was caused due to diabetes. All the dataset used for the project is gathered from Kaggle and Messidor. Around six Machine learning algorithms that fall under supervised learning techniques are executed. Among the many models, the Random Forest model has a high accuracy of 73% for DR prediction. Simultaneously Glaucoma detection is performed using different algorithms showing that Naive Bayes has the highest accuracy of 98%.

Chapter 12: Internet of Things-Empowered Next-Generation Healthcare Systems

IoT is diverse in many fields such as civil engineering, consumer goods, oil and gas fields, smart cities, agriculture apart from these it is applicable to medical field. So, it became important in the health sector to mitigate the challenges of health problems. This chapter of the book mainly highlights upon possibilities of further empowerment of healthcare systems using IoT or in other words IoMT (Internet of Medical Things). Internet of Nano Things (IoNT) has become an added advantage in healthcare applications. IoNT with IoMT is another exciting research prospect of near future. This chapter introducing a technique used in health care applications is PUF (Physical unclonable function) and it is a technique for solving many problems related to privacy and security. Italso focuses upon these issues and feasible solutions viewing from the dimension of technology driven health care cost in modern world and economic implications. One such solution is Cognitive IoMT. The applications of these systems in purview of present Covid-19 pandemic is also discussed.

Chapter 13: Information Science in Analytics of Healthcare Data

This chapter gives ideas on how information science is applied in Healthcare Data analytics. Information Science is an interdisciplinary field which deals with the effective collection, storage, retrieval and use of information for better decision making through related technologies. Today, healthcare organizations are looking for more efficient and sophisticated means of collecting, managing, analyzing data and delivering medical information to physicians, clinicians and nurses. The role of Information Science in healthcare domain is to improve the quality of patient care, reduce operational cost and make the entire internal management process well organized for better decision-making. Through the application of Technology, Data analytics and Information Science practitioners help drive data-informed health care decisions. Hence this chapter covers the techniques that are useful for data analytics and information management in healthcare such as Data Mining, Machine Learning, Cloud Computing and Data Visualization.

Chapter 14: Smart Healthcare IoT Applications Using AI

Globally, Healthcare professionals strive hard to diagnose, monitor, and save human lives. An application that advances the medical field to the next level is the need of the hour. Smart Healthcare systems using IoT helps in the process of monitoring human health by minimizing human intervention. Taking care and monitoring of human health has a significant contribution in declining the mortality rate as well. IoT in healthcare has aided smarter communications and prompt treatment to save lives. Patient's data are sensed by sensors/microcontrollers, sent over the internet, stored in the cloud, and received by healthcare professionals during emergencies. Applications of such smart health care using IoT are blood glucose meters, medical vehicles, sphygmomanometer, Pulse oximeter, Holter Monitor, etc. This chapter elucidates several Smart healthcare IoT applications using Artificial Intelligence and Cloud computing technology. The chapter also elaborates the importance and functions of various cloud and AI components in designing a Smart healthcare application.

Chapter 15: Futuristic Research Perspectives of IoT Platforms

This chapter deals with details on Future IoT innovation patterns will assist offices with getting a greatest proficiency and efficiency out of their hardware and assembling parts. IoT has gowned to be an essential element of digital transformation enterprises in business and industrial sections. Service suppliers and utilities have been also taking on IoT revelation to get underway pioneering services to keep on competitive. services with security, power management, asset presentation, health care effectiveness, and threat and agreement management must be resolved properly in order to enhance the IoT effectively and efficiently. As new tech turns up, hackers prepared to capture the benefits of its potential flaw and this is precisely why enhancing the precautions of associated strategy is the top IoT technology developments. objectives of this chapter are to analyze and access the Future of IoT in healthcare, security, education and agriculture. This chapter will focus on Edge computing, a hybrid approach to process the data that allows connected devices to distribute, compute, examine, and maintain data locally.

The book has 15 chapters each of which provides in depth details on the current status of the Healthcare data analytics on the cloud with IoT and AI/ML. Surely, this book shall be an eye opener for several researchers who are working in healthcare domain and also fruitful for the graduate students to get an idea on how they can prepare a proposal in IoT data analytics on the cloud especially for healthcare applications using ML algorithm.

Acknowledgment

At the foremost, I thank the Lord Almighty who lifts up the poor from the dust and the needy from their misery for giving me the wisdom, knowledge and courage to complete this book project as a successful one.

I sincerely acknowledge Fatima College, Madurai, Tamil Nadu, India for providing all the support in making this book project a successful one.

I thank IGI Global Publishers, USA for providing an opportunity to edit a book on "Integrating AI in IoT Analytics on the Cloud for Healthcare Applications" which is a collection of ideas from various authors working in this area.

I thank the authors for their timeless efforts and prompt submissions to make this book a useful one.

I solemnly thank all the Editorial Board Members, Reviewers and institute colleagues for providing all the support for the successful completion and publishing of this book.

This acknowledgement will not be fulfilled without my family; I thank my family members for rendering their support and patience in the success of this project.

Chapter 1
Virtual Digital Twins: A Renaissance in Precision Nutrition Approach

Anto Cordelia Tanislaus Antony Dhanapal
https://orcid.org/0000-0002-7136-9310
Universiti Tunku Abdul Rahman, Malaysia

Sylvia Subapriya M.
Avinashilingam Institute for Home Science and Higher Education for Women, India

Kavitha Subramaniam
Universiti Tunku Abdul Rahman, Malaysia

Mahenderan Appukutty
Universiti Teknologi MARA, Malaysia

ABSTRACT

Healthy ageing and disease prevention depends on nutritional and lifestyle changes. Available evidence accentuates the influence of genetic, metabolic, and host gut microbiota characteristics on how individuals respond to each nutrient leading the way for the stratification of dietary guidelines. In recent days, state-of-the-art changes are pursued in therapeutic nutrition services integrating information and communication technologies (ICT) such as big data analytics, artificial intelligence (AI), and deep learning. Furthermore, we live in the 'omics' era, where individuals' dietary needs can be tailored according to their gene pattern. Digital twin typifies virtual representation that provides real-time digital technology counterpart of a physical process or object. This chapter discusses how to converge genetic information with other biochemical parameters to conceptualize a digital replica of oneself that may well be a reference tool to guide personalized nutrition.

DOI: 10.4018/978-1-7998-9132-1.ch001

Copyright © 2022, IGI Global. Copying or distributing in print or electronic forms without written permission of IGI Global is prohibited.

INTRODUCTION

Precision Nutrition: A New Face Lift to Dietary Approaches

Nutritional Science is facing a rapid transformation in this "omics" era ever since the completion of Human Genome project in 2003. The past and current dietary guidelines originally based on population requirement is slowly being replaced by tailored diets that fits individual requirements based on gene pattern, dietary intake, food behavior, physical activity, environmental factors, and stressors. Precision nutrition (PN) is the fulcrum that bonds precision medicine, precision health and precision prevention together (Kirk et.al., 2021)

PN typifies a therapeutic model that proffers tailored diet, with better nutritional outcomes, dietary behavior or food products customized to fit the nutritional needs of the individual. This therapeutic model encompasses the selection of pertinent nutritional components that reckon on biochemical markers, genesiology or other cellular and molecular test results. Examples include selecting specially formulated anti-diabetic, anti-inflammatory foods with great importance to immune-boosting supplements (Myung, 2012), foods rich in omega-3 fatty acids for individuals with poor omega-3 index (Minihane et.al., 2016), recommending zinc and phytonutrients to prevent macular degeneration with evidence based genetic data (Rojas-Fernandez & Tyber, 2016).

PN thus offers set of dietary interventions that are reliable, effortless (Özdemir & Kolker, 2016), applicable, uncomplicated, and straight forward to avert disease and repress morbidity (Fuellen et al., 2015). Functional foods and nutraceuticals are, next to physical workout, the unassailable interventions apprehensible. Tailored to precision, biomarker-combined nutritional interventions are blueprinted as "just fit for you". With immensity of compliance, majority of dietary interventions are reputable, tested, and proven, along with positive results backed by observational studies, making these personalized diet modifications affordable and accessible.

Virtual Digital Twin - Definition

A digital twin is a virtual depiction of a physical object or the organization of a system that can stretch its life cycle which is interminably fed with real-time data, employing simulation, machine learning and artificial intelligence to prognosticate the subsequent events of their corresponding physical counterpart. In simple terms, it is the conceptualization of a highly complex identical digital version (twin) of a physical object (thing). This replication of physical object helps in decision making (Gkouskou et al., 2020). This computational technology is set to transform the healthcare system in a multitude way starting from diagnosis, disease treatment, follow-up, streamlining preventive measure and promoting new approaches for planning and implementation of health care facilities.

Integrating Virtual Digital Technology in Precision Nutrition

Precision nutrition, as an integral part of precision medicine is also gaining equal attention especially during physical examinations. The main focus of precision nutrition is to offer a protective and decisive intervention techniques to control and manage disorders and diseases with due consideration to gene pattern, lifestyle behavior (dietary intake, physical activity and other lifestyle choices like smoking, alcohol consumption etc.) their metabolic condition, gut microbiota and physiological state (nutritional status and disease status) of individuals. The three main core components to be given due consideration in precision nutrition is depicted in Figure 1.

In clinical medicine it is believed that many inborn and chronic metabolic diseases can be prevented and effectively controlled using precision nutritional management. This requires artificial intelligence (AI) and deep-learning techniques to generate customized dietary recommendation and algorithms to address these diet-related chronic diseases. Since there exists a difference in lifestyle, food intake, genetic factors, and environmental exposures between individuals in a healthy population, precision nutrition can help to promote physical activity and thereby ameliorate disease risk (Sak & Suchodolska, 2021).

Machine Learning can be introduced into Precision Nutrition research for better performance. Incorporating Machine Learning into their assessment and evaluation methods can facilitate the amalgamation of many complex processes, making way for the advancement of novel high-performance Precision Nutrition approaches (kirk et.al., 2021). Advanced machine-learning (ML) techniques will be dominating the future generation of personalized medicine, both at clinical and genomic levels.

Constructing a Biologically Detailed Digital Remodelling in Precision Nutrition

A digital twin is far more advanced than a digital model. This disparity is trapped by the word 'living' in the definition above which reiterates that a digital twin is akin to the real-life counterpart than a mere model is not (Kritzinger et al., 2018). The continuous remodelling of the twin to the real-life counterpart is driven by various technologies such as biochemical sensors, high-speed communication, cloud computing, artificial intelligence, and deep learning (Raden, 2020). The digital twin can therefore be claimed as a technological cocktail. Recently the digital twins have been acclaimed the "ten most stra-

Figure 1. Core components to be considered in precision nutrition

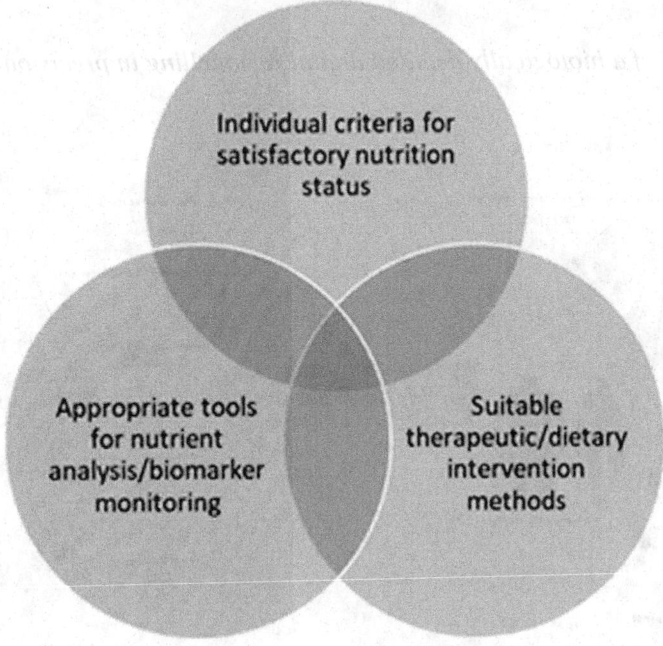

tegic emerging concepts for the near future" and it is estimated that this technology will lead to invest $10.96 billion in 2022 (Digital twins: Advantages & issues of a powerful emerging technology', n.d.)

In precision nutrition to configure a biological digital model for diet-related non-communicable disease, simulation models for diagnosis and intervention, an integrated approach using the 'omics': metabolomics, biomics, genomics, proteomics and lipidomics along with physical markers, environment exposure, demographic, and lifestyle data across the life span of an individual, in-silico approaches in drug delivery ('organ -on-a-chip') and clinical trials (Shugalo, 2019) should be considered.

Integrating Artificial Intelligence in Digital Twins for Precision Nutrition

Artificial intelligence (AI), under the umbrella of computer science, mimics thought processes, initiate learning abilities and advocates knowledge management, with a dearth to invent numerous applications in empirical and precision medicine. The last two decades saw the evolution of AI application in precision medicine and its component precision nutrition. AI application dominated medical diagnostics, predicting disease susceptibility, and supported therapeutic techniques. The introduction of AI gave nutrient research a whole new dimension and assisted with diet related non-communicable disease technology (Heydarian et al., 2019).

Artificial Neural Networks (ANN) in the Field of AI

ANN which imitates the natural neurons of human brain is the most widely used modelling technique in AI field. ANNs are mathematically designed models created to align and calculate input signals received from chains of processing elements, called artificial neurons, interconnected through artificial synapses. They constitute three types of layers: The input layer which receives and relays the raw data to the hidden layer. The second layer is connected to learning process and the third layer performs all analysis received

Figure 2. Construction of a biologically detailed digital remodelling in precision nutrition

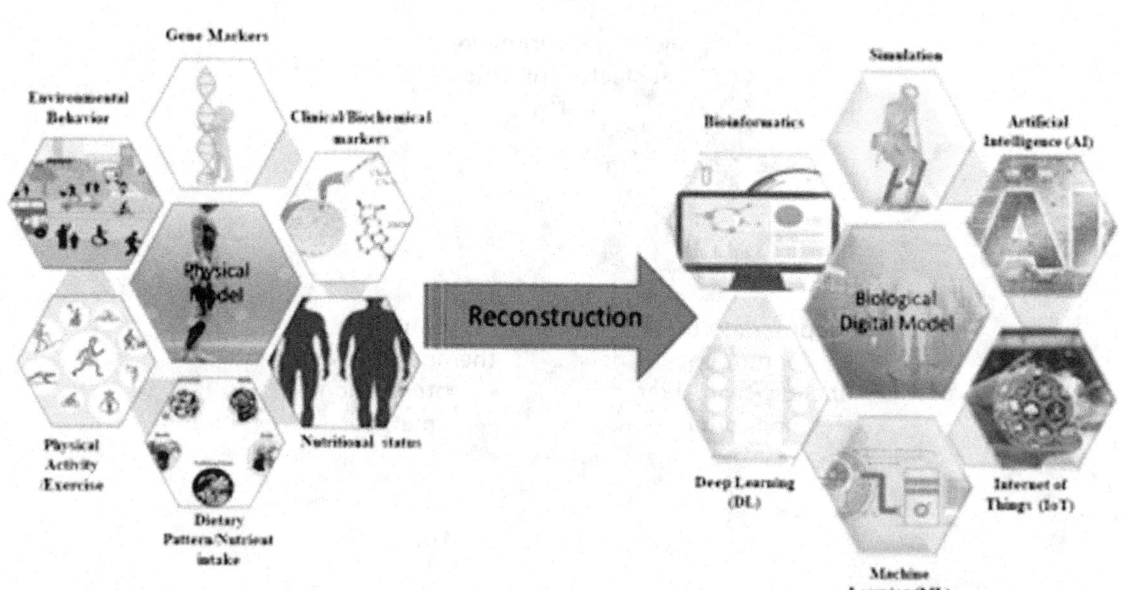

at the output layer and generates output data. A neural network is a parameterized system, composed of hundreds of single units where weights are considered as adjustable parameters. ANNs requires large training sets to estimate these parameters. It detects pattern not using programming but through experience. It is preferred when there is a requirement for modelling datasets with non-linear dependent variables. Both literature and experimental data can be used to analyse nutritional biomarkers. It was one of the profound techniques to design an experimental decision algorithm model to evaluate biochemical parameters confronted with clinical and reference values (Demirci et al., 2016). ANN was used to create prediction model in a Mediterranean study to explain the complex relationship between dietary, clinical, and cognitive functions (Gallucci et al., 2019). It was also used to analyse body composition with clearly non-linear characteristics (Cui et al., 2010). It can be of help in clinical dietetics to create predictive models that assist in interventions. Fuzzy logic methodology (FLM) combined with ANN can produce break-through techniques which can result in greater accuracy, dimensionality, and simplified structure. Feasibility to develop a creative fuzzy neural network and turn them into FLM-based models in neural networks is in progress.

Integration of Machine Learning (ML) in Digital Twins

Machine Learning is connected to algorithms that have potential to build simulation models to be involved in decision making constructed using large sets of training data without programming. This branch of AI has significant operations in biomedical, clinical as well as nutritional sciences. ML can be applied in health care to develop risk models and predictive models. The ML algorithms train and learn from the past data and produce predictive models with very high accuracy (Deo, 2020; Rajkomar et al., 2019)

It is envisaged that ML will dominate computer-assisted diagnostics, biomedical research, and personalized medicine in the near (Handelman et al., 2018). ML techniques have set foot in diabetes research as well by predicting blood glucose as well as creating a model of artificial pancreas to predict its function (Woldaregay et al., 2019).

The large data sets available from gut microbiota studies also seeks the application of ML algorithms (Danneskiold-Samsøe et al., 2019). Liu et al., (2020) reported that an ML algorithm integrated to baseline microbial signatures sampled from gut microbiota can be a better predictor of glycaemic response in relation to physical activity in the patient.

Deep learning (DL) is a subclass of ML, and an integral part of AI domain is enroute to image and voice recognition. DL is used in medical diagnostics in assembling sets of features used in recognition.

Internet of Things (IoT) in Digital Twins

The concept of IoT is that objects (devices) can generate, mine, or exchange data directly or indirectly through a computer network or an intelligent electrical installation. Internet of Everything (IoE) is used to explain a network of people, methods, data, and objects that are in conjunction with Internet. In clinical nutrition, IoT finds significant use in relation to telemedicine procedures (Olivia Li et al., (2020); Sadoughi et al., (2020), that finds wide usage lately especially during the COVID-19 pandemic. One of the key applications of IoT is to provide detailed description of food products available on the market (Jæger & Mishra, 2020).

'Omics' Data Sets in Constructing a Digital Model

Latest introduction of modern high throughput 'omics' technology serves to elucidate the connections that exist between dietary exposure and disease risk at the genetic level (Yu et al., 2014). The comprehensive 'omics' approach centres around the four explicit pathways namely genomics, transcriptomics, proteomics, and metabolomics that redefine nutritional science. They introspectively deduce the whole set of molecular data present in a cell tissue or the organism as a whole which includes DNA, RNA, proteins, and metabolites (Devika & Raman, 2019). The beginning of 21st century marked the emergence of high-throughput technologies, superior quality data, single-cell approaches, micro-array techniques, mass spectrometry, simulation, bioinformatics, and cloud computing technologies. These assessment tools are highly practised to study molecular events that address the impacts of nutritional chemicals in diet-related diseases (Shima et al., 2017).

Genomics probes the genes response under different conditions that utilizes various technologies to scrutinize vast nucleotide sequences, genes, and proteins (DeBusk, 2010). Nutrigenomics examines how common nutrients (i.e., macronutrients, micronutrients and antinutrients) can influence nutritional status and disease state by modifying the gene expression or altering genetic genome, transcriptome, proteome, and metabolome (Kaput & Rodriguez, 2004). In contrary, nutrigenetics addresses how the genetic variation respond differently to different nutrients. Next generation sequencing (NGS), or 'second-generation sequencing', enables to read the code of large numbers of DNA or RNA small fragments in line, with rapid and superior sequencing at reduced costs. Clubbing together NGS and genome-wide integral research could identify novel genomic variants to understand complex disease pathobiology and unlock the effects of nutrient exposure and genetic variants in individuals. In the postgenomic era 'omics' data sets (genomics, transcriptomics, proteomics, and metabolomics) are combined with computational bioinformatics and chemometrics to effectively manage and express them as a complex data configuration known as "functional genomics" or "system biology" (Ordovas et al., 2018). The concept of nutrition-metabolism virtual model stems from systems biology that laid the foundation for the modern gene-nutrient interaction, to concurrently estimate a sizable fraction of all regulated genes and metabolites (Wang & Hu, 2018). The data generated helps to identify and characterize gene variants which helps to propose a unique and specific diet recommendation tailored to meet the individual's dietary requirements termed as 'personalized nutrition' (Zeevi et al., 2015; Berry et al., 2020).

The limitations in epidemiological research with gene variants affecting the metabolism of nutrients or bioactive components from a food source can be overcome by introducing genetic polymorphisms into nutritional epidemiological studies (Noecker & Borenstein, 2016). NGS and omics-driven readouts related to nutrigenetics, can generate crucially significant information that can complement data sets to support physicians in recommending the preventive diet tailored to meet the requirements of the patients (Tachibana, 2015).

Transcriptomics studies are now a normal routine with the advancement of Real -Time -PCR and Robust microarrays. RNA sequencing has replaced transcriptome investigation as they possess the ability to sequence a broad spectrum of RNAs with very detailed information ((Liu & Qian, 2011; Zhao et al., 2014; Midha et al., 2019). Transcriptomics profiling allows to analyse for a specific nutritional condition, by providing a more comprehensive visualization of intracellular RNA expression (Slatko et al., (2018); Gong et al., 2019). Nutri-miromics probes the effect of diet on gene expression as an outcome of microRNAs (miRNAs). epigenetic processes which further indicates the risk for chronic diseases (Bronze-da-Rocha, 2014).

Nutritional epigenomics aims to assess the action of nutrients and bioactive components that regulate gene activity and expression through global epigenetic mechanisms that encompasses DNA methylation, modification in histone function, remodelling chromatin structures, and noncoding RNAs. The pathogenesis of several disease those including auto immune disorders have been associated to epigenetic modulations (Kura et al., (2019); Kraft & Kurth, 2019). Nutritional-epigenomics backed by novel technologies has transpired as an up-and-coming approach in the field of nutritional research and for precision nutrition (Oikonomopoulos et al., 2020). In recent years, novel and high-throughput technologies that sequence longer strands of nucleic acids by reading single DNA or RNA molecules have emerged as the most sought-after technologies (Sarda & Hannenhalli, 2014). These new technologies, defined as 'third generation sequencing', along with advanced bioinformatics tools and single-cell sequencing, will acquiesce to decipher human genome, transcriptome, microbiome, and epigenome to a greater aquity (Giacconi et al., 2019). The influence of dietary interventions on human microbiome has been successfully applied in nutritional sciences (Brandt et al., 2019).

Metabolomics aims to study the metabolome which includes the full metabolites set of biological samples. Metabolomic studies employs Nuclear Magnetic Resonance (NMR), Proton Nuclear Magnetic Resonance (1HNMR) Spectroscopy, and Mass Spectrometry (MS) as prime technologies. The advancement in these precision technologies, (Matrix-Assisted Laser Desorption Ionization Time of Flight (MALDI-TOF), Secondary Ion Mass Spectrometry (SIMS), and Fourier transform ion cyclotron resonance MS), for elucidation and compound identification (van Dijk et al., 2018) have launched greater opportunities to extensively apply both quantitative and non-invasive methods for metabolites that responds differently to food. Nutritional metabolomics serves to be the most sensitive method for deducing biochemical pathways (Singh, 2020). Also, it helps to assess metabolite profiles regarding specific nutrient intake (McGee et al., 2019) and different metabolic perturbations were identified.

Dietary biomarkers are a new complementary tool that replace the conventional approach in nutrition studies. More recently, metabolomics has emerged as a significant approach to screen new dietary biomarkers (Raiten et al., 2011). On the other hand, proteomics involves, high-throughput technique at large scale to decipher the expression, elucidate structure, analyse function, check modifications, and probe the interaction of proteins, present in a biological sample. The techniques followed in proteomic studies are microarray-based tools, mass-spectrometry, NMR, modern single-cell, and high-sensitivity protein analyses (de Vries et al., 2013). Since birth, humans co-inhabit and interact with trillions of microbes known as human microbiota, living in most body surfaces and cavities. Advancement in 'omics' and computational data sciences have taken the lead in investigating the microbiota's role in human health and disease.

Microbiomics is a fast-growing area of omics science wherein the microbiota of a specific community like the host gut microbiota are examined together, enhancing 'omics' application and technologies. The exponential growth of sequencing technologies accounts for novel strain-level findings attained by establishing a causal relationship between gut microbiota, nutrient, and human (Picó et al., 2019). Nutritional microbiomics and metabolomics studies ensure promising discoveries of metabolic pathways that are attached to disease processes. Hence Nutritional microbiomics can be considered a novel approach to investigate interrelationships that prevail between gut microbiota and diet and the necessity of bridging these linkages for preventive medicine (Palou M., Torrens J.M., Castillo P., Sánchez J., Palou A., Picó C. 2019).

Nutritional Biomarkers in Precision Nutrition

There arises a need for analytical determinants to measure the nutritional status of an individual objectively and quantify more precisely. Nutritional biomarkers extend a greater proximal assessment of nutrient status than dietary intake. It is a compound that can be quantified in different biological samples which serve as a reliable indicator of nutritional status with reference to dietary intake or the way the dietary chemicals are metabolised (Potischman, 2003).

In PN, dietary biomarkers are considered as the pillar of research that bridges the gap between functional aspects of nutrition to disease-health attributes. Due to the complexity of relationship that persist between dietary intake and health/disease status, it is essential to have in-depth understanding of integrative nutritional biomarker pertaining to the nutritional status and health, by shifting focus on nutritionally regulated biomarkers. This underlines the concept that food intake is not only quantified in terms of consumption but also measures the elicited biological response. For example, the circulating lipid profiles not only indicate intake but also genotype and health status (Gomez-Delgado et al., 2014). A modification in specific protein may also trigger a physiological response that reflects food intake. The development of such a new type of nutritional biomarker with an integrative trait, explains the close relationship between nutrition and metabolism (Ramos-Lopez et al., 2017).

The fact that nutrition and metabolism are interconnected turns to be an advantage rather than a disruption or a source of variation when it comes to integrative nutritional biomarkers. They may be designated by a single, or a set of parameters linked directly. When combined with integrating algorithm, each represent a specific aspect of metabolism, nutrient exposure, and availability (Elmadfa & Meyer, 2010). These analytical indicators could be quantified and can act as an intake indicator (short or long term) and/or denoting the status of a specific nutrient or food component and their impact on the body. In addition, they can be utilized to accurately measure the food intake, help to validate, or support the existing food intake questionnaires, explains the physiological or pathological reactions to certain food behaviours, follow-up with therapeutic and nutritional recommendations for a more personalised health care and inform us on inter-individual differences in action to the prescribed diet (Thompson et al., 2010).

Furthermore, these biomarkers can assist in tailored nutritional recommendations for optimal health based on phenotypes and genotypes (Corella & Ordovás, 2012). The inter-individual differences that originate from genetic basis which are associated with concrete polymorphisms or on epigenetic basis and relate to the genotype, exhibit different response on exposure to environmental characteristics (including diet) that span across their life. Thus, the understanding of nutritional biomarkers follow a holistic approach to be applied in precision nutrition (Figure 3). Therefore, biomarkers explain the impact of nutrient intake or deficiency and can also be used as an intermediate biomarker which highlights the potential risk of developing a pathology accompanied by an excess or deficient nutrient it belongs to.

Dietary Intake Measurement – Traditional vs. Novel Assessment Methods

The diet history is the record of the patient's food habits and choices, cultural and religious food practices, special diets for specific health condition, food allergies and intolerances. It is necessary to record their fluid as well as alcohol consumption (Figure 4).

Collecting quantitative food intake data is by far the best approaches to evaluate nutritional risk at individual levels. The protein and energy nutrition along with energy balance (energy intake and energy output) emulate the present nutrition status whether they are at positive or negative energy balance. There

Figure 3. Omics integrated nutritional biomarkers in precision nutrition

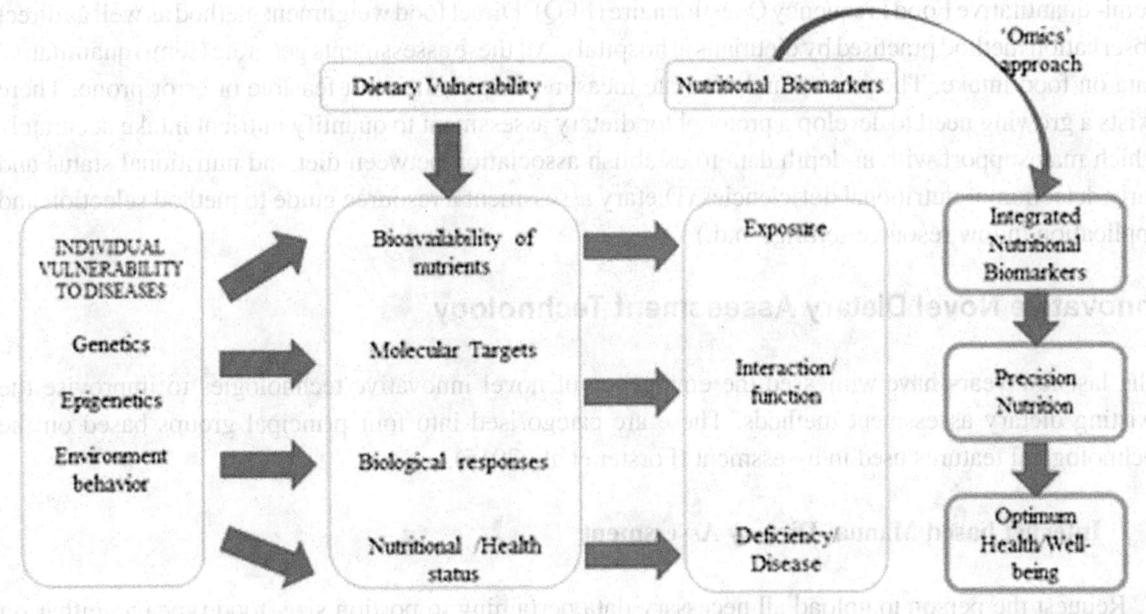

Figure 4. Components of dietary history

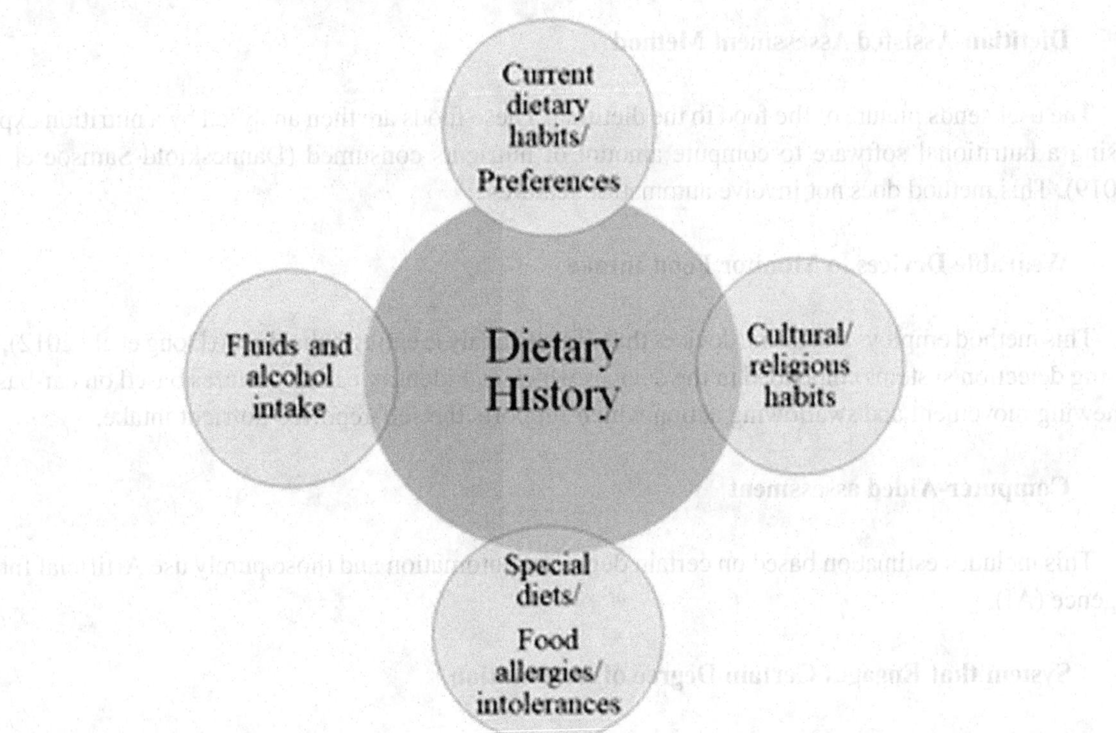

are numerous standard procedures to measure the food intake namely 24-hour dietary recall method, Semi- quantitative Food Frequency Questionnaire (FFQ), Direct food weighment method as well as direct observation method practised by dietitians at hospitals. All these assessments generate (semi) quantitative data on food intake. The precise and accurate measurement is often not feasible or error prone. There exists a growing need to develop a protocol for dietary assessment to quantify nutrient intake accurately which may support with in-depth data to establish association between diet and nutritional status and early detection of nutritional deficiencies (Dietary assessment a resource guide to method selection and application in low resource settings, n.d.)

Innovative Novel Dietary Assessment Technology

The last few years have witnessed the emergence of novel innovative technologies to improvise the existing dietary assessment methods. These are categorised into four principal groups based on the technological features used in assessment (Forster et al., 2015).

- **Internet based Manual Dietary Assessment**

Request the person to upload all necessary data pertaining to portion size, food type etc. either on a webpage or on a smartphone app (Archundia Herrera & Chan, 2018). This assessment uses photos, texts or voice recordings which transforms paper based dietary assessment into an electronic format and does not engage automatic features.

- **Dietitian-Assisted Assessment Method**

The user sends picture of the food to the dietitian. These foods are then analysed by a nutrition expert using a nutritional software to compute amount of nutrients consumed (Danneskiold-Samsøe et al., 2019). This method does not involve automation features.

- **Wearable Devices to Monitor Food Intake**

This method employs electronic devices that directly analyse eating behaviour ((Dong et al., 2012), by using detection systems embedded in the devices which can identify eating gestures based on ear-based chewing movement and swallowing action which supports the self-reported nutrient intake.

- **Computer-Aided assessment**

This includes estimation based on certain degree of automation and those purely use Artificial Intelligence (AI).

- **System that Engages Certain Degree of Automation.**

This system uses bar-code readers to read packaged food labels automatically (Archundia Herrera & Chan, 2018) or use an automatic recognition of food items on a smartphone app. Here again, the user will feed the system with images of food consumed for it to recognize the type of food. The volume/

portion of the food items is sent to the system for it to translate the perceived data into macronutrients amounts and energy (Kawano & Yanai, 2014).

- **System Based on Artificial Intelligence (AI).**

In this method, the food he consumes is captured and sent to the system in turn automatically recognise them and in real-time, identifies the various food items the type of each of them and generate a 3D model of each of them (Identification, labelling and 3D construction) (Bally et al., (2016); Dehais et al., (2017); Rhyner et al., (2016); Vasiloglou et al., 2018). Then with the support of food composition databases, the system then converts the food images to nutrient values (Bally et al., 2016)

Comparisons between the traditional and innovative dietary assessment technologies have been reported by various researchers from time to time. Some of the studies supported the use of electronic records stating that it could be a best alternative to traditional methods that are time consuming and can be a better tool for studies involving both large-scale epidemiological research as well as relevant to individuals in a clinical setting (Ambrosini et al., 2018). Others suggested that the apps could be a better replacement for 24-h dietary recall method and utilized as a more feasible tool field investigators and dietitians (Bucher Della Torre et al., 2017). They conclude that the longer the app recording time, the better is the output in terms of correlation between the traditional and new methods (Recio-Rodriguez et al., 2019). However, shortcomings in terms of small-sample sizes and short duration employed in most of the studies that used innovative technologies make them inconclusive. Hence there arise a need for well-designed longitudinal studies that involve large population to further explore the combination of using both traditional and novel technological tools which can transform the current dietary assessment methods.

Mobile applications using Ai are gaining popularity in the field of nutritional prophylaxis. The electronic photographic image processing to measure portion size was proposed by Sun et al., (2010).

Figure 5. Components of novel innovative dietary assessment technologies

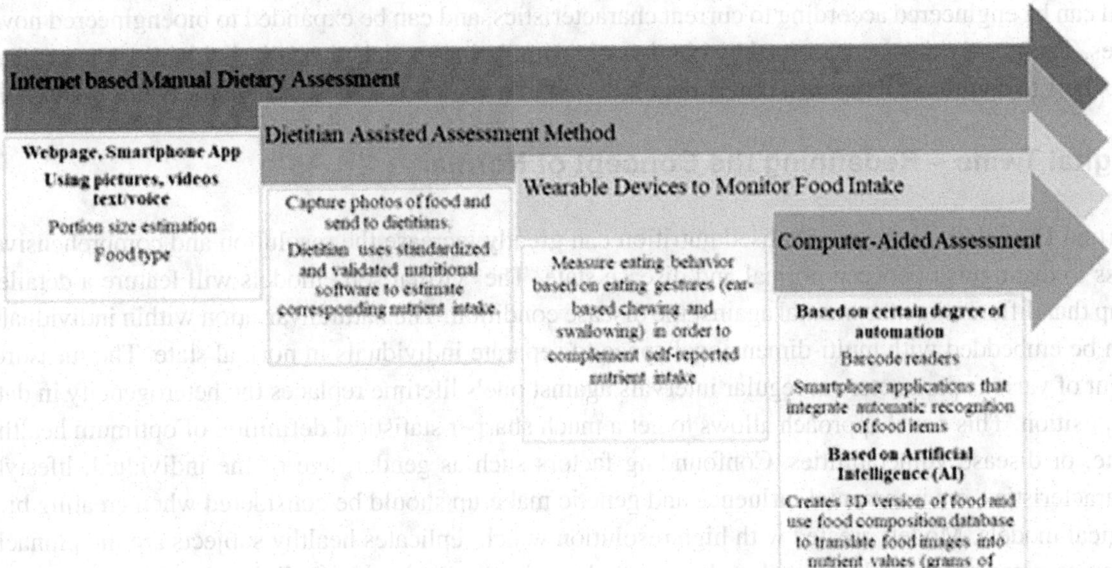

Go FOOD^{TM} is new Ai based dietary assessment system developed by Lu et al., (2020) to estimate macronutrient and calorie content of a based solely based on food images captured using a smart phone. A novel methodological approach known as Ontology for Nutritional Epidemiology (ONE) was put forward by Yang et al., (2019) which automates the process of data integration browsing and searching. ONE approach can find application in reporting completeness in the field of nutritional epidemiology. An objective dietary assessment designed by Lo et al., (2018) introducing distinct artificial neural networks wherein a in-depth image, a full 3D cloud map together with iterative closest point (ICP) algorithms were used to modify the dietary behaviour action. Another image and generative adversarial network (GAN) architecture-based estimate for food energy was used by Fang et al., (2019). A fuzzy decision model was built which applied a web-based control system that search food composition databases to calculate calorie and nutrient intake (Hsu et al., 2011).

Data Driven Digital Twins for Precision Nutrition

The data-driven precision health is gaining popularity worldwide. The introduction of this novel engineering and science design in health care focus on a dynamic digitalized biological counterpart built using molecular, clinical, biochemical, physiological, and behavioural pattern of individuals (Telenti et al., 2016). Reconstructing digital twin model of human heart imitates the engineering of artifacts (Scoles, 2016). A clearer multidimensional molecular design of normal pattern can be built at individual level with the aid of high-end sequencing technologies and electronic wearable devices. The idea of Digital Twins is to conceptualize a very reliable instrument to evaluate the effect of personalised in silico models on the core concepts in clinical nutrition and health. Probabilistic models that replicate human beings for use in precision medicine targets to substantiate the engineered model of a healthy state that use an analogy similar to predictive maintenance in industry. With the help of molecular biomarkers early diagnosis of predisposed diseases are made possible even before the disease manifest. This is advantageous in planning early interventions to regain back the healthy state. Furthermore, it enables us to understand that humans are biophysical system, and its components can be well understood in terms of mechanistic processes, and can be engineered according to current characteristics, and can be expanded to bioengineered novel ones. These activities are governed by big data and simulation models that is individualistic or artifact. It is best to combine all types of omics-data rather than using one individual data for better prediction.

Digital Twins – Redefining the Concept of Normal

Virtual Digital Twins in personalised nutrition can greatly increase the resolution and comprehensiveness to distinguish between normal and disease state. The 'virtual self' models will feature a detailed map that differentiate the normal against the disease condition. The natural variation within individuals, can be embedded with multi-dimensional space to separate individuals in normal state. The measurement of various parameters at regular intervals against one's lifetime replaces the heterogeneity in data acquisition. This novel approach allows to get a much sharper statistical definition of optimum healthy state, or disease vulnerabilities. Confounding factors such as gender, age of the individual, lifestyle characteristics, environmental influence and genetic make-up should be considered when creating biological models. Models created with high resolution which replicates healthy subjects are the pinnacle of customized nutritional approaches. It gives a clear picture of a healthy individual and lead to a better diagnosis of current disease states that requires remediation. To be more precise, it allows the assessment of biologically active ingredient or signature nutrients that is effective in treating or preventing cancer in a particular patient to classify type of cancer driven by mutations. This helps to understand better what happens when a healthy genome deviates from normal to unhealthy conditions.

This novel technology in precision medicine and nutritional care depends largely on a very intricate picture of the ideal health status of an individual, and not merely dependent on a disease report. In this context, 'normal' addresses the general molecular, physiological, behavioural and food intake patterns seen in a single person, generalised against the same backdrop present in the larger population. For example, BP measurement is taken with the aid of sphygmomanometer that is in practise for more than a century. Yet, there is no exact definition for 'normal' blood pressure. This traditional BP method generates sparse readings taken over time. (Steinhubl et al., 2016). This cuff-based measurement deny access to the factors that can interfere with the measurement like the time (day or night), age, healthy or disease state, stress conditions, physical level, caffeine consumption which may not be imperative of the exact state that can end up with ineffective management of hypertension. Wearable devices are now available which allows to monitor blood pressure continuously in an individual which proposes a "virtual medical assistant" that involve machine learning techniques to store these measurement data and observe the trends in BP significant to that specific person. This data could substantiate a personalised idea of normal BP, as against the similar patterns observed in persons of similar age group, gender, lifestyle etc. (Steinhubl et al., 2016). The same approach can be applied for molecular and nutritional biomarkers. Prediction of chronic heart disease risks can be advantageous when incorporating serial measurements of biomarkers over time, as against single values (Miller & Jaffe, 2015). The digitalized version of the physical model must be constantly updated with all types of information that span across the lifetime of a person. This helps to distinguish normal patterns that are statistically significant for that individual for a wide range of parameters. In comparison, the so-called normal patterns appear deviates to the ones followed up in large epidemiological studies. Therefore, the normal will be personalized (de Moraes Lopes et al., 2020).

Thirdly, digital biological twins can pave way for a transparent accessibility to an individual's genetic and physiological pattern which at present is difficult to access. This allows opportunity to compare between normal patterns across individuals with more detailed information effortlessly. Also, this allows to form cluster of similar individuals based on the multidimensional properties across Digital Twins. Till date, the normal range is only compared based on gender differences and age. With the help of digital twins, it is expected that a high-resolution image may allow for a heterogeneity of different types of humans, with distinct characterization of individuals within normal patterns. This phenomenon is already visible at genomic level. Referring to genomic sequence data of high resolution collected from a multitude of individuals showed that there exists a huge human genomic variation expected (Telenti et al., 2016). The multiple variation in genomics that was originally considered as junk was later looked up as a functional significance with a large data set. The existence of a multitude of healthy individuals with respect to human microbiomes are high, and diet therapy demands shifting the composition of the microbiome towards one of these healthy states (Lloyd-Price et al., 2016). Lastly, against the backdrop of a Digital Twin model, the healthy state not necessarily turn out to be the unproblematic natural state, but rather appear as an arbitrary configuration, that popped out of many probable configurations. Given the current situation, one seeks the help of a physician when the normal turns to be a problem and warrants for immediate action and intervention which contrasts with the Digital Twin supported health care practices, where the normal is the one who always approach for an action.

Virtual Digital Twins – From Personalized Nutrition to Precision Nutrition

The food we consume are to be used for various purposes for which the components present in foods must be metabolized. Numerous metabolic pathways govern the system converting food constituents into energy or into simpler structures within cells and organs. The individuality of people depends on how efficiently they mobilize food components using any of these metabolic pathways. This metabolic heterogeneity account for differences between people the way they react to different nutrients or bioactive food compounds (Scoles, 2016).

If we strive to perceive the cause of this nutrition-relevant metabolic heterogeneity, we will be able to interpret these variations early and apply this knowledge to calculate individual's dietary requirements and formulate better dietary principles and nutritional interventions. This is the foundation for 'precision nutrition'. It allows one to identify population clusters that can be of targets based on nutritional well-being as they exhibit same metabolic inefficiencies. However, it will take time before we can study in detail all the metabolic inefficiencies that prevails in a single person and use this data to advocate personal diet recommendations; hence the better choice to designate this emerging field of nutritional science would be "precision" rather than "personalized" nutrition.

Both precision and personalised nutrition implies personalizing an individual's diet taking into consideration one's DNA makeup, but precision nutrition displays a stronger appreciation of filling in the evidence gaps. As an example, a precision nutrition approach may present personalized recommendations for a certain number of nutrients where there is strong evidence to support and not the entire diet. On the other hand, personalized nutrition can imply nutritional recommendations that are exhaustively personalized, which might appear surreal and may never be possible.

Virtual Digital Twins – Can it Scale Up Precision Nutrition?

The emergence of virtual digital twins has witnessed the blooming of numerous mobile applications and digital wearables that promote real-time evaluation of individual's nutrient intake and give suggestions on one's bodily functions, such as blood glucose level, heart rate, or even blood pressure. The data collected from these devices amalgamated with -omics methodologies, with special focus on our genome, transcriptome, proteome, microbiome, and metabolome can relate to big data to render tailored nutritional guidance. Zeevi et al., (2015) reported interpersonal variation in post meal glucose levels, there was significant blood glucose responses in individuals who were on a personalized diets developed using machine learning algorithms that included dietary habits, lifestyle activity and gut microbiota.

A machine learning model was created in the PREDICT-1 study which predicted both triglyceride and glycaemic responses in response to food intake (Woldaregay, Årsand (2019), Walderhaug, et al., (2019). The findings also revealed the probability (48%) of inheriting elevated post-prandial blood glucose, highlights the modifying effect of genetic variation (Wolever, 2016). High throughput 'omics' technologies integrated with traditional study designs can be employed to monitor the effects of diet on disease states.

The use of computational tools for analysing large data sets would make health-care providers depend on electronic clinical decision support decide appropriate treatment and interventions. AI may turn out to be a daily essential in planning the right nutrition for physical well-being and menu planning (Ashman et al., 2017). Its high time we harness the functionality and accessibility of AI for precision nutrition by developing AI-based diet and supplements, affordable and precision genetic tests for individualized nutrition and physical fitness, nutritional therapeutic menu planning for specific disease condition and recovery such as cancer, cardiovascular diseases, obesity, type-2 diabetes and AI-based nutrition and health support systems and apps (Ohlhorst et al., 2013). Digital Twin Technology can create a bridge across bio-physical techniques and programming language. They can be a significant technical platform for supporting such techno-moral companionship. The data fed displays the operational character of reality, and they are generated from the metabolic constituents of blood collected at a given point of time, the genomic code, the ambulatory BP measurements, recordings of various physical movements and so on. All these data sets are intermediates that stem from the functional domain of biophysical reality, and the read-outs of symbols. This helps to graft specific symbols to decipher what structures exactly mean and how they constitute the bio-physical world (Sak & Suchodolska, 2021).

In general, virtual digital twin technology allow us to capture a glimpse into what is happening within our body, or what can happen when exposed to various factors, with physical assets we now have and lead us far into the future.

Virtual Digital Twins – The Future of Precision Nutrition

It might take another two decades for virtual digital twins in achieving precision nutrition to be accessible to all population groups alike. The birth of Virtual Digital Twin technology is still in its infancy stage and need voluminous data sets to conceptualize the physical model. A holistic approach to integrate 'omics', biochemical, physical movement, dietary intake, gut microbiota, environmental factors across lifetime is the biggest challenge currently faced by nutritional research. 'One-size-fits-all 'model can no longer be an effective recommendation for dietary interventions. The use of high-throughput novel technologies keeps evolving which are set to replace the traditional assessment methods with more precise and in-depth data. The emergence of AI, ML, DL, ANN, IoT and cloud mapping in evaluating nutritional status, nutritional biomarkers, clinical biomarkers, body composition, physical activity, environmental,

Figure 6. Addressing challenges and moving forward

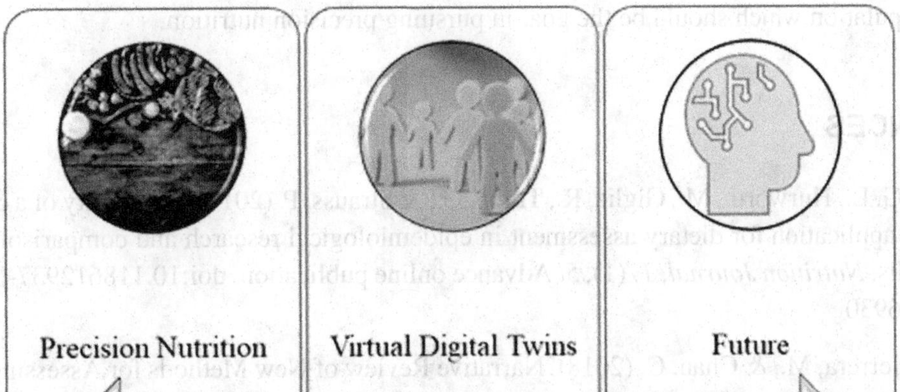

psychological, genotyping, phenotyping and deep phenotyping have made researchers conduct in-depth analysis and study the different pathways to develop better interventions.

CONCLUSION – MOVING FORWARD

Currently there are barriers in translating the evidence from genomics into meaningful dietary recommendations starting from measurements to implementation of intervention. 1. There is paucity in developing an accurate, precise, minimally invasive or non-invasive technique to collect and repeat data from human sample across the life span. 2.There arise a need for more dynamic and sophisticated dietary intervention approaches to ensure long-term compliance and adaptability. 3. Appropriate bioinformatic and biostatistical tools for integrating multi-omics datasets with dietary, clinical, environmental, and behavioural to unleash mechanism of action and explore robust biomarkers for clinical and nutritional translation to diversified population. To fully achieve this, an integrated and holistic approach involving multidisciplinary collaborations across fundamental and applied physical and chemical sciences, engineering and technology, Genetics and bioinformatics, Information technology, behavioural, clinical and nutrition sciences, biostatistics, and social sciences. In the future, a digital twin of our genetic profile could be developed for each and every one right at birth. This virtual self can be treated with a multitude of nutrient rich foods to ensure preventive nutrition. This may also set foot to discover which medical conditions oneself is predisposed to enabling us to intervene and prevent diseases before they take effect. The renaissance brought about by this virtual twin technology can help to solve the problems of higher health care costs and enable us to better understand our body system, monitor and maintain our health along the life span.

To move forward, the data gaps in each area of nutritional science must be narrowed down and should be considered when constructing biological models and need to be tested and validated for effectiveness of the software programming. Fusion of both traditional and novel technologies can be considered for better understanding. Above all, the novel tools should be accessible, affordable, and available to all sector of population which should be the goal in pursuing precision nutrition.

REFERENCES

Ambrosini, G. L., Hurworth, M., Giglia, R., Trapp, G., & Strauss, P. (2018). Feasibility of a commercial smartphone application for dietary assessment in epidemiological research and comparison with 24-h dietary recalls. *Nutrition Journal*, *17*(1), 5. Advance online publication. doi:10.118612937-018-0315-4 PMID:29316930

Archundia Herrera, M., & Chan, C. (2018). Narrative Review of New Methods for Assessing Food and Energy Intake. *Nutrients*, *10*(8), 1064. doi:10.3390/nu10081064 PMID:30103401

Ashman, A., Collins, C., Brown, L., Rae, K., & Rollo, M. (2017). Validation of a Smartphone Image-Based Dietary Assessment Method for Pregnant Women. *Nutrients*, *9*(1), 73. doi:10.3390/nu9010073 PMID:28106758

Bally, L., Dehais, J., Nakas, C. T., Anthimopoulos, M., Laimer, M., Rhyner, D., Rosenberg, G., Zueger, T., Diem, P., Mougiakakou, S., & Stettler, C. (2016). Carbohydrate Estimation Supported by the GoCARB System in Individuals with Type 1 Diabetes: A Randomized Prospective Pilot Study. *Diabetes Care*, *40*(2), e6–e7. doi:10.2337/dc16-2173 PMID:27899490

Berry, S. E., Valdes, A. M., Drew, D. A., Asnicar, F., Mazidi, M., Wolf, J., Capdevila, J., Hadjigeorgiou, G., Davies, R., Al Khatib, H., Bonnett, C., Ganesh, S., Bakker, E., Hart, D., Mangino, M., Merino, J., Linenberg, I., Wyatt, P., Ordovas, J. M., ... Spector, T. D. (2020). Human postprandial responses to food and potential for precision nutrition. *Nature Medicine*, *26*(6), 964–973. doi:10.103841591-020-0934-0 PMID:32528151

Brandt, B., Rashidiani, S., Bán, Á., & Rauch, T. A. (2019). DNA Methylation-Governed Gene Expression in Autoimmune Arthritis. *International Journal of Molecular Sciences*, *20*(22), 5646. Advance online publication. doi:10.3390/ijms20225646 PMID:31718084

Bronze-da-Rocha, E. (2014). MicroRNAs Expression Profiles in Cardiovascular Diseases. *BioMed Research International*, *2014*, 1–23. doi:10.1155/2014/985408 PMID:25013816

Bucher Della Torre, S., Carrard, I., Farina, E., Danuser, B., & Kruseman, M. (2017). Development and Evaluation of e-CA, an Electronic Mobile-Based Food Record. *Nutrients*, *9*(1), 76. doi:10.3390/nu9010076 PMID:28106767

Corella, D., & Ordovás, J. M. (2012). Interactions between dietary n-3 fatty acids and genetic variants and risk of disease. *British Journal of Nutrition*, *107*(S2), S271–S283. doi:10.1017/S0007114512001651 PMID:22591901

Cui, X. R., Abbod, M. F., Liu, Q., Shieh, J.-S., Chao, T. Y., Hsieh, C. Y., & Yang, Y. C. (2010). Ensembled artificial neural networks to predict the fitness score for body composition analysis. *The Journal of Nutrition, Health & Aging*, *15*(5), 341–348. doi:10.100712603-010-0260-1 PMID:21528159

Danneskiold-Samsøe, N. B., Dias de Freitas Queiroz Barros, H., Santos, R., Bicas, J. L., Cazarin, C. B. B., Madsen, L., Kristiansen, K., Pastore, G. M., Brix, S., & Maróstica Júnior, M. R. (2019). Interplay between food and gut microbiota in health and disease. *Food Research International*, *115*, 23–31. doi:10.1016/j.foodres.2018.07.043 PMID:30599936

de Moraes Lopes, M. H. B., Ferreira, D. D., Ferreira, A. C. B. H., da Silva, G. R., Caetano, A. S., & Braz, V. N. (2020). Use of artificial intelligence in precision nutrition and fitness. *Artificial Intelligence in Precision Health*, 465–496. doi:10.1016/B978-0-12-817133-2.00020-3

de Vries, J., Antoine, J.-M., Burzykowski, T., Chiodini, A., Gibney, M., Kuhnle, G., Méheust, A., Pijls, L., & Rowland, I. (2013). Markers for nutrition studies: Review of criteria for the evaluation of markers. *European Journal of Nutrition*, *52*(7), 1685–1699. doi:10.100700394-013-0553-3 PMID:23955424

DeBusk, R. (2010). The Role of Nutritional Genomics in Developing an Optimal Diet for Humans. *Nutrition in Clinical Practice*, *25*(6), 627–633. doi:10.1177/0884533610385700 PMID:21139127

Dehais, J., Anthimopoulos, M., Shevchik, S., & Mougiakakou, S. (2017). Two-View 3D Reconstruction for Food Volume Estimation. *IEEE Transactions on Multimedia*, *19*(5), 1090–1099. doi:10.1109/TMM.2016.2642792

Demirci, F., Akan, P., Kume, T., Sisman, A. R., Erbayraktar, Z., & Sevinc, S. (2016). Artificial Neural Network Approach in Laboratory Test Reporting. *American Journal of Clinical Pathology, 146*(2), 227–237. doi:10.1093/ajcp/aqw104 PMID:27473741

Deo, R. C. (2020). Machine Learning in Medicine. *Circulation, 142*(16), 1521–1523. doi:10.1161/CIRCULATIONAHA.120.050583 PMID:33074761

Devika, N. T., & Raman, K. (2019). Deciphering the metabolic capabilities of Bifidobacteria using genome-scale metabolic models. *Scientific Reports, 9*(1), 18222. Advance online publication. doi:10.103841598-019-54696-9 PMID:31796826

Dietary assessment a resource guiDe to method selection and application in low resource settings. (n.d.). https://www.fao.org/3/i9940en/I9940EN.pdf

Dong, Y., Hoover, A., Scisco, J., & Muth, E. (2012). A New Method for Measuring Meal Intake in Humans via Automated Wrist Motion Tracking. *Applied Psychophysiology and Biofeedback, 37*(3), 205–215. doi:10.100710484-012-9194-1 PMID:22488204

Elmadfa, I., & Meyer, A. L. (2010). Importance of food composition data to nutrition and public health. *European Journal of Clinical Nutrition, 64*(S3), S4–S7. doi:10.1038/ejcn.2010.202 PMID:21045848

Fang, S., & Kerr, B. (2019). An End-to-End Image-Based Automatic Food Energy Estimation Technique Based on Learned Energy Distribution Images: Protocol and Methodology. *Nutrients, 11*(4), 877. doi:10.3390/nu11040877 PMID:31003547

Forster, H., Walsh, M. C., Gibney, M. J., Brennan, L., & Gibney, E. R. (2015). Personalised nutrition: The role of new dietary assessment methods. *The Proceedings of the Nutrition Society, 75*(1), 96–105. doi:10.1017/S0029665115002086 PMID:26032731

Fuellen, G., Schofield, P., Flatt, T., Schulz, R.-J., Boege, F., Kraft, K., Rimbach, G., Ibrahim, S., Tietz, A., Schmidt, C., Köhling, R., & Simm, A. (2015). Living Long and Well: Prospects for a Personalized Approach to the Medicine of Ageing. *Gerontology, 62*(4), 409–416. doi:10.1159/000442746 PMID:26675034

Gallucci, M., Pallucca, C., Di Battista, M. E., Fougère, B., & Grossi, E. (2019). Artificial Neural Networks Help to Better Understand the Interplay Between Cognition, Mediterranean Diet, and Physical Performance: Clues from TRELONG Study. *Journal of Alzheimer's Disease, 71*(4), 1321–1330. doi:10.3233/JAD-190609 PMID:31524170

Giacconi, R., Malavolta, M., Bürkle, A., Moreno-Villanueva, M., Franceschi, C., Capri, M., Slagboom, P. E., Jansen, E. H. J. M., Dollé, M. E. T., Grune, T., Weber, D., Hervonen, A., Stuetz, W., Breusing, N., Ciccarone, F., Zampieri, M., Aversano, V., Caiafa, P., Formentini, L., ... Cardelli, M. (2019). Nutritional Factors Modulating Alu Methylation in an Italian Sample from The Mark-Age Study Including Offspring of Healthy Nonagenarians. *Nutrients, 11*(12), 2986. doi:10.3390/nu11122986 PMID:31817660

Gkouskou, K., Vlastos, I., Karkalousos, P., Chaniotis, D., Sanoudou, D., & Eliopoulos, A. G. (2020). The "Virtual Digital Twins" Concept in Precision Nutrition. *Advances in Nutrition, 11*(6), 1405–1413. doi:10.1093/advances/nmaa089 PMID:32770212

Gomez-Delgado, F., Alcala-Diaz, J. F., Garcia-Rios, A., Delgado-Lista, J., Ortiz-Morales, A., Rangel-Zuñiga, O., Tinahones, F. J., Gonzalez-Guardia, L., Malagon, M. M., Bellido-Muñoz, E., Ordovas, J. M., Perez-Jimenez, F., Lopez-Miranda, J., & Perez-Martinez, P. (2014). Polymorphism at the TNF-alpha gene interacts with Mediterranean diet to influence triglyceride metabolism and inflammation status in metabolic syndrome patients: From the CORDIOPREV clinical trial. *Molecular Nutrition & Food Research*, *58*(7), 1519–1527. doi:10.1002/mnfr.201300723 PMID:24753491

Gong, L., Wong, C.-H., Idol, J., Ngan, C. Y., & Wei, C.-L. (2019). Ultra-long Read Sequencing for Whole Genomic DNA Analysis. *Journal of Visualized Experiments*, *145*(145). Advance online publication. doi:10.3791/58954 PMID:30933081

Handelman, G. S., Kok, H. K., Chandra, R. V., Razavi, A. H., Lee, M. J., & Asadi, H. (2018). eDoctor: Machine learning and the future of medicine. *Journal of Internal Medicine*, *284*(6), 603–619. doi:10.1111/joim.12822 PMID:30102808

Heydarian, H., Adam, M., Burrows, T., Collins, C., & Rollo, M. E. (2019). Assessing Eating Behaviour Using Upper Limb Mounted Motion Sensors: A Systematic Review. *Nutrients*, *11*(5), 1168. doi:10.3390/nu11051168 PMID:31137677

Hsu, C.-Y., Huang, L.-C., Chen, T. M., Chen, L.-F., & Chao, J. C.-J. (2011). A Web-Based Decision Support System for Dietary Analysis and Recommendations. *Telemedicine Journal and e-Health*, *17*(2), 68–75. doi:10.1089/tmj.2010.0104 PMID:21385024

Jæger, B., & Mishra, A. (2020). IoT Platform for Seafood Farmers and Consumers. *Sensors (Basel)*, *20*(15), 4230. doi:10.339020154230 PMID:32751365

Kaput, J., & Rodriguez, R. L. (2004). Nutritional genomics: The next frontier in the postgenomic era. *Physiological Genomics*, *16*(2), 166–177. doi:10.1152/physiolgenomics.00107.2003 PMID:14726599

Kawano, Y., & Yanai, K. (2014). FoodCam: A real-time food recognition system on a smartphone. *Multimedia Tools and Applications*, *74*(14), 5263–5287. doi:10.100711042-014-2000-8

Kirk, D., Catal, C., & Tekinerdogan, B. (2021). Precision nutrition: A systematic literature review. *Computers in Biology and Medicine*, *133*, 104365. doi:10.1016/j.compbiomed.2021.104365 PMID:33866251

Kraft, F., & Kurth, I. (2019). Long-read sequencing in human genetics. *Medizinische Genetik*, *31*(2), 198–204. doi:10.100711825-019-0249-z

Kritzinger, W., Karner, M., Traar, G., Henjes, J., & Sihn, W. (2018). Digital Twin in manufacturing: A categorical literature review and classification. *IFAC-PapersOnLine*, *51*(11), 1016–1022. doi:10.1016/j.ifacol.2018.08.474

Kura, B., Parikh, M., Slezak, J., & Pierce, G. N. (2019). The Influence of Diet on MicroRNAs that Impact Cardiovascular Disease. *Molecules (Basel, Switzerland)*, *24*(8), 1509. doi:10.3390/molecules24081509 PMID:30999630

Liu, B., & Qian, S.-B. (2011). Translational Regulation in Nutrigenomics. *Advances in Nutrition*, *2*(6), 511–519. doi:10.3945/an.111.001057 PMID:22332093

Liu, Y., Wang, Y., Ni, Y., Cheung, C. K. Y., Lam, K. S. L., Wang, Y., Xia, Z., Ye, D., Guo, J., Tse, M. A., Panagiotou, G., & Xu, A. (2020). Gut Microbiome Fermentation Determines the Efficacy of Exercise for Diabetes Prevention. *Cell Metabolism*, *31*(1), 77–91.e5. doi:10.1016/j.cmet.2019.11.001 PMID:31786155

Lloyd-Price, J., Abu-Ali, G., & Huttenhower, C. (2016). The healthy human microbiome. *Genome Medicine*, *8*(1), 51. Advance online publication. doi:10.118613073-016-0307-y PMID:27122046

Lo, F., Sun, Y., Qiu, J., & Lo, B. (2018). Food Volume Estimation Based on Deep Learning View Synthesis from a Single Depth Map. *Nutrients*, *10*(12), 2005. doi:10.3390/nu10122005 PMID:30567362

Lu, Y., Stathopoulou, T., Vasiloglou, M. F., Pinault, L. F., Kiley, C., Spanakis, E. K., & Mougiakakou, S. (2020). goFOODTM: An Artificial Intelligence System for Dietary Assessment. *Sensors (Basel)*, *20*(15), 4283. Advance online publication. doi:10.339020154283 PMID:32752007

McGee, E. E., Kiblawi, R., Playdon, M. C., & Eliassen, A. H. (2019). Nutritional Metabolomics in Cancer Epidemiology: Current Trends, Challenges, and Future Directions. *Current Nutrition Reports*, *8*(3), 187–201. doi:10.100713668-019-00279-z PMID:31129888

Midha, M. K., Wu, M., & Chiu, K.-P. (2019). Long-read sequencing in deciphering human genetics to a greater depth. *Human Genetics*, *138*(11-12), 1201–1215. doi:10.100700439-019-02064-y PMID:31538236

Miller, W. L., & Jaffe, A. S. (2015). Biomarkers in heart failure: The importance of inconvenient details. *ESC Heart Failure*, *3*(1), 3–10. doi:10.1002/ehf2.12071 PMID:27774262

Minihane, A. M., Armah, C. K., Miles, E. A., Madden, J. M., Clark, A. B., Caslake, M. J., Packard, C. J., Kofler, B. M., Lietz, G., Curtis, P. J., Mathers, J. C., Williams, C. M., & Calder, P. C. (2016). Consumption of Fish Oil Providing Amounts of Eicosapentaenoic Acid and Docosahexaenoic Acid That Can Be Obtained from the Diet Reduces Blood Pressure in Adults with Systolic Hypertension: A Retrospective Analysis. *The Journal of Nutrition*, *146*(3), 516–523. doi:10.3945/jn.115.220475 PMID:26817716

Myung, S.-K. (2012). Efficacy of Omega-3 Fatty Acid Supplements (Eicosapentaenoic Acid and Docosahexaenoic Acid) in the Secondary Prevention of Cardiovascular Disease. *Archives of Internal Medicine*, *172*(9), 686. doi:10.1001/archinternmed.2012.262 PMID:22493407

Noecker, C., & Borenstein, E. (2016). Getting Personal About Nutrition. *Trends in Molecular Medicine*, *22*(2), 83–85. doi:10.1016/j.molmed.2015.12.010 PMID:26776092

Ohlhorst, S. D., Russell, R., Bier, D., Klurfeld, D. M., Li, Z., Mein, J. R., Milner, J., Ross, A. C., Stover, P., & Konopka, E. (2013). Nutrition research to affect food and a healthy lifespan. *Advances in Nutrition*, *4*(5), 579–584. doi:10.3945/an.113.004176 PMID:24038264

Oikonomopoulos, S., Bayega, A., Fahiminiya, S., Djambazian, H., Berube, P., & Ragoussis, J. (2020). Methodologies for Transcript Profiling Using Long-Read Technologies. *Frontiers in Genetics*, *11*, 606. Advance online publication. doi:10.3389/fgene.2020.00606 PMID:32733532

Olivia Li, J.-P., Liu, H., Ting, D. S. J., Jeon, S., & Chan, R. V. P., Kim, J. E., Sim, D. A., Thomas, P. B. M., Lin, H., Chen, Y., Sakomoto, T., Loewenstein, A., Lam, D. S. C., Pasquale, L. R., Wong, T. Y., Lam, L. A., & Ting, D. S. W. (2020). Digital technology, tele-medicine and artificial intelligence in ophthalmology: A global perspective. *Progress in Retinal and Eye Research, 100900*. Advance online publication. doi:10.1016/j.preteyeres.2020.100900

Ordovas, J. M., Ferguson, L. R., Tai, E. S., & Mathers, J. C. (2018). Personalised nutrition and health. *BMJ*, k2173. doi:10.1136/bmj.k2173

Özdemir, V., & Kolker, E. (2016). Precision Nutrition 4.0: A Big Data and Ethics Foresight Analysis—Convergence of Agrigenomics, Nutrigenomics, Nutriproteomics, and Nutrimetabolomics. *OMICS: A Journal of Integrative Biology*, *20*(2), 69–75. doi:10.1089/omi.2015.0193 PMID:26785082

Palou, M., Torrens, J. M., Castillo, P., Sánchez, J., Palou, A., & Picó, C. (2019). Metabolomic approach in milk from calorie-restricted rats during lactation: A potential link to the programming of a healthy phenotype in offspring. *European Journal of Nutrition*, *59*(3), 1191–1204. doi:10.100700394-019-01979-6 PMID:31069458

Picó, C., Serra, F., Rodríguez, A. M., Keiper, J., & Palou, A. (2019). Biomarkers of Nutrition and Health: New Tools for New Approaches. *Nutrients*, *11*(5), 1092. doi:10.3390/nu11051092 PMID:31100942

Potischman, N. (2003). Biologic and Methodologic Issues for Nutritional Biomarkers. *The Journal of Nutrition, 133*(3). doi:10.1093/jn/133.3.875S

Raden, N. (2020). *Digital twins for personalized medicine - a critical assessment*. Diginomica. Retrieved from https://diginomica.com/digital-twins-personalized-medicine-critical-assessment

Raiten, D. J., Namasté, S., Brabin, B., Combs, G., L'Abbe, M. R., Wasantwisut, E., & Darnton-Hill, I. (2011). Executive summary—Biomarkers of Nutrition for Development: Building a Consensus. *The American Journal of Clinical Nutrition, 94*(2). doi:10.3945/ajcn.110.008227

Rajkomar, A., Dean, J., & Kohane, I. (2019). Machine Learning in Medicine. *The New England Journal of Medicine*, *380*(14), 1347–1358. doi:10.1056/NEJMra1814259 PMID:30943338

Ramos-Lopez, O., Milagro, F. I., Allayee, H., Chmurzynska, A., Choi, M. S., Curi, R., De Caterina, R., Ferguson, L. R., Goni, L., Kang, J. X., Kohlmeier, M., Marti, A., Moreno, L. A., Pérusse, L., Prasad, C., Qi, L., Reifen, R., Riezu-Boj, J. I., San-Cristobal, R., ... Martínez, J. A. (2017). Guide for Current Nutrigenetic, Nutrigenomic, and Nutriepigenetic Approaches for Precision Nutrition Involving the Prevention and Management of Chronic Diseases Associated with Obesity. *Journal of Nutrigenetics and Nutrigenomics*, *10*(1-2), 43–62. doi:10.1159/000477729 PMID:28689206

Recio-Rodriguez, J. I., Rodriguez-Martin, C., Gonzalez-Sanchez, J., Rodriguez-Sanchez, E., Martin-Borras, C., Martínez-Vizcaino, V., Arietaleanizbeaskoa, M. S., Magdalena-Gonzalez, O., Fernandez-Alonso, C., Maderuelo-Fernandez, J. A., Gomez-Marcos, M. A., Garcia-Ortiz, L., & Investigators, E. (2019). EVIDENT Smartphone App, a New Method for the Dietary Record: Comparison with a Food Frequency Questionnaire. *JMIR mHealth and uHealth*, *7*(2), e11463. doi:10.2196/11463 PMID:30735141

Rhyner, D., Loher, H., Dehais, J., Anthimopoulos, M., Shevchik, S., Botwey, R. H., Duke, D., Stettler, C., Diem, P., & Mougiakakou, S. (2016). Carbohydrate Estimation by a Mobile Phone-Based System Versus Self-Estimations of Individuals with Type 1 Diabetes Mellitus: A Comparative Study. *Journal of Medical Internet Research, 18*(5), e101. doi:10.2196/jmir.5567 PMID:27170498

Rojas-Fernandez, C. H., & Tyber, K. (2016). Benefits, Potential Harms, and Optimal Use of Nutritional Supplementation for Preventing Progression of Age-Related Macular Degeneration. *The Annals of Pharmacotherapy, 51*(3), 264–270. doi:10.1177/1060028016680643 PMID:27866147

Sadoughi, F., Behmanesh, A., & Sayfouri, N. (2020). Internet of things in medicine: A systematic mapping study. *Journal of Biomedical Informatics, 103*, 103383. doi:10.1016/j.jbi.2020.103383 PMID:32044417

Sak, J., & Suchodolska, M. (2021). Artificial Intelligence in Nutrients Science Research: A Review. *Nutrients, 13*(2), 322. doi:10.3390/nu13020322 PMID:33499405

Sarda, S., & Hannenhalli, S. (2014). Next-Generation Sequencing and Epigenomics Research: A Hammer in Search of Nails. *Genomics & Informatics, 12*(1), 2. doi:10.5808/GI.2014.12.1.2 PMID:24748856

Scholes, S. (2016). Politics, Business, Technology, and the Arts. *Slate Magazine*. http://www.slate.com

Shima, H., Masuda, S., Date, Y., Shino, A., Tsuboi, Y., Kajikawa, M., Inoue, Y., Kanamoto, T., & Kikuchi, J. (2017). Exploring the Impact of Food on the Gut Ecosystem Based on the Combination of Machine Learning and Network Visualization. *Nutrients, 9*(12), 1307. doi:10.3390/nu9121307 PMID:29194366

Shugalo, I. (2019, April 29). *Digital Twin Technology: Should Healthcare Jump on the Bandwagon?* https://hitconsultant.net/2019/04/29/digital-twin-technology-should-healthcare-jump-on-the-bandwagon/#.Xsy9OGj7RPZ

Singh, A. (2020). Tools for metabolomics. *Nature Methods, 17*(1), 24–24. doi:10.103841592-019-0710-6 PMID:31907484

Slatko, B. E., Gardner, A. F., & Ausubel, F. M. (2018). Overview of Next-Generation Sequencing Technologies. *Current Protocols in Molecular Biology, 122*(1), e59. doi:10.1002/cpmb.59 PMID:29851291

Steinhubl, S. R., Muse, E. D., Barrett, P. M., & Topol, E. J. (2016). Off the cuff: Rebooting blood pressure treatment. *Lancet, 388*(10046), 749. doi:10.1016/S0140-6736(16)31348-4 PMID:27560266

Sun, M., Fernstrom, J. D., Jia, W., Hackworth, S. A., Yao, N., Li, Y., Li, C., Fernstrom, M. H., & Sclabassi, R. J. (2010). A Wearable Electronic System for Objective Dietary Assessment. *Journal of the American Dietetic Association, 110*(1), 45–47. doi:10.1016/j.jada.2009.10.013 PMID:20102825

Tachibana, C. (2015). Transcriptomics today: Microarrays, RNA-seq, and more. *Science, 349*(6247), 544–546. doi:10.1126cience.349.6247.544

Telenti, A., Pierce, L. C. T., Biggs, W. H., di Iulio, J., Wong, E. H. M., Fabani, M. M., Kirkness, E. F., Moustafa, A., Shah, N., Xie, C., Brewerton, S. C., Bulsara, N., Garner, C., Metzker, G., Sandoval, E., Perkins, B. A., Och, F. J., Turpaz, Y., & Venter, J. C. (2016). Deep sequencing of 10,000 human genomes. *Proceedings of the National Academy of Sciences of the United States of America, 113*(42), 11901–11906. doi:10.1073/pnas.1613365113 PMID:27702888

Thompson, F. E., Subar, A. F., Loria, C. M., Reedy, J. L., & Baranowski, T. (2010). Need for Technological Innovation in Dietary Assessment. *Journal of the American Dietetic Association, 110*(1), 48–51. doi:10.1016/j.jada.2009.10.008 PMID:20102826

van Dijk, E. L., Jaszczyszyn, Y., Naquin, D., & Thermes, C. (2018). The Third Revolution in Sequencing Technology. *Trends in Genetics, 34*(9), 666–681. doi:10.1016/j.tig.2018.05.008 PMID:29941292

Vasiloglou, M., Mougiakakou, S., Aubry, E., Bokelmann, A., Fricker, R., Gomes, F., Guntermann, C., Meyer, A., Studerus, D., & Stanga, Z. (2018). A Comparative Study on Carbohydrate Estimation: GoCARB vs. Dietitians. *Nutrients, 10*(6), 741. doi:10.3390/nu10060741 PMID:29880772

Wang, D. D., & Hu, F. B. (2018). Precision nutrition for prevention and management of type 2 diabetes. *The Lancet. Diabetes & Endocrinology, 6*(5), 416–426. doi:10.1016/S2213-8587(18)30037-8 PMID:29433995

Woldaregay, A. Z., Årsand, E., Botsis, T., Albers, D., Mamykina, L., & Hartvigsen, G. (2019). Data-Driven Blood Glucose Pattern Classification and Anomalies Detection: Machine-Learning Applications in Type 1 Diabetes. *Journal of Medical Internet Research, 21*(5), e11030. doi:10.2196/11030 PMID:31042157

Woldaregay, A. Z., Årsand, E., Walderhaug, S., Albers, D., Mamykina, L., Botsis, T., & Hartvigsen, G. (2019). Data-driven modelling and prediction of blood glucose dynamics: Machine learning applications in type 1 diabetes. *Artificial Intelligence in Medicine, 98*, 109–134. doi:10.1016/j.artmed.2019.07.007 PMID:31383477

Wolever, T. M. S. (2016). Personalized nutrition by prediction of glycaemic responses: Fact or fantasy? *European Journal of Clinical Nutrition, 70*(4), 411–413. doi:10.1038/ejcn.2016.31 PMID:27050901

Yang, C., Ambayo, H., De Baets, B., Kolsteren, P., Thanintorn, N., Hawwash, D., Bouwman, J., Bronselaer, A., Pattyn, F., & Lachat, C. (2019). An Ontology to Standardize Research Output of Nutritional Epidemiology: From Paper-Based Standards to Linked Content. *Nutrients, 11*(6), 1300. doi:10.3390/nu11061300 PMID:31181762

Yu, D.-J., Hu, J., Yan, H., Yang, X.-B., Yang, J.-Y., & Shen, H.-B. (2014). Enhancing protein-vitamin binding residues prediction by multiple heterogeneous subspace SVMs ensemble. *BMC Bioinformatics, 15*(1), 297. Advance online publication. doi:10.1186/1471-2105-15-297 PMID:25189131

Zeevi, D., Korem, T., Zmora, N., Israeli, D., Rothschild, D., Weinberger, A., Ben-Yacov, O., Lador, D., Avnit-Sagi, T., Lotan-Pompan, M., Suez, J., Mahdi, J. A., Matot, E., Malka, G., Kosower, N., Rein, M., Zilberman-Schapira, G., Dohnalová, L., Pevsner-Fischer, M., ... Segal, E. (2015). Personalized Nutrition by Prediction of Glycemic Responses. *Cell, 163*(5), 1079–1094. doi:10.1016/j.cell.2015.11.001 PMID:26590418

Zhao, S., Fung-Leung, W.-P., Bittner, A., Ngo, K., & Liu, X. (2014). Comparison of RNA-Seq and Microarray in Transcriptome Profiling of Activated T Cells. *PLoS One, 9*(1), e78644. doi:10.1371/journal.pone.0078644 PMID:24454679

Chapter 2
Smart Medical Kit in Chronic Kidney Disease Management

Pitchumani Angayarkanni Sekaran
Sri Ramachandra Institute of Higher Education and Research, India

ABSTRACT

Internet of things (IoT)-enabled devices perform remote monitoring of patients and keep them healthy. They also facilitate physicians to provide high-quality care to their patients with accurate data. Chronic disease involves a wide range of health issues like diabetics, asthma, heart disease, kidney disease, and other disorders. To avoid disease progression, the IoT-based smart medical kit helps in episodic patient monitoring, continuous patient monitoring in acute conditions, and patient alarm monitoring. The chapter focuses on the deployment of interconnected devices (sensors, actuators, monitors, detectors, and camera systems) to collect data from heterogeneous systems. The output is connected to a think speak dashboard for monitoring the variation over the period. The smart kit provides more accurate and reliable recommendations to assist patients in controlling their chronic disease and assists in remote monitoring of a patient's health conditions.

INTRODUCTION

Internet of Things (IoT) is used to interconnect gadgets using Internet of computing devices embedded in everyday objects, enabling them to send and receive data. One of the use cases of IoT is the effective monitoring of health care sectors which had enhanced the safety and health of the patients by providing superlative care. IoT has transformed the health care industry by providing an efficient health care solution. IoT devices had been devised for both patients and physicians. For example, wearable devices like smart fitness band watch, blood pressure and heart rate monitor provide personal attention to patients. The IoT devices were used to remind the patients about their calorie count, doctor's appointment, blood pressure variation etc. by constantly monitoring their health conditions. Any change in the routine activity will automatically send an alert signal to the physicians and family members. IoT for physicians helps to keep track of their patients' health condition more effectively. It helps the physicians to keep track of the patient's health condition and provide timely care to them. Data collected through IoT devices helps

DOI: 10.4018/978-1-7998-9132-1.ch002

Copyright © 2022, IGI Global. Copying or distributing in print or electronic forms without written permission of IGI Global is prohibited.

the physicians to identify best and timely treatment plans to the patients. IoT are very useful devices in hospitals these devices tagged with sensors helps in real time tracking of the patient's location in case of emergency through the sensors fixed in the wheelchair, nebulizer, defibrillators, oxygen pumps etc. Spread of infectious disease can also be monitored effectively through hygiene monitoring IoT devices. This can help in effective hospital management by tracking the supply chain management. The impact of IoT in health care domain can transform health experience by increasing the patient outcome and quality of care. Global IoT health market will increase by 20.4% from 2014 to 2024 as per IoT trends statistic 2020. It clearly stated that IoT market will raise from $22.5 billion to $72.02 billion in 2021. The Internet of Medical Things (IoMT) which is a network of connected devices which can collect data in real time. It is the key application of IoT in health care which has created a positive impact in solving medical issues. In this chapter we focus on how IoT can be used to monitor the patients with Chronic Kidney Disease (CKD) and help in health management in an effective and efficient manner.

BACKGROUND

Today we are in an information era. The advancement of technology and scientific theories gradually began to digitize and to informatize. Smart health care is a simple technological advancement at multi-level changes. As healthcare technologies are advancing, there is a need for high and effective engagement with patients. The demand for remote health care through the advent of technology will provide a real time update of patient's information. The basic foundation for our smart health solutions involves:

1. Sensors to collect patient data
2. Cloud enabled data storage, process and analyze data
3. Web and mobile based applications for care givers and users
4. A gateway to transmit data

Chronic diseases include diabetics, kidney, heart, cancer, obesity, arthritis and stroke are most common among people. It is difficult for doctors to visit them regularly. Therefore, the proposed IoT handy smart kit will help doctors to track the patient's health status remotely. The Internet enabled devices can store patients' health data on cloud and can be accessed by medical professionals anytime, anywhere. These data can be captured daily and can be uploaded and visualized in cloud to monitor the changes in the health data.

REVIEW OF RELATED LITERATURE

Dharani et. al. (2020) developed an Automated Peritoneal Dialysis (APD) device as a vital treatment option for patients suffering from renal failure. The life span was improved day by day than the patient's undergoing hemodialysis. The hyperkalaemia that is K ion is monitored by this device, the increase of which might lead to severe heart damage to patients like arrhythmia, shock, heart attack and sometimes to even death. The K range is measured continuously and the value is shared to the medical team and care taker of the patient by Remote Patient Monitoring (RPM) system.

Mohammed Al-khafajiy et. al. (2019), IoT based technology to track a person's physiological data to detect specific disorders which can aid in Early Intervention Practices. This is achieved by accurately processing and analysing the acquired sensory data while transmitting the detection of a disorder to an appropriate career. The finding reveals that the proposed system can improve clinical decision supports while facilitating Early Intervention Practices.

Nishant Singh et. al (2021) proposed the use of cloud services integrated with IoT allows the collection, analysis, and provisioning of support and solution at a rapid rate. This facilitates remote patient-monitoring and safeguards healthcare providers from coming in direct contact with the patient and highly infectious and contagious work environment. It also brings in great potentials for smart-health solutions with enhanced patient observation, monitoring, support, and prediction of vital needs essential in emergency situations.

IOT HEALTH CARE ARCHITECTURE

IoT in health care is considered as four-step architecture. At each stage the data captured and processed is given as input to the next stage for delivering dynamic business prospects (Rajkamal, 2017).

Step 1: Deployment of interconnected devices like sensors, actuators, monitors, detectors, camera system etc. for collecting data.

Step 2: Data received from sensors and other devices are analog and are aggregated together and converted to digital for data processing

Step 3: The digitized data are aggregated, pre-processed, standardized and transferred to the cloud.

Step 4: The resultant data are monitored and analyzed at each level by performing analytics providing effective business insight with decision-making process.

CASE STUDY OF IOT IN CHRONIC KIDNEY DISEASE MONITORING

IoT has redefined the health care sector by ensuring effective patient care, enhanced treatment, reduced cost, improved patient experience and better workflow. Now we are going to see how the IoT device implemented using CC3200 Launchpad with appropriate sensors helps in monitoring of Chronic Kidney Disease in patients.

Chronic Kidney Failure Causes and Symptoms

Chronic Kidney Disease (CKD) also called as Chronic kidney failure results from the gradual loss of kidney functions. Kidney is used to filter wastes and excess fluids from the blood which are excreted through urine. CKD at the advanced stage results in building dangerous level of fluids. Electrolytes and wastes. In its early stage the signs and symptoms are very less. Complications related to CKD are high blood pressure, anemia, bone weakness, poor nutrition and nerve damage. These problems result slowly over the period of time. CKD may also be caused by diabetes, high blood pressure and other disorders. Early diagnosis and treatment can prevent the CKD progression (Alkhazaali, 2020).

Other Conditions that Affect the Kidneys Are:

- Glomerulonephritis, a group of diseases that cause inflammation and damage to the kidney's filtering units. These disorders are the third most common type of kidney disease.
- Inherited diseases, such as polycystic kidney disease, which causes large cysts to form in the kidneys and damage the surrounding tissue.
- Malformations that occur as a baby develops in its mother's womb. For example, a narrowing may occur that prevents normal outflow of urine and causes urine to flow back up to the kidney. This causes infections and may damage the kidneys.
- Lupus and other diseases that affect the body's immune system.
- Obstructions caused by problems like kidney stones, tumors or an enlarged prostate gland in men.
- Repeated urinary infections. (**Source:** https://www.kidney.org/atoz/content/about-chronic-kidney-disease)

Symptoms of CKD

The symptoms for chronic kidney disease include Itching, Muscle cramps, Nausea and vomiting, Not feeling hungry, swelling in your feet and ankles, Too much urine (pee) or not enough urine, Trouble catching your breath and Trouble sleeping. Acute kidney failure symptoms include Abdominal (belly) pain, Back pain, Diarrhoea, Fever, Nosebleeds, Rash and Vomiting.There are 5 stages of CKD starting from a very mild damage to complete kidney failure respectively. Stages of kidney disease are based on the basic functions of kidney to filter waste and extract the fluid out of blood.

Attributes to Monitor CKD

The two important attributes for CKD are urine albumin and eGFR. A blood test that checks how well your kidneys are filtering your blood is called GFR. GFR stands for glomerular filtration rate. A urine test to check for albumin content in urine also plays a vital role in monitoring CKD. Estimation of glomerular filtration rate (eGFR) and assessment of albuminuria (or proteinuria) plays a vital role in CKD. Key attributes in laboratory test for CKD includes creatinine, eGFR, urine albumin-to-creatinine ratio and urine protein-to-creatinine ratio with the use of appropriate reporting units. Other factors which need to be monitored are high blood pressure and heart rate.

Internet of Things in Health Care

The term Internet of Things was coined by the British technology pioneer Kevin Ashton in 1999; he gave this title for his presentation on how to use RFID tags for Supply chain management. Internet of Things (IoT) is defined as a concept which enables communication between interconnecting devices and applications whereby physical object or things communicate through Internet (Raj Kumar, 2017). There is no common definition for IoT. It is also defined as a network of objects or physical things sending, receiving or communicating information using Internet or other communication technologies and network just as the computer, tablets and mobiles do and thus enabling monitoring, coordinating or controlling process across the Internet or another data network. Internet of Things is a vision where things like wearable watches, home devices and surrounding objects become smart and functions like a living entity by sensing, computing and communicating embedded devices with server, cloud services, applications and processes or person through Internet or Near Field Communication. This kind of IoT Vision plays a vital role in monitoring and diagnosis of chronic diseases in medical field along with the physicians and other health care officials. New advances in machine learning and IoT are used in health care sector to screen the therapeutic conditions and other related patients' details. In this we are going to see the use of IoT in chronic kidney disease monitoring. The microcontroller and the sensors to be used for monitoring the Blood pressure level, urine albumin content, glomerular filtration rate and heart beat using cloud IoT in detail. The health care professionals get connected with the patients more proactively through IoT technology. Some of the examples of IoT used in health care sectors include

- Kinect HoloLens Assisted Rehabilitation Experience (KHARE) platform created by Microsoft Enterprise Services in conjunction with the National Institute for Insurance Against Accidents at Work (INAIL) assists mirror neuron therapy.
- Smart Fridge by Weka for vaccine is used to addresses mainstay issues in vaccine management such as storing vaccines at a recommended temperature, the reliability of electrical power, and inventory errors leading to spoilage.

Next, we will see the IoT kit CC3200 Lauchpad and its architecture which is connected with appropriate sensors for monitoring chronic kidney disease.

CC3200 Launchpad Architecture and Sensors used for CKD Monitoring

The CC3200 is a programmable Wi-Fi MCU that enables true, integrated IoT development. The CC3200 device has the same Wi-Fi Network Processor (NWP) sub-system as the CC3100 device (TI, n.d.). This NWP integrates all protocols for Wi-Fi and Internet, greatly minimizing MCU software requirements. It is a low-cost evaluation platform. It uses ARM® Cortex™-M4-based CC3200 Wi-Fi MCU. The CC3200 Launch has a temperature sensor and a three-axis accelerometer included on the board. Sensors to be used in the design of the Kit includes AMS 5915AN03 sensor for monitoring blood pressure, TCS3200 color sensor for detection of albumin in a mixture of human urine, INA219 glucose sensor to monitor blood sugar level, 16×2 LCD and KY039 Heartbeat Sensor Module is designed here which can calculate the heart rate of a person Heartbeat Sensor are embedded with the CC3200 Launchpad. Each of these sensors are represented diagrammatically in figures 1,2,3,4 and 5 respectively.

The block diagram in figure 8 clearly explains proposed CKD monitoring system. The CC3200 Launchpad is connected to monitor the patients with Chronic kidney disease and send the health details like blood pressure level, heart beat level, glucose level and albumin content in urine to the doctors mobile. If there is a variation or abnormality detected it will make an alarm in the doctor's mobile. These health monitoring sensors are used to acquire data from the patients and transmit wirelessly by the CC3200 controller over the Internet. The data processing is done in the server and displayed in the ThinkSpeak followed by sending message to the website designed for the doctors to view the patient's details. The SimpleLink™ Wi-Fi® CC3200 LaunchPad™ development kit (with QFN-packaged device) is an evaluation development platform for the CC3200 wireless microcontroller (MCU), the industry's first single-chip programmable MCU with built-in Wi-Fi

Figure 1. CC3200 launchpad

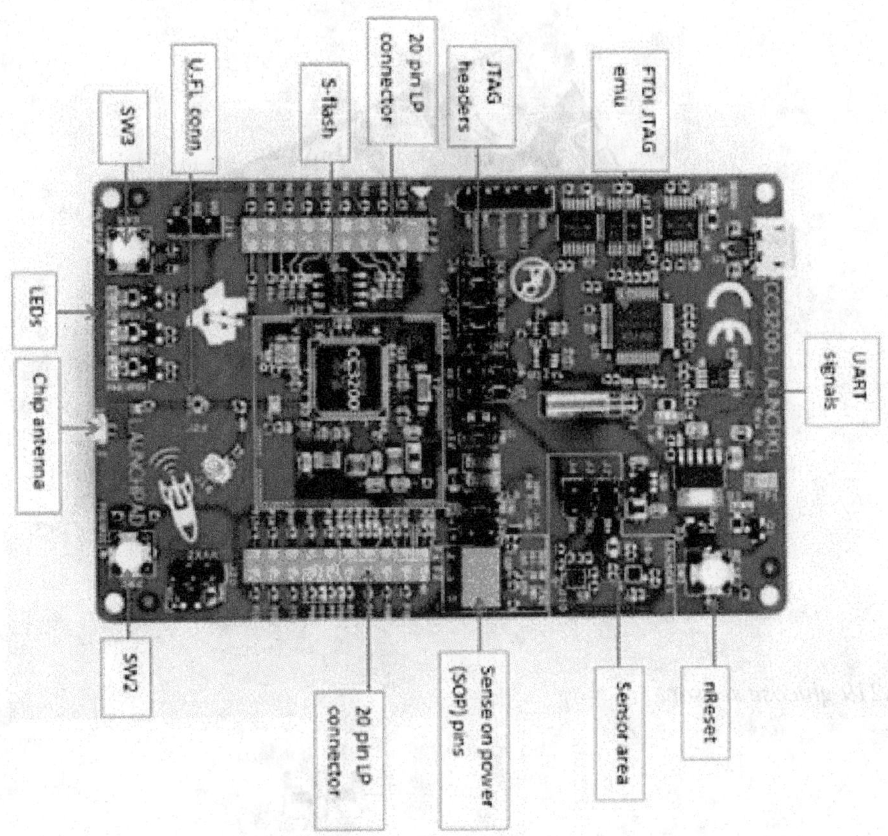

Figure 2. Measurement setup using an AMS 5915, Arduino Nano, the AMS 5915Arduino Nano kit[4] and an inflatable cuff

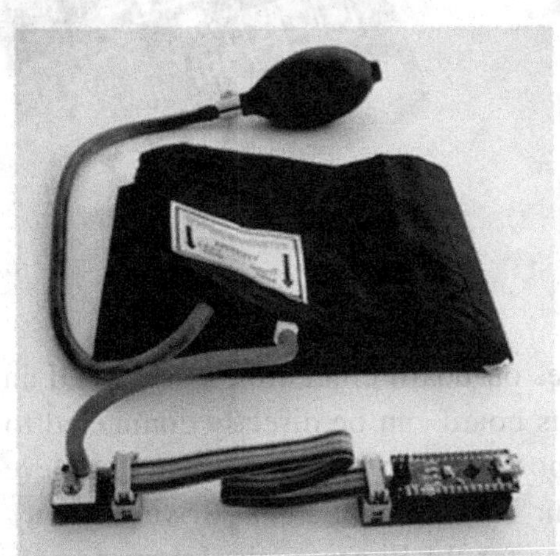

Figure 3. TCS 3200 urine sensor

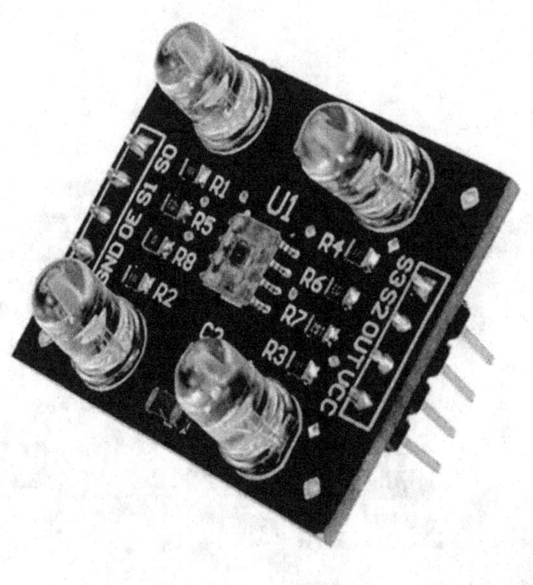

Figure 4. INA219 glucose sensor

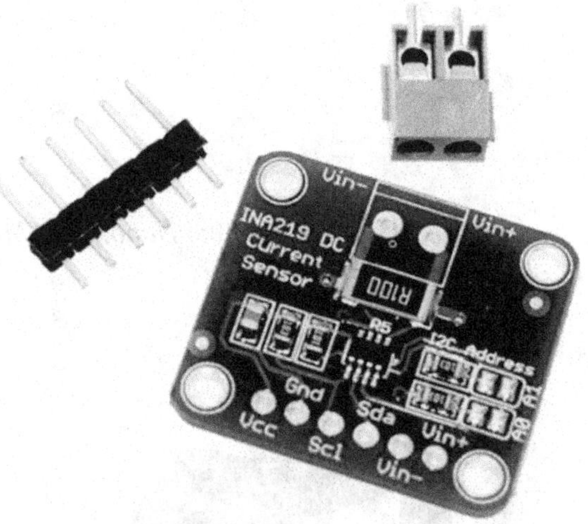

connectivity. The board features on-board emulation using FTDI and includes sensors for a full out-of-the-box experience. This board can be directly connected to a PC for use with development tools such as Code Composer Studio™ Cloud integrated development environment (IDE) and IAR Embedded Workbench. This LaunchPad has driver support and a software development kit (SDK) with 40+ applications for Wi-Fi protocols, Internet applications and MCU peripheral examples. CC3200 is supported in v7.20 of IAR (Townsend & Term, 2001).

Figure 5. KY039 heartbeat sensor

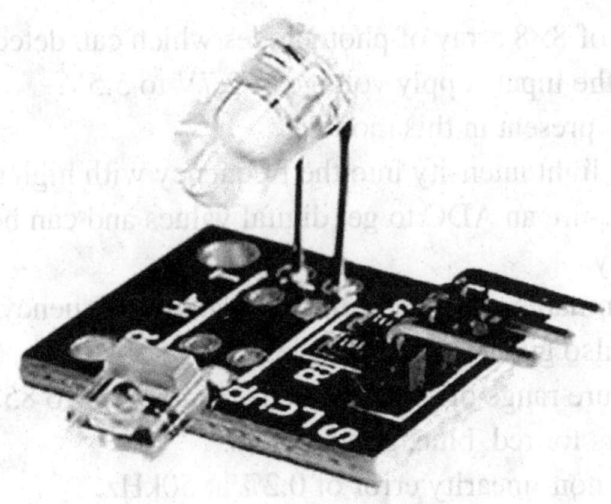

Measurement Setup using an AMS 5915, Arduino Nano, the AMS 5915Arduino Nano Kit[4]and an Inflatable Cuff

One of the well-known methods for non-invasive blood pressure measurement is the oscillometer principle (Townsend & Term, 2001). Currently it is the most popular measurement method in automatic blood pressure monitors. It uses an inflatable cuff with inflation and deflation mechanism, a pressure sensor and an evaluation unit like an Arduino Nano. After the cuff was inflated to a certain pressure it is slowly deflated while the pressure sensor measures the pressure inside the cuff. As soon as the pressure in the cuff decreases below a certain pressure the intra-arterial blood pulsation caused by the pulse induces pressure oscillations in the cuff. The amplitude of these oscillations depends on the cuff's pressure and can be used to estimate the systolic and diastolic blood pressure (Azbeg et al., 2011). The blood pressure is measured against air pressure; therefore, a differential/ relative pressure sensor is necessary. In most cases the systolic blood pressure is lower than 180 mmHg (= 239.98 mbar). In our setup we chose AMS 5915-0350-D for the blood pressure measurement with a minimum pressure of 0 mbar and a maximum pressure of 350mbar.

Blood pressure is caused by the force created through the heart's pumping action that drives blood into the arteries and circulating system when the blood flows through the arteries they provide resistance to blood flow which results in blood pressure. Early detection of hypertension can reduce the risk of kidney failure. Normal pressure for a healthy person ranges from 90/60mmHg and 120/80mmHg and below this range is considered as low blood pressure. The high blood pressure ranges from 140/90mmHg or higher (Gahan, 2019).

B. G. Gahan *et al.*, (2019) proposed a TCS3200 sensor and a urine strip a portable urine analysis system to detect CKD. The sensor detects the change in color on the strip when the sample is introduced. Change in color of the strip is due to the presence of albumin in urine, which is the primary biomarker considered to detect the early stage of kidney dysfunction.

Some of the specifications of TCS3200 are as follows:

- The main blocks of this module are TCS3200 RGB sensor chip and 4 white LEDs.
- The four LEDs are given to provide sufficient lighting conditions for the sensor during color detection.
- TCS3200 chip consists of 8×8 array of photodiodes which can detect red, blue, green colors.
- This module works on the input supply voltage of 2.7V to 5.5V.
- Digital TTL interface is present in this module.
- TCS3200 chip converts light intensity into the frequency with high resolution.
- This module doesn't require an ADC to get digital values and can be connected to digital pins of microcontrollers directly.
- TCS3200 has a programmable color and full-scale output frequency.
- Power down feature is also given to this module.
- The operating temperature range of this module is from -40°C to 85°C.
- TCS3200 contains filters for red, blue, green colors.
- This module contains a non-linearity error of 0.2% at 50kHz.
- TCS3200 module has a stable 200 ppm/°C temperature co-efficient.

The sensor TCS3200 senses light using an 8x8 array of photodiodes, which converts light energy to current. The current is then converted into square wave frequencies using a current to frequency converter whose frequency is directly proportional to light intensity. Finally, by exploiting the Arduino Board, a square wave is observed as a result. This exemplifies color detection by means of a sensor. The photodiodes have 3 different color filters - Red, green and blue, each of which are sixteen in number. The other sixteen photodiodes are clear with no filters. Each of the sixteen photodiodes is arranged in a parallel manner. The required photodiode type can be derived by using the two control pins S2 and S3. Consider an example to detect green color, both pins are set to high based on the logic table given below.

The TCS 3200 is a color sensor used to detect 3 colors red, blue and green. Urine test strips are used to detect the presence of albumin in urine. In the proposed system the sensor is used to detect a change in color which indicates the presence of albumin in the urine. A multi parameter urine test strip is used. Egg white is used to detect the presence of protein for the experimentation purpose. The TCS 3200 color sensor was able to detect the change in color from yellow to green. The results are shown in the table below

A **glucose sensor** is an electrochemical diagnostic strip which used **glucose** oxidizes enzymes; **INA219** current sensing module converts signals from **glucose sensor** (milliamp) to voltage interfaces with the **CC3200**. LCD module is used to display the measured value of the blood **glucose**. Ahmed S. Abd El-Hamid, Amani E. Fetohi, R.S. Amin, R.M. Abdel Hameed. This is based on an electronic system to perform a measurement of the blood glucose based onArduino UNO. A glucose sensor is an electrochemical diagnostic strip which used glucose oxidizes enzymes; INA219 current sensing module converts signals from glucose sensor (milliamp) to voltage interfaces with the Arduino UNO. LCD

Table 1. Color detection using sensor

Parameters	Color Detected	Result
EGG WHITE	GREEN	ALBUMIN PRESENT
WATER	YELLOW	ALBUMIN ABSENT

module is used to display the measuredvalue of the blood glucose. Software is developed in C language (Townsend & Term, 2001).

With this sensor module, which contains a phototransistor and an infrared diode, you can measure a pulse. For that, you have to put a finger between the diode and the transistor. Explanation: exactly like you know it from a flashlight, the light can shine through your skin. If you hit a vein with the light, you can see the pumping of the blood a little bit. You can see it because the blood concentration is different on different areas in the vein, which means you can see brightness differences in the blood flow. Exactly these differences can be measured with the sensor module and with that you will get the pulse. You can see it clear at the oscilloscope picture. This shows the changes of the voltage at the phototransistor – and with it the brightness change which comes from the flowing blood. The peaks above show the heartbeat. If you calculate the measured beats per recorded time, you will nearly get 71 beats per minute (bpm). Additionally, to that, you can see that the signal from the transistor is really low or the transistor is really sensitive to measure the small signal. For optimal results, we advise to prepare the module like it is shown in the pictures below in figure 6.

Figure 6 shows a thumb-sized heart rate monitor which is DFRobot. This monitors the pulse and detects blood volume by changing the microvascular bed of tissues. This sensor is easy to detect the pulsatile components of the cardiac cycle. It has two holes one to be attached to the belt, another to warp on the finger, wrist, earlobe or other skin contact areas. The output of the heart beat monitored using the sensor is displayed in ThingSpeak as shown in figure 7.

Figure 8 clearly depicts the conceptual framework of the Smart Chronic Kidney disease monitoring system. The proposed IoT architecture is based on the ITU-T five-layer model. The conceptual framework is based on the equation depicted below:

Gather + Consolidate + Connect + Collect + Assemble + Manage and Analyse = IoT with Connectivity to Cloud Services

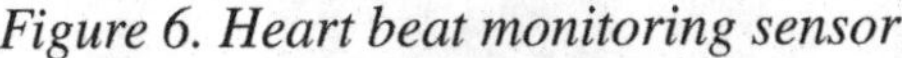

Figure 6. Heart beat monitoring sensor

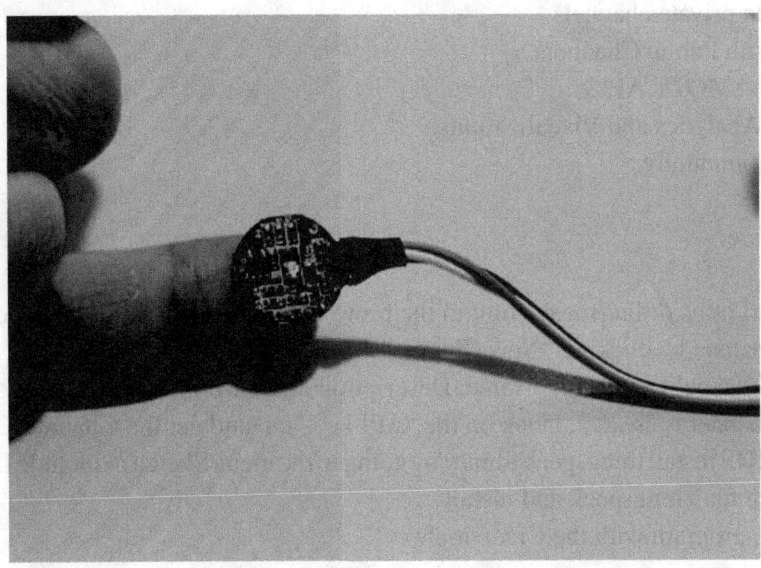

Figure 7. Result of the heartbeat monitored through the sensor on ThingSpeak

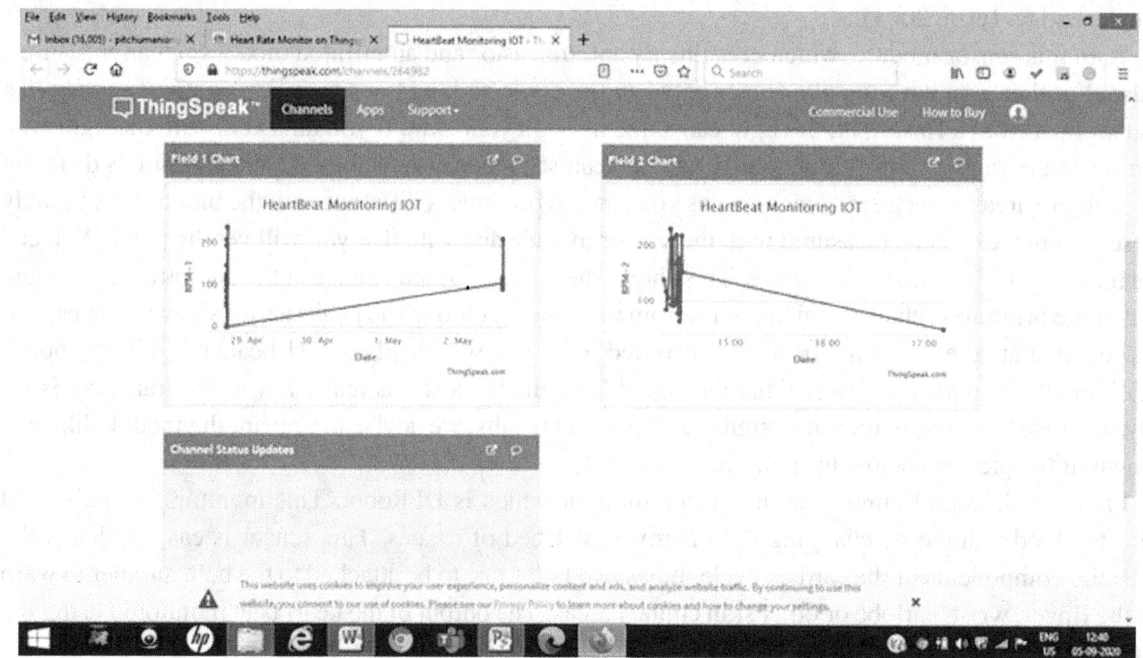

Thinspeak is an open-source IoT application and API. It is used to store and retrieve data from Hardware devices and sensors using HTTP protocol over the Internet or LAN communication. Channels are created for each and every sensor data. They can be set as private or public channels (Al-khafajiy et al., 2019).

The variation in the heartbeat, blood pressure and the albumin content detected data are transferred to the Thingspeak cloud and the results are displayed in a graphical format with day wise variations are shown in Figure 9. Features of Thingspeak are:

- Collect data in private channels.
- Share Data with Public Channels
- REST API and MQTT APIS
- MATLAB® Analytics and Visualizations.
- Worldwide Community

Steps involved are:

Step 1: Type the url https://thingspeak.com/ in the browser and create a thingspeak account
Step 2: Create a channel by clicking "New Channel"
Step 3: Enter the Channel Details like Name, Description and Save the settings
Step 4: Now the channel is created. Click on the "API key" tab and get the ChannelID and API keys
Step 5: In ArduinoIDE install thingspeak library by going to the menu Sketch->Include Library->Manage Library search for Thingspeak and install
Step 6: Modify the program with the Credentials

Figure 8. Block diagram of the proposed architecture

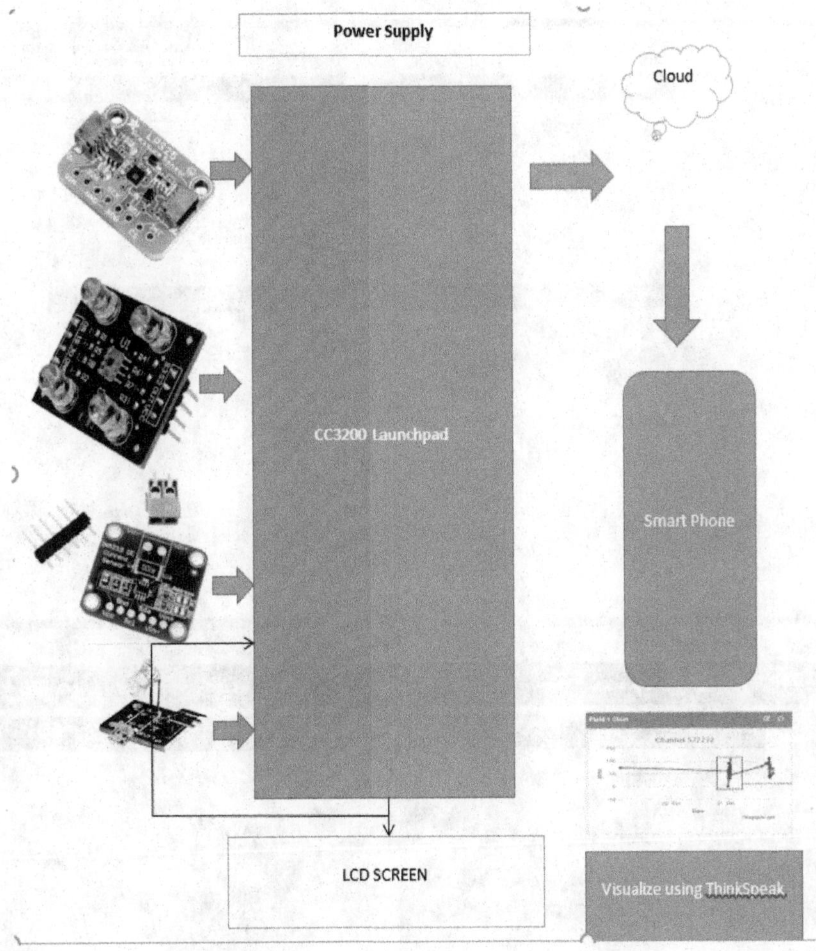

The data and information obtained from the sensors are stored in cloud server for future purpose and can be accessed by the physicians for monitoring the patients' health condition effectively. This chapter provides the simple IoT architecture to help and support kidney transplant patients in after care process (). Figure 9 shows the output of the sensors displaying the health condition of the patients in ThingSpeak cloud followed by figure 14 indicating a mobile app displaying the output from the sensors.

FUTURE RESEARCH DIRECTIONS

Many IoT healthcare companies are working on new ways to use this technology to help our medical world. According to the IoT healthcare market trends, the industry is expected to grow to $8.9 trillion in the year 2020. IoT can enhance patients care through Real time monitoring, IoT smart pills, Controlling Diabetes, Smart watches to cure major neuro disorder, Monitor and provide proper health care through early detection, diagnosis and management for neuro degenerative disorder, Monitoring of blood pressure etc., Jaimon et. al.(2020) stated in his research that enablers of IoT in

Figure 9. Patients health monitored using Thingspeak channel

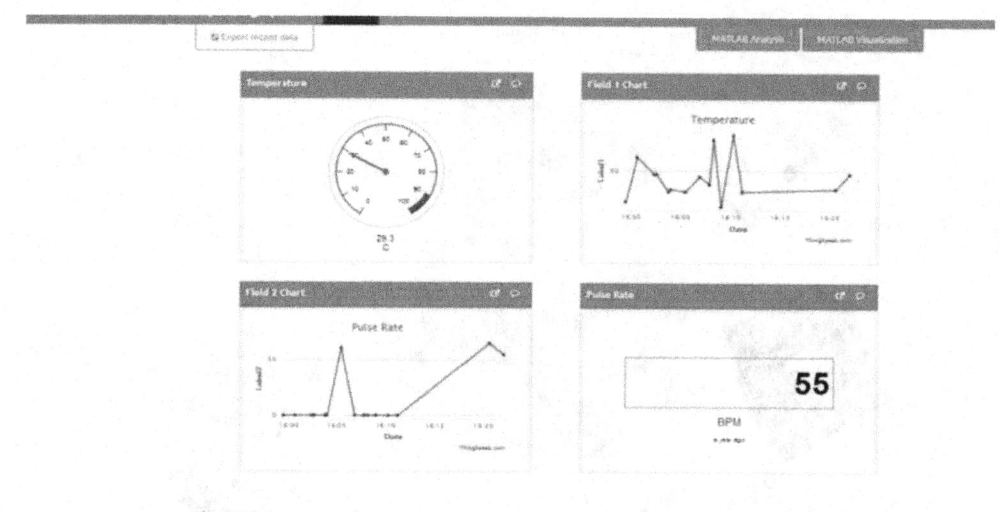

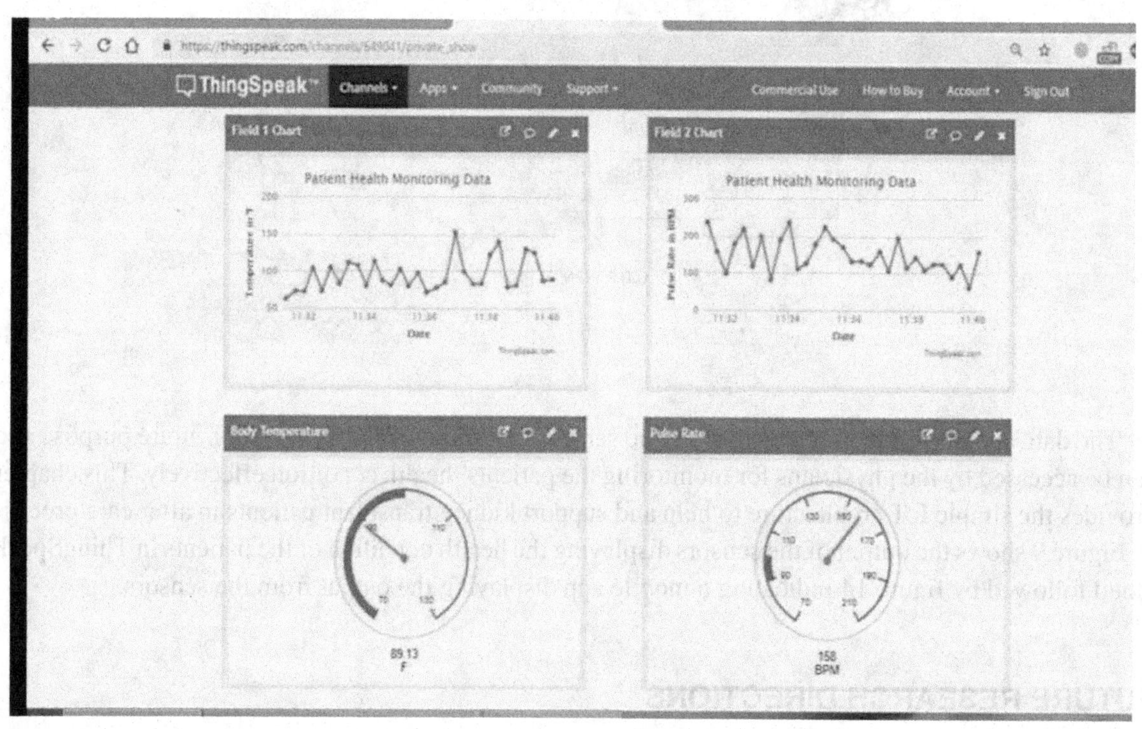

current health care will rely on policy support, cybersecurity-focused guidelines, careful strategic planning, and transparent policies within health care organizations. IoT-based health care has great potential to improve the efficiency of the health system and improve population health(Albahri et al., 2020). There will be a wider uptake of IoT, which can ultimately save health care dollars and improve patient-centered care.

Figure 10.

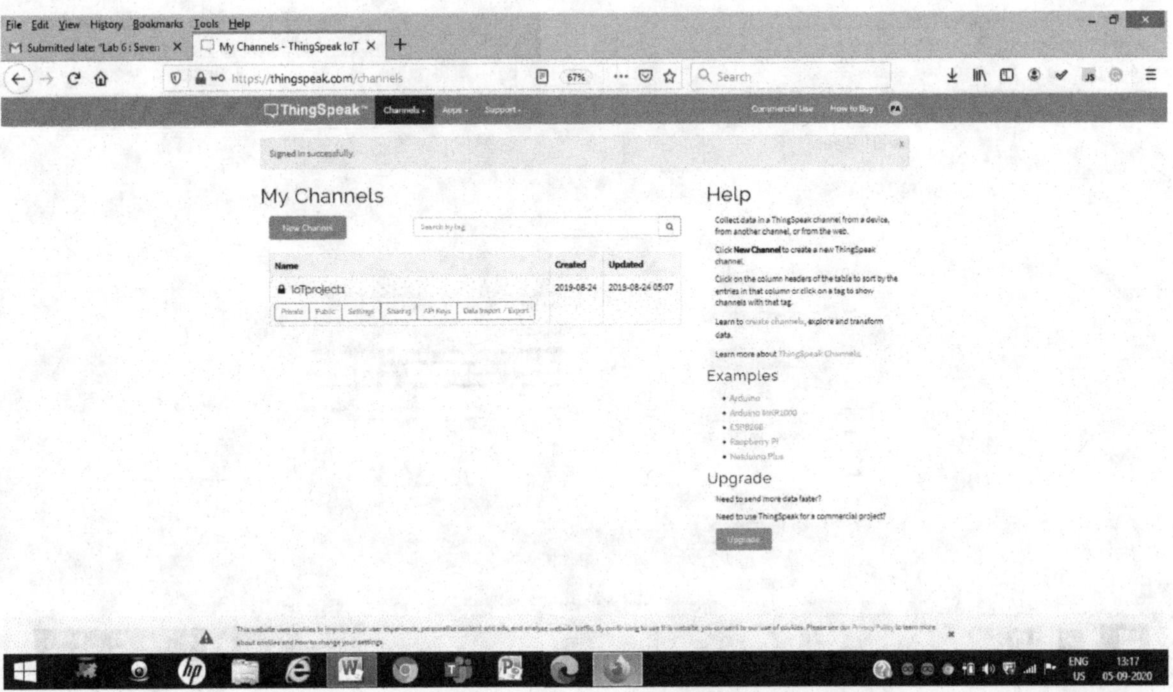

Figure 11.

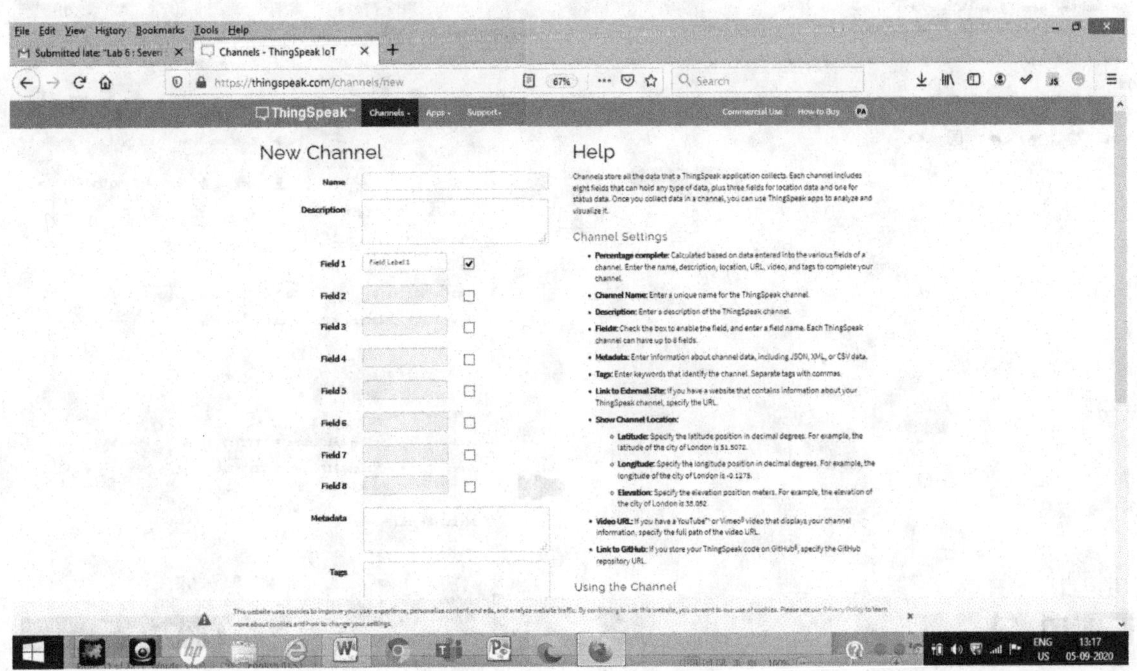

Figure 12.

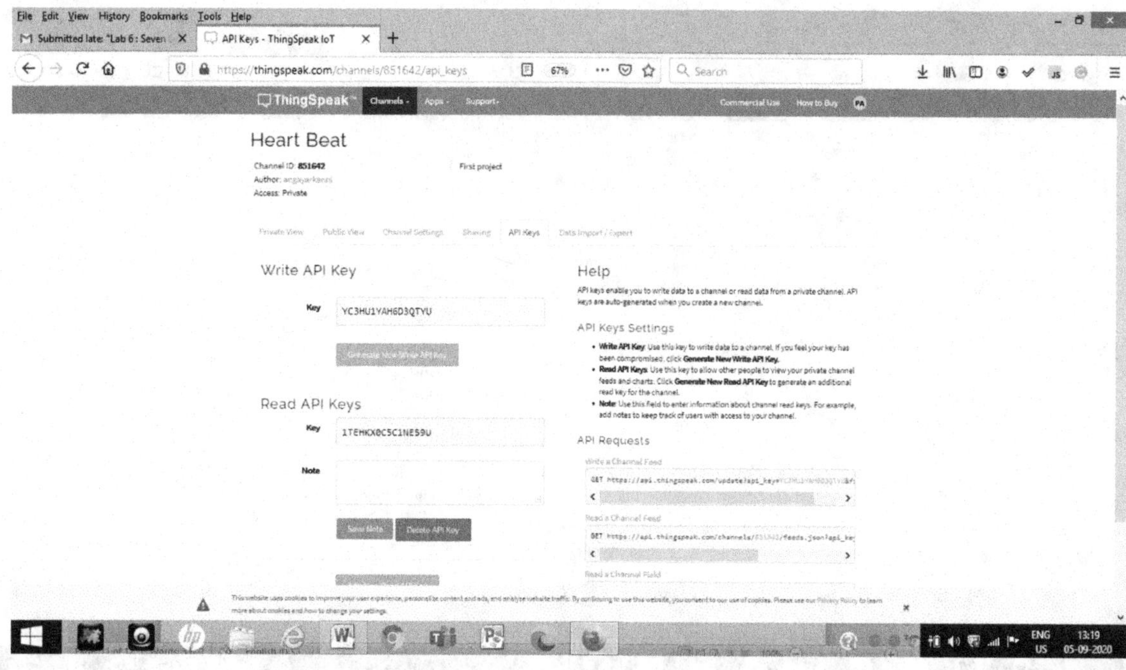

Figure 13.

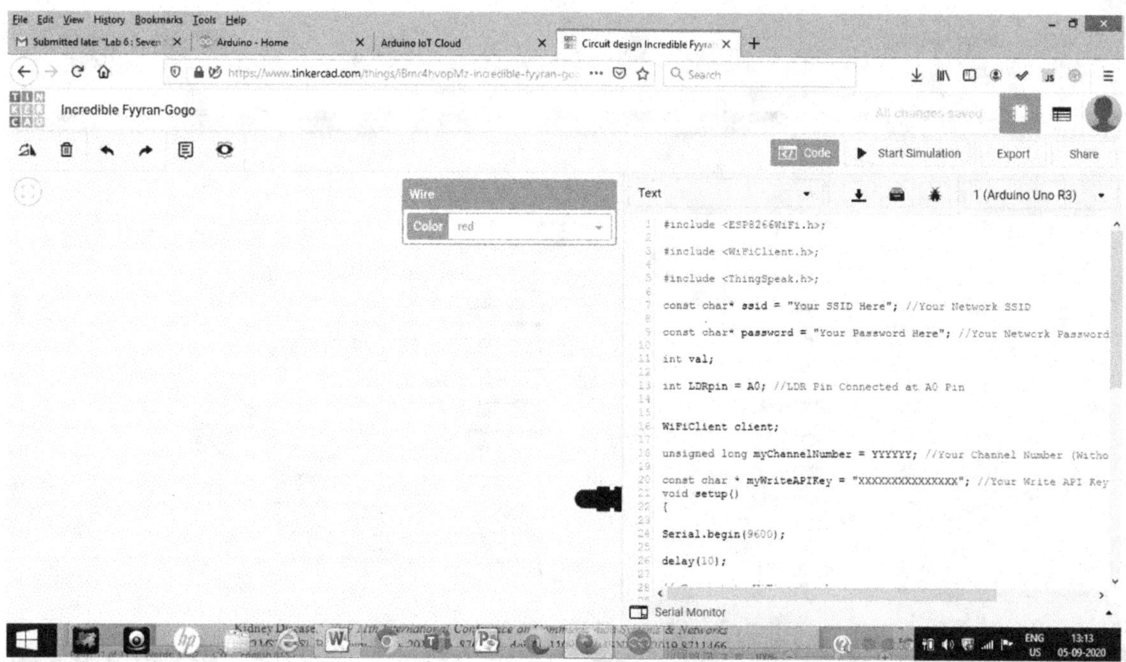

Figure 14. Mobile app to display the patients health data from sensor

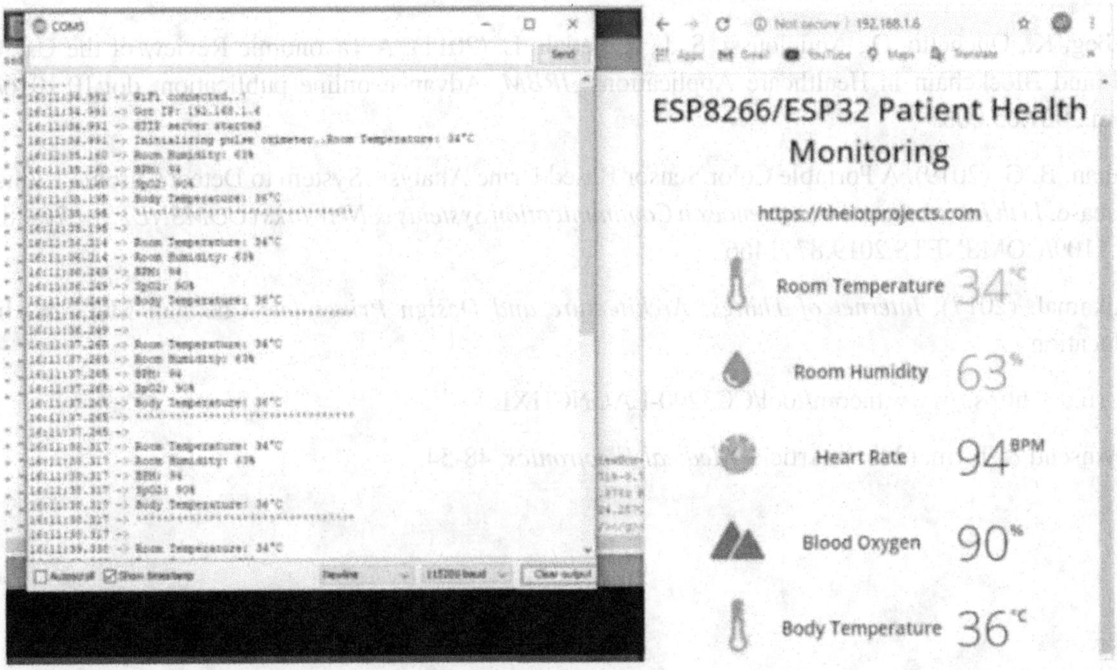

CONCLUSION

The proposed IoT Architecture can be used for remote dialysis patient monitoring from home thereby enhancing the patient care, reduce health care cost and enhance the quality of treatment. It is a valuable tool to improve the clinical outcome by enabling effective and easy connectivity between patients and the clinicians. With the advancement of the technology early monitoring of the symptoms and giving timely care is enhanced through IoT. Monitoring conditions like blood pressure, temperature, EGC, fluid overload, heart failure, peritonitis or sepsis through leveraging the emerging computational techniques in machine learning and artificial intelligence could help prevent or postpone hospitalization and avert the related costs.

REFERENCES

Al-khafajiy, M., Baker, T., Chalmers, C., Asim, M., Kolivand, H., Fahim, M., & Waraich, A. (2019). Remote health monitoring of elderly through wearable sensors. *Multimedia Tools and Applications, 78*(17), 24681–24706. doi:10.100711042-018-7134-7

Albahri, Alwan, Taha, Ismail, Hamid, Zaidan, Albahri, Zaidan, Alamoodi, & Alsalem. (2020). IoT-based telemedicine for disease prevention and health promotion: State-of-the-Art. *Journal of Network and Computer Applications*, (102873). Advance online publication. doi:10.1016/j.jnca.2020.102873

Alkhazaali, A. H. (2020). *International Congress on Human-Computer Interaction, Optimization and Robotic Applications (HORA)*. 10.1109/HORA49412.2020.9152923

Azbeg, K., Ouchetto, O., Andaloussi, S. J., & Fetjah, L. (2011). A Taxonomic Review of the Use of IoT and Blockchain in Healthcare Applications. *IRBM*. Advance online publication. doi:10.1016/j.irbm.2021.05.003

Gahan, B. G. (2019). A Portable Color Sensor Based Urine Analysis System to Detect Chronic Kidney Disease. *11th International Conference on Communication Systems & Networks (COMSNETS)*, 876-881. 10.1109/COMSNETS.2019.8711466

Rajkamal. (2017). *Internet of Things: Architecture and Design Principles*. Chennai: McGraw-Hill Education.

TI. (n.d.). https://www.ti.com/tool/CC3200-LAUNCHXL

Townsend & Term. (2001). Article. *Medical Electronics*, 48-54.

Chapter 3
Application of Machine Learning in Data Analytics on COVID-19 First Wave in India:
COVID-19 First Wave Analytics on the Cloud

Jeya Mala Dharmalingam
https://orcid.org/0000-0002-2100-8218
Jain University, Bangalore, India

Pradeep Reynold A.
GEMS Polytechnic College, India

ABSTRACT

As there are several data sets available, this chapter gives insight on which regions of India have been heavily impacted during the first wave of COVID-19 and the classification of patient status using an ML-based data analytics algorithm. The chapter provides a greater insight on the background work and the reports generated based on the analytical results gathered from the data set. In this pandemic situation, such reports will be a great benefit to assess the history of occurrence and the current status of the COVID-19 situation in India.

INTRODUCTION

As India is the second heavily populated country in the World, the impact of Covid-19 has also been alarming. It is time to revisit the impact of first wave in India so that, the lessons learnt from that, shall help understand the insights on distribution of the deadly disease.

DOI: 10.4018/978-1-7998-9132-1.ch003

Copyright © 2022, IGI Global. Copying or distributing in print or electronic forms without written permission of IGI Global is prohibited.

Based on several inputs from various sources related to the first wave, this chapter provides information on how ML is applied in the Covid-19 dataset to provide analytical reports in order to gain valuable insights on the available data.

Prior to Data Analytics, 'Data analysis' has ruled the World. It has the ability to spot patterns in a set and make predictions about past events accounts for a large part of its value. 'Data mining' is the term used to describe the act of finding patterns in data sets in order to better understand trends. Despite the many advantages that data analysis and big data provide, much of its potential is untapped because employees lack quick and reliable access to the information (Difference-data-analytics-data-analysis, 2020).

According to Gartner, 85 percent of Fortune 500 organizations do not fully profit from their big data analytics using data analysis due to a lack of data access, causing them to miss out on opportunities to better engage with and satisfy the demands of their customers.

Data analysis becomes more available as analysis goes to cloud drives, as corporate personnel may access company information remotely from any location, liberating them from being tethered to local networks and making data more accessible (Difference-data-analytics-data-analysis, 2020).

According to the dictionary definition, "analytics" is a systematic computational analysis that additionally includes the word "analysis". Data analytics methods also uses analysis to discover past information, apart from logical, systematic, and deductive reasoning to offer insights on how to act in the future (Difference-data-analytics-data-analysis, 2020).

Hence, Data Analytics now rules the World by means of applying several Machine Learning algorithms in it to process the raw data and to derive useful reports from it.

Machine learning has its backbone in Data Analytics; without it, models fail. Relevant data improves predictions. After the data, we must select an algorithm to solve the problem. Finance, retail, health care, and social data are some of the industries that machine learning can be applied to.

There are different types of learning algorithms available in Machine Learning. They are: Supervised Learning, Unsupervised Learning, Semi-Supervised Learning, Reinforced Learning etc (Caesar Wu et.al. 2016).

In the case of IoT in healthcare, the data needs to be collected from the sensors present in these devices. Sensor data is made up of sensor data such as time series signals, ordered sequences of pairs, simple numerical or categorical values, or more complex data, can be processed by computing devices. Data streams from wearable sensors could be used to identify people who have Parkinson's disease (Caesar Wu et.al. 2016).

According to research, the longer time, the people have to wait for treatment; the less likely they are to maintain their health. The treatment also depends on the results of the diagnostics. So it may be a lengthy process to interpret a large number of results (Guoguang Rang et.al. 2020).

In this chapter, we are going to provide the healthcare analytics reports based on the dataset taken from the public dataset pool Kaggle which is a part of Google's research dataset. As the dataset is larger, it is recommended to perform the analytics on the cloud by applying ML algorithm on the dataset.

BACKGROUND

Cloud Analytics

Cloud computing is the cornerstone of data analytics. Cloud computing is based on a series of hardware and software that can be remotely accessed using any web browser. Files and software are typically shared and worked on by several users, and all data is centralized remotely rather than being saved on individual users' hard discs (R.Maheshwari et.al, 2020). Analytics in cloud computing, such as social media engagement tracking and statistics, is essentially applying analytics ideas to data stored on cloud storage, instead of on individual servers or hard drives.

Cloud computing is the most important and emerging field in computer science that helps to do analytics in streamlining the business intelligence process. It helps in business decision making by gathering data, integrate them based on the pattern and then processing them using some analytical algorithms. The general idea is shown in Figure 1.

There are several cloud tools and platforms available for cloud analytics in order to provide relevant reports from huge data generated in a problem domain. Say for instance; consider a manufacturing unit which wants to improve their quality need to analyze the data collected from their processing units to find the quality breaches in order to fix them. As the data is voluminous, it is time to think about placing this analytics on the cloud in order to get the reports faster and based on the need. Compared to the traditional analytics platforms, the cloud analytics' performance will be faster in order to gets accurate decision making (Altexsoft, 2021, Comparing Machine Learning as a Service: Amazon, Microsoft Azure, Google Cloud AI, IBM Watson, 2021).

Some of the advantages of Cloud Analytics are: efficient processing, collaborative working, quick generation of reports using business intelligence.

Some of the other important advantages of Cloud Analytics are:

- Scalability

One of the benefits of cloud analytics is its scalability in terms of user and data volume. Another advantage is the ability to narrow down the search for data processing. Cloud computing gives the flexibility to scale up data storage and analysis capabilities on need basis. Through insights that reflect changing market conditions, firms may most efficiently scale the storing, processing, and generating reports on the data.

- Efficient Data Processing

Cloud analytics can give an efficient approach to data processing, by providing an organization's decision-makers to quickly access critical business data. This includes having access to various sorts

Figure 1. Data analytics on the cloud

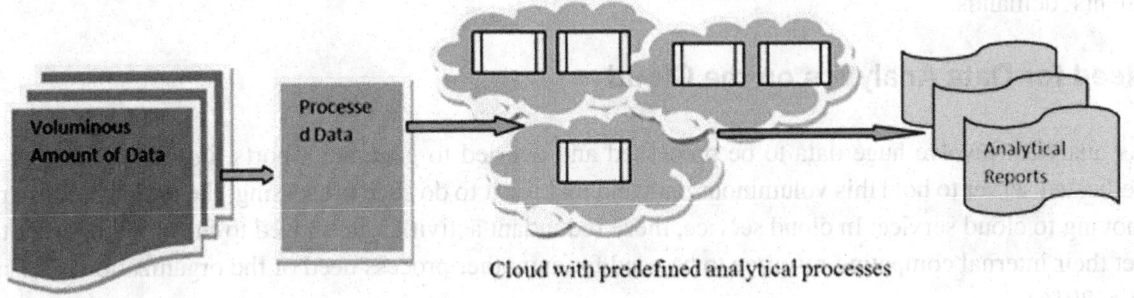

of data as well as data from various sources. You can quickly examine, test, and review data to uncover key insights that help a company to grow.

- Decomposition of data

When an organization uses cloud analytics, it may efficiently integrate data across departments and organizations. Using a cloud analytics system to combine data from many parts of a firm might provide daily insights. These insights might provide an organization a competitive advantage and help it grow. Data saved and analyzed in the cloud enables employees of all types to instantly access data and share insights, facilitating effective communication, collaboration, and decision-making.

- Quick insights

The platform that helps cloud analytics helps businesses to collect, integrate and analyze data in a much faster manner so that, intelligence decision making can be done at that moment.

- Collaborative working

Businesses that employ a cloud analytics platform obtain a central location to access data and connect to shared information when it's needed or given proactively. This common link and quick access to data improve collaboration across the organization.

- Data Security

A cloud-based analytics platform can offer a centralized and secure data access point. A cloud analytics platform also improves data governance by providing more precise access controls for who has access to what data, as well as auditing capabilities to see who has viewed what data.

Ideally data analytics helps eliminate much of the guesswork involved in trying to understand clients, instead systemically tracking data patterns to best construct business tactics and operations to minimize uncertainty. Analytics not only identifies what can attract new customers, but it also discovers current patterns in data to assist better serve existing clients, which is often less expensive than developing new business. In an ever-changing business world subject to countless variants, analytics gives companies the edge in recognizing changing climates so they can take initiate appropriate action to stay competitive. Along with analytics, cloud computing is helping organizations become more efficient, and combining the two could help firms store, understand, and process their big data in order to better satisfy their clients' demands.

Need for Data Analytics on the Cloud

As analytics involve huge data to be processed and queried to generate reports, instead of placing a dedicated server to hold this voluminous data and making it to do such processing, the organizations are moving to cloud service. In cloud service, these redundant activities are moved to the cloud in order to get their internal computing resource to be used for any other process need of the organization (Caesar Wu, 2016).

Big data which by its name has huge data set and has scalability as one of its primary attributes, it is necessary to keep this data to the cloud by means of IaaS (Infrastructure as a Service). Using this cloud service, the organizations are free from setting up a dedicated infrastructure to do this analysis (Hayk Gharagyozyan, 2019).

As in several of the cases, if the organization failed to properly estimate the computing resource, it will be tedious to keep the data which may cause issues while doing the processing part. The computational power of cloud service can also be leveraged to meet the real time requirements such as ML based data processing (Hayk Gharagyozyan, 2019).

If it appears random and from vastly different fields that data is processed and available on cloud drives, it could strain the magnet drives on cloud servers and cause them not to work with large data sets fully. Diversifying data across several cloud servers to avoid overburdening individual servers can help cloud networks function more like traditional networks, allowing them to remain competitive.

Because of the extent of big data, some clouds, regardless of their size or competence, are nevertheless unable to host or analyze specific kinds of data. Understanding the demands and scale of big data, as well as how it will be processed, is crucial to reaping the benefits of cloud based data analytics (Caeser Wu, 2016).

Another common purpose for cloud data analysis is Software-as-a-Service(SaaS). It allows users to access cloud-based software from any web browser, removing the requirement for users to use specific machines to complete tasks. Companies charging consumers a membership or monthly fee to access software on their website are common examples of Saas applications (Caeser Wu, 2016).

Users only have access to the programme as long as they pay their dues, and the software is never fully installed on their computers' hard drives. While SaaS allows users to access their applications from any location, it also limits their options if they do not have internet access or desire to work offline. More software companies are likely to utilise SaaS in the future in order to increase profitability and maintain complete control over their product. For software users, this means that they can either save money by not having to buy software if it is only needed for a short period of time, or they can spend more money in the long run as the expenses of software subscription build up.

MACHINE LEARNING (ML) IN DATA ANALYTICS

Data science is very broad, and it involves many diverse roles and functions. Data science work is typically comprised of the tasks of working with unstructural data, implementing machine learning (ML) concepts and techniques, and generating insights. After the visual presentation of data-driven insights, this process usually ends (Caeser Wu, 2016).

Machine learning is a critical element of the process, but training ML models is often a time-consuming process that requires a lot of resources. In the past, gaining access to ML resources was difficult and expensive. Today, many cloud computing vendors offer resources for data science in the cloud (K.Shailaja, 2018).

The number of iterations required to train machine learning and deep learning models may range from a hundred to thousand and these are part of machine learning and deep learning training. Accurate models can only be produced through a large number of iterations

Another way to look at this is that if you only have 1TB of training data, 10 training iterations will require 10TB of I/O. The dataset size that computer vision algorithms work with must be quite large in order to process high-resolution images. In many cases, removal of associated network latency can help reduce processing time. This will help you keep the source data's I/O performance at its peak (Arwinder Dhillan and Ashima Singh, 2019).

Cloud computing lets you scale the processing and storage capacity at the same time. Let's say, for example, that AWS is offering GPUs with 8–256GB of memory capacity. Each of these incidents has an hourly rate associated with it. GPUs are specifically designed processors for the more demanding image-processing requirements. The NC-series high performance GPU is available on Azure for high performance computing applications and algorithms (Moongu Jeon et.al., 2017).

Some of the ML service providers on the cloud are:

There are a number of machine learning tools and services available at Amazon, Microsoft Azure etc (Altexsoft, 2021). By implementing these services, organizations and developers can make computer-intensive and high performance computing models run better (Altexsoft, 2021 - Comparing Machine Learning as a Service: Amazon, Microsoft Azure, Google Cloud AI, IBM Watson, 2021).

These services are:

1. The Amazon SageMaker machine learning platform, which is available to anyone with machine learning expertise. If Elastic Compute Cloud (EC2) is used in a project, then it will be able to use machine learning models, collect the data, and increase the operations scalability. In addition to voice recognition, computer vision, and recommendations, SageMaker is also used for image and speech recognition.
2. Instead of creating our own ML models, one can use models that are already available through the AWS Marketplace. Overall, the most popular frameworks for deep learning applications are Keras, TensorFlow, and PyTorch. If a person wants to configure and optimise these frameworks, SageMaker can do it. Otherwise, it can be trained based on our needs. One can also develop his/her own algorithm by creating a Docker container and writing your algorithm inside. Jupyter notebooks make it easy to build and visualise machine learning models.
3. The Lex API is created to allow chatbots to be integrated into application. Lex contains advanced natural language processing techniques such as Natural Language Processing (NLP) and automatic speech recognition. An API is capable of distinguishing speech and text. You can embed recognised inputs to many different back-end solutions by using Lex's User Interface (UI). Lex supports chatbots deployment for Slack, Facebook Messenger, and Twilio, as well as standalone apps.
4. Rekognition from Amazon- It offers services with regards to image and video recognition is perfect for prototyping applications. Companies can tailor their apps using Rekognition to meet their needs.
5. The Azure Machine Learning library has a large collection of pre-trained and pre-packaged machine learning algorithms. While Azure Machine Learning Service also offers an environment where algorithm implementations and applied to real-world scenarios can take place, One can build machine learning pipelines that combine multiple algorithms using the Azure ML UI. Using the UI for training, testing, and evaluation is possible. Azure Machine Learning also provides AI solutions (AI). This includes the process of understanding the behaviour of a model and data that can be used to assess different algorithms.
6. On the first level, Google offers machine learning and AI services to professionals. On the second level, Google offers beginner-level machine learning and AI services.
7. Automatic Machine Learning on Google Cloud - An easy-to-use machine learning platform specifically designed for users who are new to the field. Data upload, model training, and web deployment

are all available to you. AutoML incorporates all of Google's services and data is stored in the cloud. The REST API enables you to deploy trained models. AutoML software is made available to the public via a graphical user interface. This incorporates image and video processing services, a natural language processing and translation engine, and training models on structured data.

8. One can run ML training jobs and predictions at scale with the Google Cloud ML Engine. By using Google Cloud ML and GPU and Tensor Processing Unit (TPU) infrastructure, you can train a complex model. To deploy an externally trained model, use the service. Automating all of the monitoring and resource provisioning processes frees up your time to focus on running your jobs. In addition to serving as a training and hosting location, Cloud ML also serves as a platform for hyperparameter tuning that impacts predictions. If data scientists do not use automatic hyperparameter tuning, they must experiment with multiple values to evaluate the results.
9. TensorFlow is an open source software library that utilizes data flow graphs for numeric calculations. When performing mathematical operations in these graphs, nodes are used as a symbol for mathematical operations, while edges stand in for data movement from one node to another. A tensor is a multidimensional array in TensorFlow. For research and practice, TensorFlow is often used for deep learning. TensorFlow is open-source and cross-platform. The application can be used on GPU-accelerated processing, CPU-accelerated processing, TPU-accelerated processing, and mobile-device-optimized processes.

HEALTHCARE ANALYTICS ON THE CLOUD

Cloud analytics enables data collection and processing without regard to location, regardless of the physical location of the servers. In the case of health care applications, once a sample is taken from a patient from any of the geographical locations across the country, the Government is able to keep track of that person and update their status as necessary. Health care reports from nearby hospitals are not necessary when managing the patient details from cloud data automatically uploaded to the cloud drives (R. Maheshwari et.al. 2018). Data stored in the cloud gives hospitals a better understanding of their patients' status and helps them to provide their service more efficiently (Tirthajyoti Sarkar, 2020).

Cloud computing gets even more secure, reliable, and affordable. It's conceivable that an entire hospital's records could soon be stored in the cloud and available to those who need it, anywhere. Because local servers and personal computer hard drives have the ability to give rise to all data being stored remotely in data warehouses far from the physical location of a business, it is a possibility that all data could be stored remotely in data warehouses located in remote locations (Tirthajyoti Sarkar, 2020).

Application of ML in Healthcare Analytics

The crux of machine learning is the application of advanced technology to improve healthcare. Some artificial intelligence applications, such as speech recognition in voice assistants, and personalized online shopping experiences that make use of learning associations, may be familiar to many people (Guoguang Rong, 2020). While machine learning has been shown to have tremendous potential in healthcare, in particular for the detection of medical conditions (K.Shailaja et.al, 2018),

Electronically-stored medical imaging data is plentiful today, and Deep Learning algorithms can be provided with these kinds of datasets, to detect and discover patterns and anomalies (Arwinder Dhillon and Ashima Singh, 2019).

The machines and algorithms can read through the imaging data and spot suspicious spots on the skin, lesions, tumors, and brain bleeds in the same way that a highly trained radiologist can. There is considerable headroom for the use of AI/ML tools/platforms in assisting radiologists, and this trend is only going to grow (Hayk Gharagyozyan,2019).

As there is a critical shortage of well-trained radiologists around the world, in the vast majority of cases, the AI/ML integrated solutions can easily handle the flood of digital medical data and provide expected reports effectively (Hayk Gharagyozyan,2019).

Different types of data collected from the health care domains such as clinical data, sensor data, Omics data etc. All these data are generally in the raw format and cannot be used as such for getting any insights on these meta data. For instance, the sensor data is directly collected from the sensors of wearable devices, monitoring devices etc. and Omics data includes genome and proteome data etc (Nilesh Barla, 2021).

In order to process this meta-data, the Machine Learning algorithms came as a real boon to get relevant insights and to provide analytical reports.

Samuel invented machine learning in 1950 to design games like chess. A machine's ability to learn without human involvement is made possible by mechanisms. Machine Learning is focused on creating a programme that is able to use data and learn from it. Advanced algorithms and statistical techniques allow machines to better make predictions and help make data-driven systems more powerful (Tirthajyoti Sarkar, 2020).

In recent years, hospitals have started using machine learning to increase the speed at which they can analyze and diagnose patients. As of now, doctors are now supported in both the diagnosis and treatment phases to shorten the time to recovery (Nilesh Barla, 2021).

The level of perfection that machine learning can reach when it's used to examine CT scans or diagnosis reports is astonishing. An expert doctor reviews reports and suggestions created by machine learning models to ensure that the patients' needs are met (S.Vollmer et.al, 2020).

By categorizing patients into separate categories based on their health conditions, doctors can direct their efforts toward those patients who have the most serious issues, increasing their treatment success.

A lot of research is going on in predictive health analytics. Using historical data, one can train a machine learning model to identify patterns and generate accurate predictions. Symptoms, habits, diseases, and predictions are correlated and associated, which is how it finds correlations and associations. Using

Figure 2. AI/ML embedded healthcare data analytics on the cloud

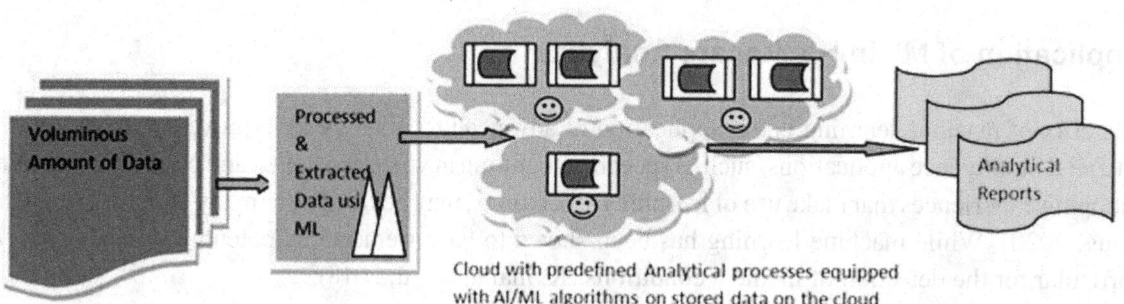

patient's behavior, eating habits, and various activities, doctors can now use this prediction model to foresee various diseases (Sebastian Vollmer et.al, 2020).

Supply chains and pharmaceutical logistics are enhanced with the use of predictive analytics. To avoid having medicine or injection shortages in the event of an emergency, pharmaceutical logistics models in particular hospitals can be used to forecast the local demand for the product (Moongu Jeon et.al, 2017).

Especially during the pandemic situation of Covid-19, where there was a huge shortage of vaccines has lead to several chaos in many places of India. In these kind of situations, a predictive analytics help in properly planning and identifying the worst affected areas and prioritize them to give vaccines.

The health of patients can be predicted and preventive measures, like starting an early treatment, can be put in place to reduce the risk of their condition worsening.

Predictive analytics is commonly used by larger companies, such as Apple or Nike, in their Wearables, such as heart rate, breathing rate, sleep cycles, and many more.

The virtual healthcare assistants that the data scientists build can provide assistance to patients using both disease predictive modelling and advancements in natural language processing (NLP) (Nilesh Barla, 2021).

Patients can input their symptoms, and through these platforms and machine learning algorithms, receive information about different possible diseases and a recommendation on which treatment they should follow.

Virtual applications can be useful to patients suffering from psychological issues like depression or anxiety, as well as diseases like Alzheimer's or Parkinson's. NLP is a powerful tool in machine learning, which allows algorithms to suggest a patient's most appropriate prescription, treatment, healthcare routine, and diet. Clinicians and other medical staff members are given the opportunity to examine the algorithm's suggested course of action and make better decisions. In addition to recommending content, a chatbot can also suggest new content for you when you are on the go (Tirthajyoti Sarkar, 2020).

Patients can interact with a chatbot by entering their issues and providing solutions. An algorithm can examine a patient's prior data, medical data, and answers to prior questions, and then evaluate the solutions that may be appropriate (Hayk Gharagyozyan, 2019).

ANALYTICAL REPORTS ON COVID-19 DATASET

Analytical Report 1 - Cloud Data Analytics for Covid-19 First Wave in India

The sample dataset related to Covid-19 first wave happened in India was taken from https://datasetsearch.research.google.com/ which has several data sets for experimentation purpose. For this chapter, the dataset "Covid 19 India Individual Patient Dataset" is taken from Kaggle website which is given with license Attribution-NonCommercial-ShareAlike 4.0 (CC BY-NC-SA 4.0).

As the dataset is open access with non-commercial license, this chapter analyses the dataset and provided a number of insights as a result.

From the results of the first dataset - covid19indiadata, 2021, (Santhoshkumar, 2021), https://www.kaggle.com/santhoshkumarv/covid19indiadata

From the next dataset given in (Ruchi, 2021) https://www.kaggle.com/ruchi798/siim-covid-19-detection-eda-data-augmentation (siim-covid-19-detection-eda-data-augmentation, 2021)

Figure 3. Kaggle Data Set Page

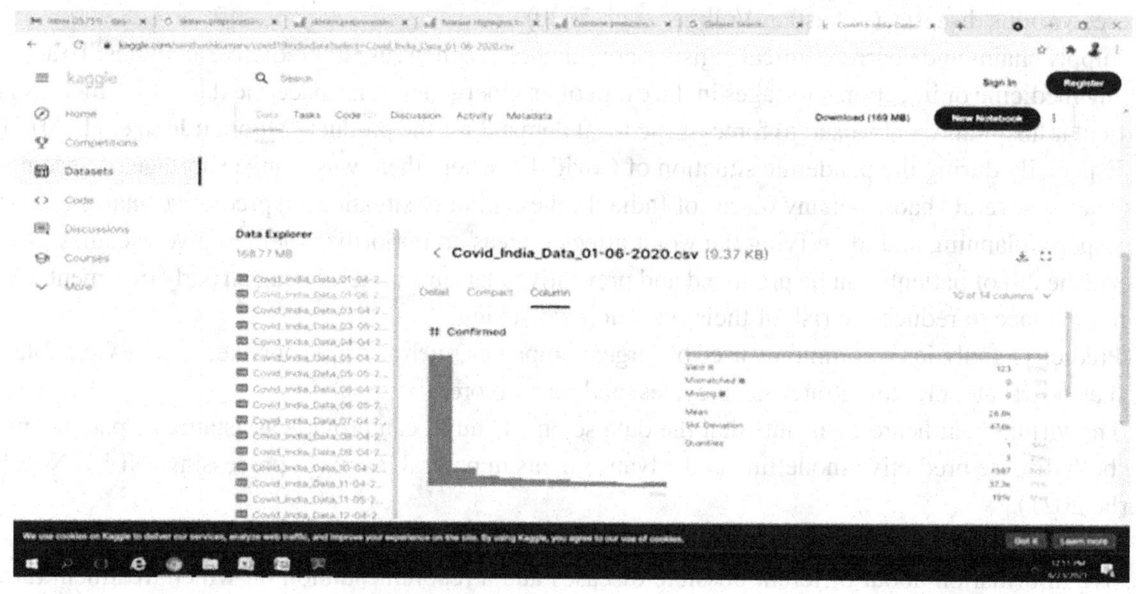

The following observations have been found:

```
params = {'legend.fontsize': 'x-large',
          'figure.figsize': (20, 32),
         'axes.labelsize': 'x-large',
         'axes.titlesize':'x-large',
         'xtick.labelsize':'x-large',
         'ytick.labelsize':'x-large'}
pylab.rcParams.update(params)
fig, ax = plt.subplots(4,2)
sns.kdeplot(train_df["Negative for Pneumonia"], shade=True,ax=ax[0,0],color="#ffb4a2")
ax[0,0].set_title("Negative for Pneumonia Distribution",font="Serif", fontsize=20,weight="bold")
sns.countplot(x = train_df["Negative for Pneumonia"], ax=ax[0,1],color="#ffb4a2")
ax[0,1].set_title("Negative for Pneumonia Distribution",font="Serif", fontsize=20,weight="bold")
sns.kdeplot(train_df["Typical Appearance"], shade=True,ax=ax[1,0],color="#e5989b")
ax[1,0].set_title("Typical Appearance Distribution",font="Serif", fontsize=20,weight="bold")
sns.countplot(x = train_df["Typical Appearance"], ax=ax[1,1],color="#e5989b")
ax[1,1].set_title("Typical Appearance Distribution",font="Serif", fontsize=20,weight="bold")
sns.kdeplot(train_df["Indeterminate Appearance"], shade=True,ax=ax[2,0],color="#b5838d")
ax[2,0].set_title("Indeterminate Appearance Distribution",font="Serif", fontsize=20,weight="bold")
sns.countplot(x = train_df["Indeterminate Appearance"], ax=ax[2,1],color="#b5838d")
ax[2,1].set_title("Indeterminate Appearance Distribution",font="Serif", fontsize=20,weight="bold")
sns.kdeplot(train_df["Atypical Appearance"], shade=True,ax=ax[3,0],color="#6d6875")
ax[3,0].set_title("Atypical Appearance Distribution",font="Serif", fontsize=20,weight="bold")
sns.countplot(x = train_df["Atypical Appearance"], ax=ax[3,1],color="#6d6875")
```

```
ax[3,1].set_title("Atypical Appearance Distribution",font="Serif", fontsize=20,weight="bold")
fig.subplots_adjust(wspace=0.2, hspace=0.4, top=0.93)
plt.show()

In [11]:
def plot_wb_bar(df,col1,col2):
    run = wandb.init(project='siim', job_type='image-visualization',name=col1,config = CONFIG)
    dt = [[label, val] for (label, val) in zip(df[col1], df[col2])]
    table = wandb.Table(data=dt, columns = [col1,col2])
    wandb.log({col1: wandb.plot.bar(table, col1,col2,title=col1)})
    run.finish()
def count_values(df,col):
    df = pd.DataFrame(df[col].value_counts().reset_index().values,columns=[col, "counts"])
    return df
plot_wb_bar(count_values(train_df,"Negative for Pneumonia"),"Negative for Pneumonia", 'counts')
plot_wb_bar(count_values(train_df,"Typical Appearance"),"Typical Appearance", 'counts')
plot_wb_bar(count_values(train_df,"Indeterminate Appearance"),"Indeterminate Appearance", 'counts')
plot_wb_bar(count_values(train_df,"Atypical Appearance"),"Atypical Appearance", 'counts')
```

Analytical Report 2 - ML Based Data Analytics on Covid-19 First Wave Dataset

The dataset for analysis on Covid-19, first wave is taken from (Sudalairajkumar, 2021),

Figure 4. Covid-19 detection EDA with data augmentation from Kaggle

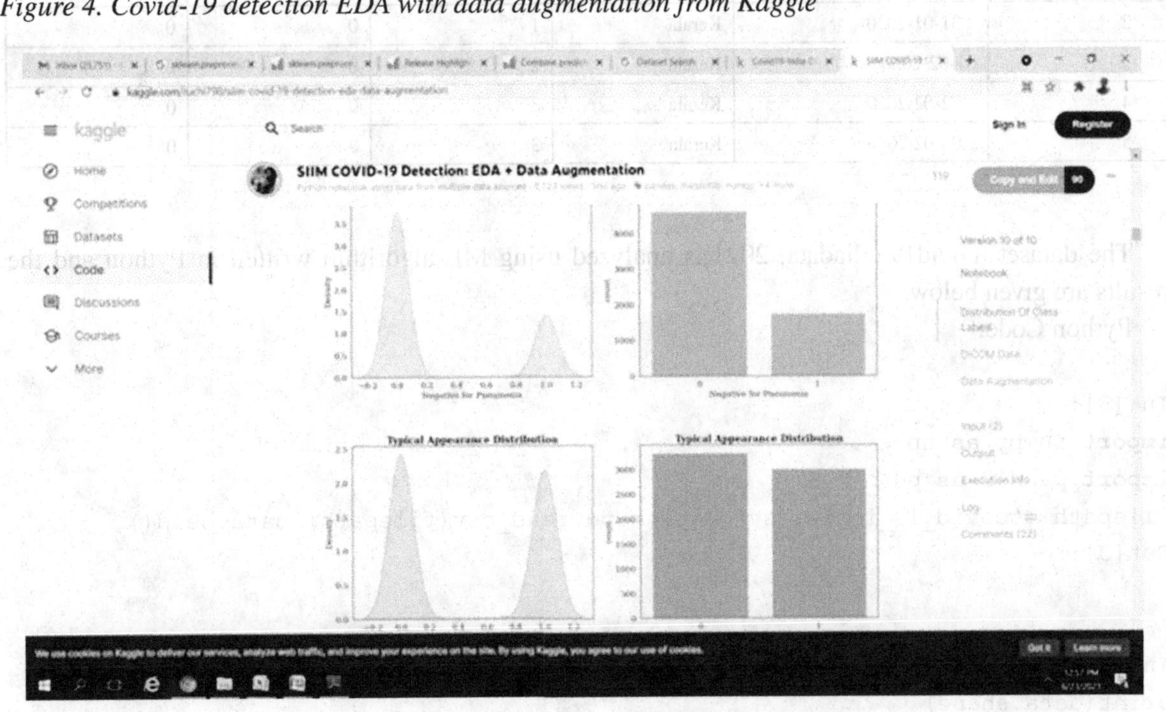

Figure 5. Analytical reports about the distribution

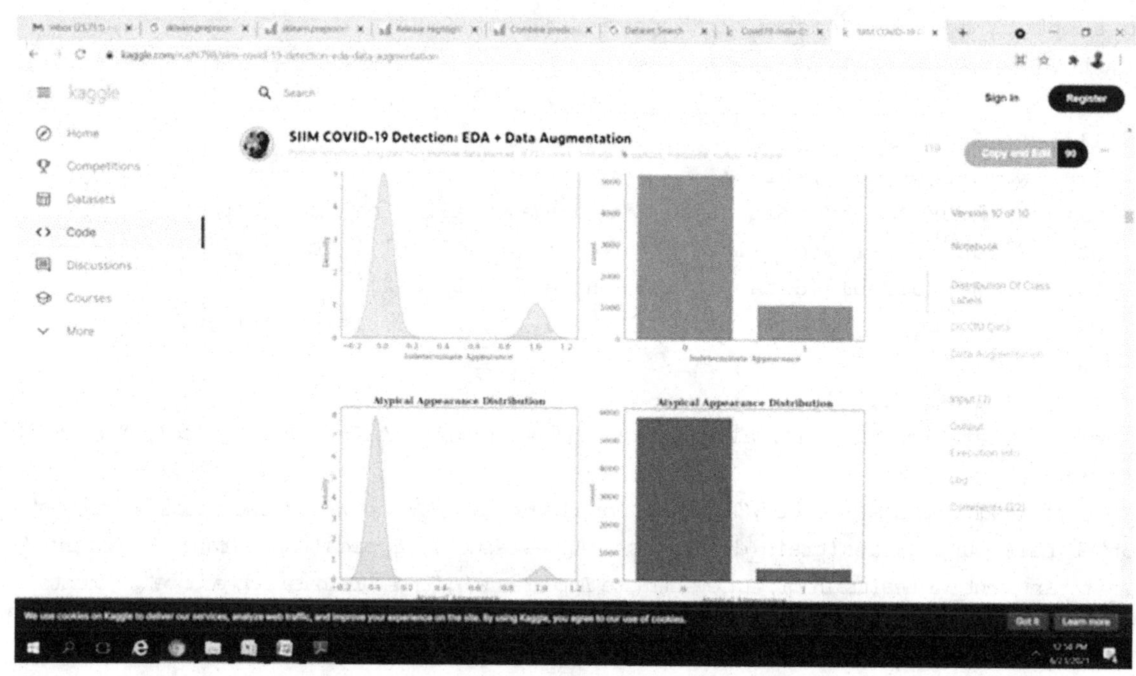

Table 1.

S.No.	Date	Region	Infected	Cure	Death
1.	30-01-2020	Kerala	1	0	0
2.	31-01-2020	Kerala	1	0	0
3.	01-02-2020	Kerala	2	0	0
4.	02-02-2020	Kerala	3	0	0
5.	03-02-2020	Kerala	3	0	0

The dataset (covid19indiadata, 2021)is analyzed using ML algorithm written in Python and the results are given below:

Python Code:

```
In [3]:
import numpy as np
import pandas as pd
filepath ='covid_19_india.csv' data = pd.read_csv(filepath) data.head()
Out[3]:
```

```
In [4]:
print(data.shape)
```

```
(2306, 9)
In [5]:
print(data.dtypes)
Sno         int64
Date       object
Time       object
Region object
Cured                        float64
Deaths                       float64
Confirmed                  int64
dtype: object
```

```
Name: Region, dtype: int64
In [7]:
st_df = data.describe()
st_df.loc['range']=st_df.loc['max']-st_df.loc['min']
out_fields =['mean','25%','50%','75%','range']
st_df = st_df.loc[out_fields]
st_df
Out[7]:
```

```
In [9]:
import matplotlib.pyplot as plt
%matplotlib inline
ax = plt.axes() ax.scatter(data.Cured,data.Deaths) ax.set(xlabel='cured',ylabe
l='death',title='cured vs death')
Out[9]:
[Text(0.5, 0, 'cured'), Text(0, 0.5, 'death'),
Text(0.5, 1.0, 'cured vs death')]
```

CONCLUSION

Many state-of-the-art technological applications began to be all the rage. Machine learning is ubiquitous and can be found in a variety of applications. It has numerous applications in the financial sector, including medical science, and in the field of security. With machine learning, the capability of discovering patterns from medical data sources and accurately predicting diseases is developed. This chapter helps to show how ML can be applied to analyze the medical data set collected from Covid-19 first wave in India. The findings have helped to find out the distribution of areas, the highly affected area and the number of cured against death count.

Table 2.

In [6]: data.Region.value_counts()	
Out[6]:	
Kerala	117
Telengana	85
Delhi	85
Rajasthan	84
Uttar Pradesh	83
Haryana	83
Tamil Nadu	80
Ladakh	80
Maharashtra	78
Jammu and Kashmir	78
Punjab	78
Karnataka	78
Andhra Pradesh	75
Uttarakhand	72
Odisha	71
Puducherry	69
West Bengal	69
Chhattisgarh	68
Chandigarh	68
Gujarat	67
Madhya Pradesh	66
Himachal Pradesh	66
Bihar	65
Manipur	63
Mizoram	62
Andaman and Nicobar Islands	61
Goa	61
Assam	55
Jharkhand	54
Arunachal Pradesh	53
Tripura	49
Meghalaya	42
Dadar Nagar Haveli	20
Cases being reassigned to states	6
Nagaland#	5
Nagaland	4
Unassigned	3
Sikkim	2
Jharkhand#	1

Table 3.

	Sno	Cured	Deaths	Confirmed
Mean	1153.50	337.618696	32.795652	1037.843018
25%	577.25	0.000000	0.000000	7.000000
50%	1153.50	12.000000	1.000000	46.000000
75%	1729.75	127.000000	9.000000	547.500000
Range	2305.00	14600.000000	1635.000000	50231.000000

Figure 6. Cured vs. death graph using ML based analytics

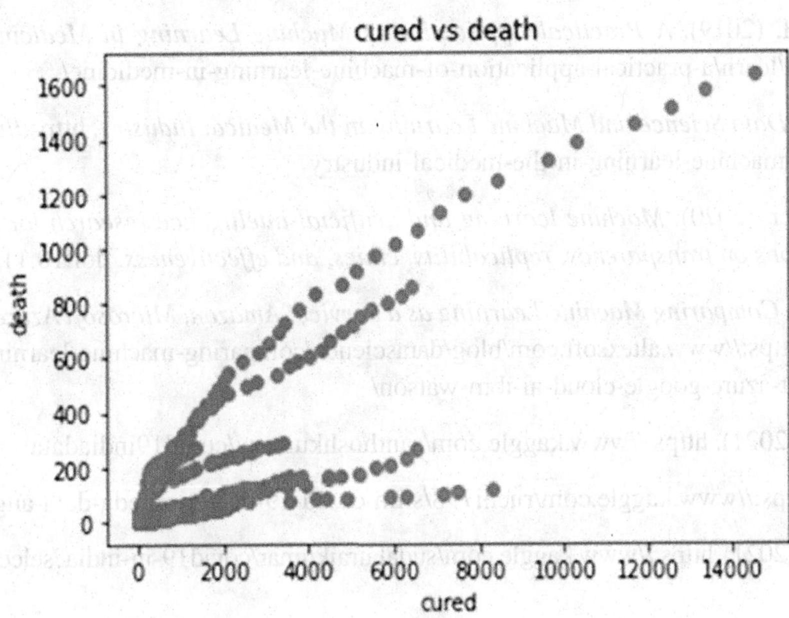

REFERENCES

Difference-data-analytics-data-analysis. (2020). *What's the Difference Between Data Analytics and Data Analysis? | FAQs*. https://www.getsmarter.com/blog/career-advice/difference-data-analytics-data-analysis/

Wu, C., Buyya, R., & Ramamohanarao, K. (2016). *Big Data Analytics = Machine Learning + Cloud Computing*. doi:10.1016/B978-0-12-805394-2.00001-5

Rong, G., Mendez, A., Bou Assi, E., Zhao, B., & Sawan, M. (2020). Artificial Intelligence in Healthcare: Review and Prediction Case Studies. Engineering, 6(3), 291-301.

Maheshwari, R., Moudgil, K., Parekh, H., & Sawant, R. (2018). A Machine Learning Based Medical Data Analytics and Visualization Research Platform. *2018 International Conference on Current Trends towards Converging Technologies (ICCTCT)*, 1-5. 10.1109/ICCTCT.2018.8550953

Shailaja, K., Seetharamulu, B., & Jabbar, M. A. (2018). Machine Learning in Healthcare: A Review. *2018 Second International Conference on Electronics, Communication and Aerospace Technology (ICECA)*, 910-914. 10.1109/ICECA.2018.8474918

Dhillon & Singh. (2019). Machine Learning in Healthcare Data Analysis: A Survey. *Journal of Biology and Today's World, 8*(6), 1-10.

Jeon, M., Sethi, I. K., & Xu, B. (2017). Machine Learning Theory and Applications for Healthcare. *Journal of Healthcare Engineering*. PMID:29090076

Sarkar, T. (2020). *AI and machine learning for healthcare article*. https://towardsdatascience.com/ai-and-machine-learning-for-healthcare-7a70fb3acb67

Gharagyozyan, H. (2019). *A Practical Application of Machine Learning in Medicine*. https://www.macadamian.com/learn/a-practical-application-of-machine-learning-in-medicine/

Barla, N. (2021). *Data Science and Machine Learning in the Medical Industry*. https://neptune.ai/blog/data-science-and-machine-learning-in-the-medical-industry

Vollmer & Bohner. (2020). *Machine learning and artificial intelligence research for patient benefit: 20 critical questions on transparency, replicability, ethics, and effectiveness*. doi:10.1136/bmj.l6927

Altexsoft. (2020). *Comparing Machine Learning as a Service: Amazon, Microsoft Azure, Google Cloud AI, IBM Watson*. https://www.altexsoft.com/blog/datascience/comparing-machine-learning-as-a-service-amazon-microsoft-azure-google-cloud-ai-ibm-watson/

Santhoshkumar. (2021). https://www.kaggle.com/santhoshkumarv/covid19indiadata

Ruchi. (2021). https://www.kaggle.com/ruchi798/siim-covid-19-detection-eda-data-augmentation

Sudalairajkumar. (2021). https://www.kaggle.com/sudalairajkumar/covid19-in-india?select=covid_19_india.csv

Chapter 4
An IoT-Based Sanitation Monitoring System Using Machine Learning for Stagnant Water to Prevent Water-Borne Diseases

G.Vinoth Chakkaravarthy
Velammal College of Engineering and Technology, India

Raja Lavanya
Thiagarajar College of Engineering, India

ABSTRACT

In low and middle-income countries, people die as a result of unhygienic water quality each year. The proposed method monitors stagnant water quality. Improving sanitation facilities by prior detection of contamination depends on both knowledge and resources (both microbiological and personnel). The proposed method uses Node MCU as core controller and various sensors to monitor the water quality. The micro controller will access the data from different sensors and then processes the data. Once the data is collected, the data is fed into machine learning models, and it is trained using machine learning algorithms (classification - SVM) or neural networks (ANN). Productive decision can be made out of the results from the model. Model will be trained using the parameters such as temperature, dissolved oxygen (D.O.), pH, biochemical oxygen demand (B.O.D), Nitrate-N and Nitrite-N, and fecal coliform. The outcome of the proposed work gives a complete report about contamination in the stagnant water and gives early alert to municipalities for preventing water-borne diseases.

DOI: 10.4018/978-1-7998-9132-1.ch004

Copyright © 2022, IGI Global. Copying or distributing in print or electronic forms without written permission of IGI Global is prohibited.

INTRODUCTION

In low and middle-income countries, over 8,20,000 people die as a result of inadequate water quality and hygiene each year, representing 61% of total diarrhoeal deaths. A major reason for the outbreak of these diseases is due to lack of sanitation in waste management, stagnant water and drinking water. Unfortunately there is no prevailing method that can effectively detect and monitor the outbreak and spreading of these diseases. In Current trend, there are a number of different possibilities that could suggest a waterborne outbreak, complaints about water quality and increase of AGI in the community, in general practices, or in hospitals (clinical surveillance) an increase of positive laboratory results indicating possible waterborne agents (laboratory surveillance).There is no technique that could detect the contamination in earlier stages and contamination /dumping of waste in water bodies is un-notified. Thus the early detection prevents the spreading of water-borne diseases thereby ensuring sanitation to create a healthy world. In this chapter, the possible solution is proposed for providing a healthy environment with a proper IOT based sanitation monitoring system using machine learning on stagnant water in various resources. The proposed monitoring system provides stable, real time, reliable and regional water quality monitoring in the stagnant water. The proposed system has IoT-enabled water sensors which can track the quality, portability, pressure, and temperature of wastewater.

Objective

The Sole objective is to monitor stagnant water quality and to improve sanitation facilities by prior detection of contamination depends on both knowledge and resources (both microbiological and personnel). This early detection prevents the spreading of water-borne diseases thereby ensuring sanitation to create a healthy world.

RELATED WORKS

The researchers developed a system for real time monitoring of the water quality parameters. In their research they measure the water parameter such as turbidity, conductivity, temperature, ph and dissolved oxygen (N. Vijayakumar, 2013). Instead of arduino they used the raspberry pi b+ model as core controller and send the sensor data on cloud platform. Cloete, Malekain and Nair in their paper they designed and developed a water quality monitoring system which measures the physicochemical parameters of water such as flow, temperature, ph, conductivity, and the oxidation reduction potential. They detect the contamination of water by measuring the parameters and then send notification to the user. Sensors are connected to a microcontroller- based measuring node which processes and analyzes the data. In their paper, they used a zigbee transmitter and receiver module for communication between the measuring and notification nodes.

The system architecture with three layers for water quality monitoring system was proposed, in that the three are nodes for data monitorization, a base station and a remote station (Barabde, 2015). They connected all the layers with wireless communication protocol and data being send to the base station from data monitoring nodes via microcontroller. Collected data was displayed on a local host PC. Matlab was used to create a GUI (graphical User Interface) for data visualization and water parameters such as ph, turbidity, conductivity were displayed. If the compared value exceeds standard value a SMS will be sent to the client.

A self configurable, reusable and energy efficient WSN- based water quality monitoring system was considered about the monitoring of water quality (Nidal Nasser, 2013). Existing frameworks though have the applicability in water monitoring system, cannot be reused in other monitoring applications because of its static nature. Moreover this dynamic framework also improves the network life time, monitor the water quality real time, and store the information in a portal.

A Water Quality Monitoring System Using IOT consists of various physiochemical sensors which can measures the physical and chemical parameters of the water such as Temperature, Turbidity, pH and Flow. By these sensors, water contaminants are detected (Ankit Sharma, 2018). The sensor values processed by Raspberry pi and send to the cloud. The sensed data is visible on the cloud using cloud computing and the flow of the water in the pipeline is controlled through IoT.

Another IoT system measures the parameter like pH, turbidity, hardness, chloride, TDS (Total dissolved solid), arsenic, iron, FC (Fecal Coliform) and TC (Total Coliform) are analysed and results are compared with the World Health Organization (WHO), Bangladesh Standard (BD) and the Indian Standard Institute (ISI) (Gulam Md. Munna, 2015).The investigation discovers that the value of turbidity and iron in the location of Christian Mission designated by S-11 crosses the all three standard.

Another low cost monitoring system to monitor water in real time using IoT is considered for survey. In this system quality parameters are measured using different sensors such as pH, turbidity, temperature and communicating data onto a platform of microcontroller system and GPRS are used (Ashwini Doni, 2018).

A Monitoring Water Quality system Using RF Module constantly monitor the water available through the taps through various sensors. The sensors which we are using are pH sensor, temperature sensor and a turbidity sensor (LED-LDR assembly). The available data is transmitted to a remote base station using a 2.4 GHz RF module which makes it convenient to monitor at a remote location and requires less man power (Dharon Joseph Edison, 2013)

A reconfigurable smart sensor interface device for water quality monitoring system in an IoT environment collects the five parameters of water data such as water pH, water level, turbidity, carbon dioxide (CO_2) on the surface of water and water temperature in parallel and in real time basis with high speed from multiple different sensor nodes (Cho Zin Myint, 2017)

SYSTEM MODEL

Problem Definition

Water pollution occurs when unwanted materials, industrial waste, human waste or animal waste, garbage, sewage effluents, etc... enter into the water, changes the quality of water which makes it harmful to the environment and also to human health. Waterborne diseases are caused by drinking water or eating food washed in water which is polluted, contains protozoa and bacteria. Lack of access to safe drinking water, together with inadequate sanitation and hygiene, is the overwhelming contributor to the greater probability of annual disease. The Sole objective is to monitor stagnant water quality and to improve sanitation facilities by prior detection of contamination depends on both knowledge and resources (both microbiological and personnel).

Figure 1. Conceptual framework

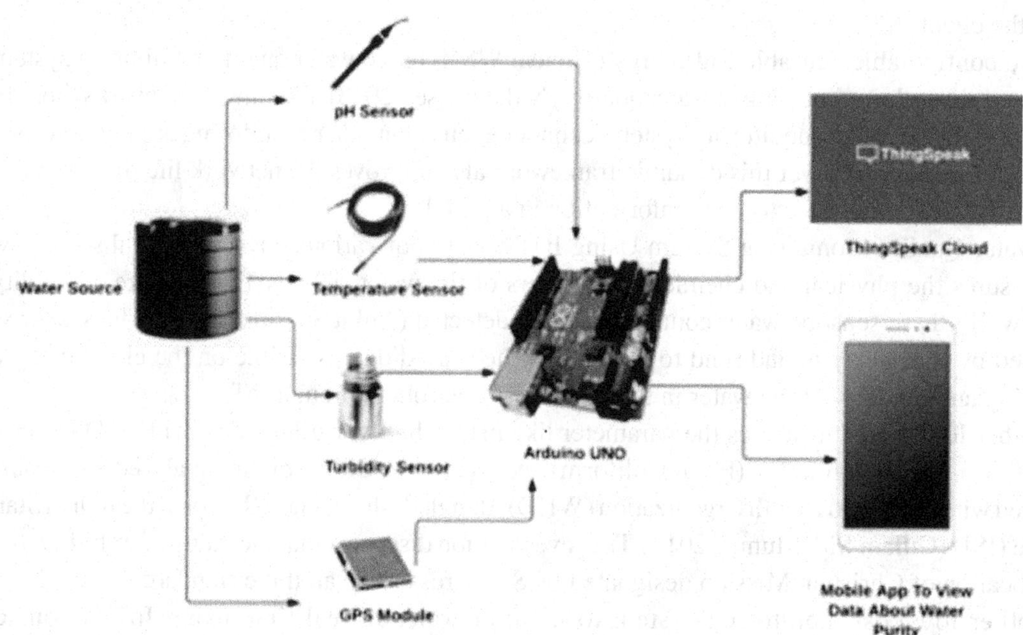

Prototype Design

The proposed method uses arduino as core controller and various sensors to monitor the water quality. The arduino will access the data from different sensors and then processes the data. The data gets analysed, normalized and performs feature selection on the water quality measures, and therefore, obtains the minimum relevant subset that allows high precision with low cost. The sensor data can be viewed on the cloud using ThingSpeak API and a mobile application. IoT-enabled water sensors can track the quality, portability, pressure, and temperature of wastewater. This solution includes dynamic sensor clusters and robust platform-driven analytics.

Properties Detection

The Sensors get fitted in the water tank used in home for drinking and also the tap in public corporation for fetching water. The properties like pH (Power of hydrogen), turbidity, temperature of the water gets measured here. pH is measured using SEN0161 sensor which should possess a pH value of 6.5-8.5. Turbidity is measured using SEN0189 sensor which should be less than 5 NTU and ideally should be less than 1 NTU for drinking purpose. Temperature gets measured using DS18B20 sensor. Core controller receives these values and sends it to the admin.

Testing of Water Quality

Once the values of pH, temperature, turbidity are received they are cross checked with their ideal values for usage and if they don't possess the ideal value, the disease that can be caused due to its usage, is returned to the user via call and an alert message using GSM module.

Location Detection

Tanks using prevention kit gets monitored regularly by admin and a GPS module gets fitted over that. Once a water tank in home or public is seemed to have the affected values, call gets generated to the corresponding user of that location and area water corporation to clean those tanks. So as to prevent the spreading of disease. By using the values received and location the probability of the disease that can be caused in that locality is sent to the users through the app.

Prevention and Waste Management

Clear instructions like storage of water, cleaning of tanks etc... will be provided in the application for user to follow that and Proper sanitation management and waste management instructions will be provided as an anime podcast in the application.

Machine Learning Process

Once the data is collected, the data is fed into machine learning model. Model is trained using machine learning algorithms (classification - SVM) or Neural networks (ANN). Productive decision can be made out of the results from the model. Model will be trained using the parameters such as Temperature, Dissolved Oxygen(D.O.), pH, Conductivity, Biochemical Oxygen Demand(B.O.D), Nitrate-N and Nitrite-N, Fecal Coliform and Total Coliform. AI system which is involved in the predictive analysis uses a Machine Learning algorithm(SVM) or Deep Learning algorithm (SSD/YOLO). The listed suitable Neural Network architectures has to be tested for its performance and its accuracy. AI system which is involved in the sanitary monitoring uses a Deep Learning algorithm (SSD/YOLO). The listed suitable Neural Network architectures has to be tested for its performance and its accuracy. The outcome of the proposed work gives the complete report about the contaminations in the stagnant water and gives early alert to municipal for preventing water-borne diseases. Using this system, the organizations can record the level of pollutants existing in the resources of water and send instant life-threatening cautions to the society or public. The outcome of this proposed work is to provide a proper monitoring of sanitation systems which aim to protect human health by providing a clean environment that will stop the transmission of disease, especially through the fecal–oral route.

Here Data mining uses information from past data to analyze the outcome of a particular problem or situation that may arise. Data mining works to analyze data stored in data warehouses that are used to store that data that is being analyzed. Naive Bayes classifiers can be trained very efficiently in a supervised learning setting. In many practical applications, parameter estimation for naive Bayes models uses the method of maximum likelihood in other words, one can work with the naive Bayes model without accepting Bayesian probability or using any Bayesian methods. An advantage of Naive Bayes is that it only requires a small amount of training data to estimate the parameters (means and variances of the variables) necessary for classification. Gaussian filter is used to fit the dataset containing ph,ldr sensor values which we provide and train the dataset in order to provide appropriate predicted values.

Figure 2. Dataset

	A	B	C
1	ph	ldr	result
2	6.5	748	yes
3	6.4	338	yes
4	7	333	yes
5	5.7	791	no
6	7	510	yes
7	5.1	125	no
8	6.8	599	yes
9	5.9	446	no
10	6.4	705	yes
11	6.9	716	yes
12	5.7	591	no
13	6.6	562	yes
14	5.7	248	no
15	13.6	544	no
16	6.2	649	yes
17	6.6	817	yes
18	11.9	195	no
19	6.6	475	yes
20	6.5	748	yes
21	6.4	417	yes

RESULTS AND DISCUSSIONS

Dataset Collection

A dataset consists of attributes and facts, which correspond to data we want to measure and the data that we want to use to segment or filter those measurements. the dataset has to be processed in a way so that our model can make sense of the information. That way the model can successfully learn from that dataset. When building a dataset, it's important to know what features to look for, so that the model can get the most benefit out of it. After acquiring the data, we need to do noise removal, to make the useful features stand out. Now the dataset is sent for classification in ths module.

First the ph and ldr values from the water are taken. These values are stored in the excel sheet. It is used as a database for further classification process

pH Calculation

A pH meter is a scientific instrument that measures hydrogen-ion activity in water based solutions indicating it's acidity or alkalinity measured as pH. The pH meter measures the difference in electrical potential between a pH electrode and a reference electrode, and so the pH meter is sometimes referred to as a "potentiometric pH meter". The difference in electrical potential relates to the acidity or pH of the solution. The pH meter is used in many applications ranging from laboratory experimentation to quality control. The dataset is given to the naïve bayes classifier to predict the purity of water and it finally predicts whether water is pure(yes) or not(no).Bayes theorem performs probabilistic prediction and it can be explained as:

$$P(H|X) = P(X|H)P(H) \mid P(X)$$

Let X be a data sample ("evidence"): class label is unknown

Let H be a hypothesis that X belongs to class C

Classification is to determine P(H|X), (i.e., posteriori probability): the probability that the hypothesis holds given the observed data sample X.

P(H) (prior probability): the initial probability

P(**X**): probability that sample data is observed

P(**X**|H) (likelihood): the probability of observing the sample **X**, given that the hypothesis holds E.g., Given that **X** will buy computer, the prob. that X is 31..40, medium income

Implementation of pH Sensor:

```
#define SensorPin 0 // the pH meter Analog output is connected with the Ardui-
no's Analog
unsigned long int avgValue; //Store the average value of the sensor feedback
float b;
int buf[10], temp;
void setup()
{
Serial.begin(9600);
Serial.println("Ready"); //Test the serial monitor
}
void loop()
{
for (int i = 0; i < 10; i++) //Get 10 sample value from the sensor for smooth
the value
{
buf[i] = analogRead(SensorPin);
delay(10);
} Serial.print(" pH:");
for (int i = 0; i < 9; i++) //sort the analog from small to large
{
for (int j = i + 1; j < 10; j++)
{
```

```
if (buf[i] > buf[j])
{
temp = buf[i];
buf[i] = buf[j];
buf[j] = temp;
}
}
}
avgValue = 0;
for (int i = 2; i < 8; i++) //take the average value of 6 center sample
avgValue += buf[i];
float phValue = (float)avgValue * 5.0 / 1024 / 6; //convert the analog into
millivolt
phValue = 3.5 * phValue; //convert the millivolt into pH value
Serial.print(" pH:");
Serial.print(phValue, 2);
Serial.println(" ");
digitalWrite(13, HIGH);
delay(800);
digitalWrite(13, LOW);
}
```

The sensor determines how far into the range of acidic or alkaline the current state of the water is. If it's in the neutral zone, then it's perfectly safe. However, the addition of various chemicals can change this at any time. It may have nothing to do with the operator of the water plant either. There could be an influx of water from a local manufacturing plant that is toxic with particular chemicals. This new mix of water will infect the entire batch of water currently in the plant. In order to determine the best treatment,

Figure 3. PH calculation

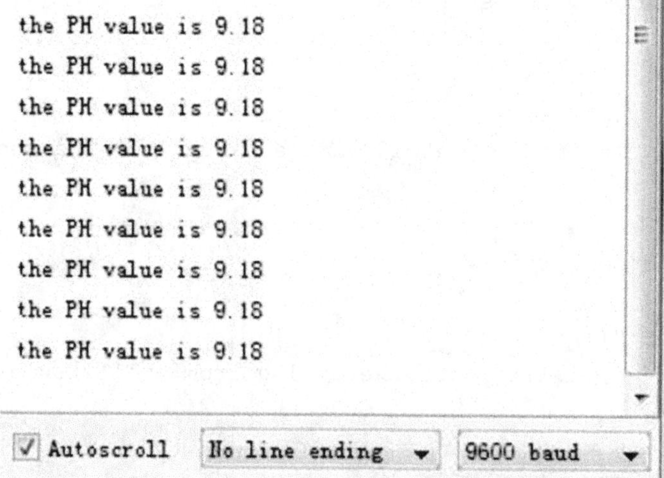

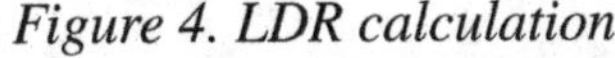

Figure 4. LDR calculation

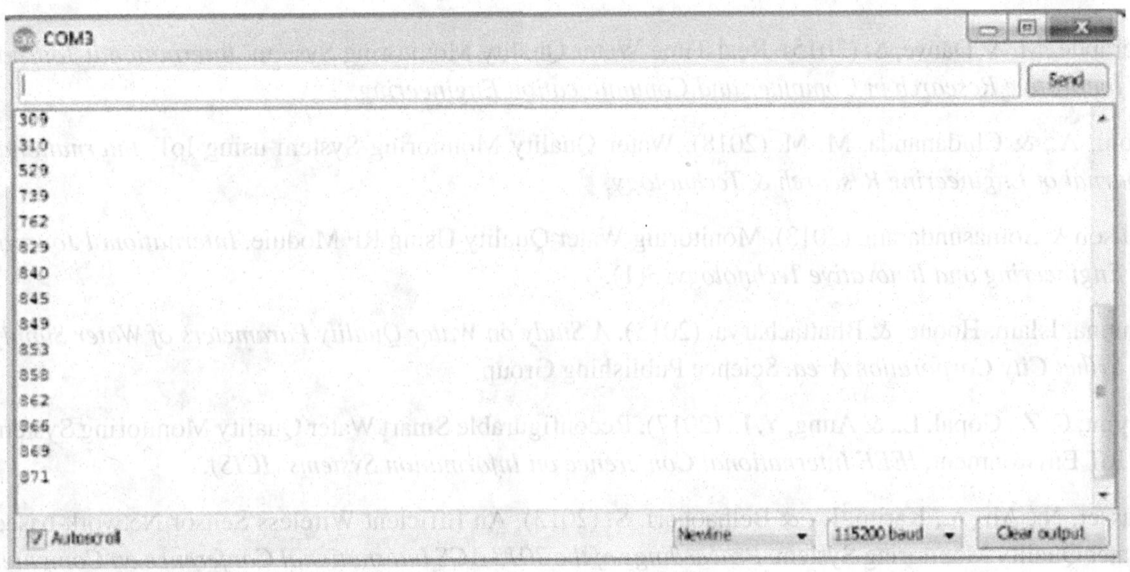

the pH sensor will be used to see whether the water is now acidic or alkaline. The about table shows the PH value of collected samples at various time. The value 9.18 in all samples stated that the water is contaminated with alkaline which leads to smell which leads to various waterborne diseases and it can also damage pipes and water-carrying appliances.

LDR Calculation

The LDR Sensor Module is used to detect the presence of light / measuring the intensity of light. The system comprises of a microcontroller (Arduino Uno), a micropump, a sensing unit and a water filter that detect changes in water and to define the turbidity value of the water. Experiments on water turbidity was conducted under two conditions, undisturbed flow and continuous flow, which will affect the measurements of the LDR. The output of the module goes high in the presence of light and it becomes low in the absence of light. The sensitivity of the signal detection can be adjusted using potentiometer. The water is tested daily and the value of ph sensor and the ldr module is updated in the excel sheet daily

Results show that the LDR readings in continuous flow require more time in between reading so that the turbidity value can be consistent.

CONCLUSION AND FUTURE WORK

The outcome of the proposed work gives the complete report about the contaminations in the stagnant water and gives early alert to municipal for preventing water-borne diseases. Using this system, the organizations can record the level of pollutants existing in the resources of water and send instant life-threatening cautions to the society or public. Thus it protects human health by providing a clean environment that will prevent the water-borne diseases

REFERENCES

Barabde, M. & Danve, S. (2015). Real Time Water Quality Monitoring System. *International Journal of Innovative Research in Computer and Communication Engineering*.

Doni, A., & Chidananda, M. M. (2018). Water Quality Monitoring System using IoT. *International Journal of Engineering Research & Technology*.

Edison & Somasundaram. (2013). Monitoring Water Quality Using RF Module. *International Journal of Engineering and Innovative Technology, 3*(1).

Munna, Islam, Hoque, & Bhattacharya. (2015). *A Study on Water Quality Parameters of Water Supply in Sylhet City Corporation Area*. Science Publishing Group.

Myint, C. Z., Gopal, L., & Aung, Y. L. (2017), Reconfigurable Smart Water Quality Monitoring System in IoT Environment. *IEEE International Conference on Information Systems (ICIS)*.

Nasser, N., Ali, A., Karim, L., & Belhaouari, S. (2013), An Efficient Wireless Sensor Network-based Water Quality Monitoring System. *Proceedings of the 2013 ACS International Conference on Computer Systems and Applications (AICCSA'13)*.

Sharma, Pawbake, Patel, & Potdar. (2018). Water Quality Monitoring System Using IOT. *International Journal of Advance Research and Innovative Ideas in Education, 4*(5). doi:10.1109/ICCPCT.2015.7159459

Vijayakumar, N., & Ramya, R. (2015). The real time monitoring of water quality in IoT environment. *International Conference on Circuits, Power and Computing Technologies*.

Chapter 5
Relevance of Artificial Intelligence in Modern Healthcare

Dhanabalan Thangam
https://orcid.org/0000-0003-1253-3587
Acharya Institute of Graduate Studies, India

Anil B. Malali
Acharya Institute of Graduate Studies, India

Gopalakrishanan Subramaniyan
https://orcid.org/0000-0002-2158-7483
Acharya Institute of Graduate Studies, India

Sudha Mariappan
Acharya Institute of Graduate Studies, India

Sumathy Mohan
Bharathiar University, India

Jin Yong Park
Konkuk University, South Korea

ABSTRACT

Artificial intelligence (AI) and machine learning (ML) are playing a major role in addressing and understanding better the COVID-19 crisis in recent days. These technologies are simulating human intelligence into the machines and consume large amounts of data for identifying and understanding the patterns and insights quickly than a human and preparing us with new kinds of technologies for preventing and fighting with COVID-19 and other pandemics. It helps a lot to notice the people who got infected by the virus and to forecast the infection rate in the upcoming days with the earlier data. Healthcare and medical sectors are in requirement of advanced technologies for taking accurate decision to manage this virus spread. AI-enabled technologies are working in a talented way to do things intelligently like human intelligence. Thus, the AI-enabled technologies are employed for attaining accurate health results by examining, forecasting, and checking present infected and possibly future cases.

DOI: 10.4018/978-1-7998-9132-1.ch005

Copyright © 2022, IGI Global. Copying or distributing in print or electronic forms without written permission of IGI Global is prohibited.

INTRODUCTION

Due to the worldwide pandemic called Coronavirus (Covid-19), the healthcare industry is need of well equipped technologies for the multipurpose usage and also for analysing and controlling the spread of Covid-19 pandemic. Artificial Intelligence (AI) is an advanced technology, which is having the capability of tracking the pattern of increasing Covid-19, and it also diagnosis the patients who are at high risk and it is helping to manage this disease in real-time. It is also forecasting the fatality risk by assessing patients' previous data thoroughly. Moreover, AI looks as if a crucial technology in searching and preparing preventive measures to manage the Covid-19 and other possible diseases. AI is a technology that simulates human intelligence into the machine and thereby it processes the real-time data for the necessary purpose. AI-enabled technologies are evolving quickly in the recent years, because of its advancement in the data processing, yes, AI processes millions of million data within few minutes with much faster and smarter, thus it predicts the happening more exactly than human. Since the present pandemic has collapsed the entire world, all the countries are trying to come up with sophisticated technologies such as AI, and Machine Learning (ML), to develop new and ground-breaking ideas to fight against Covid-19 (Vaishya, Javaid, Khan, and Haleem, 2020). AI and ML offer numerous advantages than conventional analytics and moreover they are supporting a lot in taking decisions with more accuracy and reliability. Learning algorithms can be converted into more accurate and precise as they mesh with training data, letting humans attain extraordinary insights into diagnostics, treatment variability, patient care processes, and patient outcomes (Chen, Yang, Yang, Wang, and Barnighausen, 2020). The worldwide medical field also needs well equipped technologies for taking appropriate decision immediately, to deal with this pandemic and to save the society from the spread in real-time. AI and ML technology work in a brilliant way to mimic human intelligence. It may also play an imperative role in understanding and suggesting ways and means for the developing vaccine for Covid-19. Such a wonderful result-driven real-time technology is utilized for screening, evaluating, predicting, and tracking of existing patients and expected future patients properly (Dialani, 2021).

Covid-19 pandemic has damaged the whole world drastically and slowdown the medical and systems healthcare sector. Still all countries are trying to find out the root cause for this pandemic, but unfortunately, it is getting delay and thus it leaves room for the development of advanced healthcare technologies to deal with various harms related to this pandemic. In this juncture, industry 4.0 enabled AI and ML technologies have given a tremendous support to eradicate this pandemic issue by establishing wireless technologies. These technologies are helping to improve process automation in across the industries including health sector. Thus, These technologies are linked with various stakeholders of the healthcare industry and to communicate with each other for the developing various health related products and services such as healthcare equipment, drugs, and vaccines, check-up instruments, patient care applications and so on. All these products and services are made safely, smartly, accurately, and with the lesser human contribution (Alloghani et al., 2018). As a consequence, AI enabled smart manufacturing system ensures the availability of necessary healthcare items on time, to face the Covid-19 pandemic issues. This technology also helps to design and develop healthcare necessities rapidly. Further the AI enabled digital health instruments like pressure testing kits, contact tracing applications, response systems, health rings, and so on are contributing a lot to this sector (Javaid et al., 2018). Against this backdrop, the present chapter has made an attempt to demonstrate the relevance of AI and enabled technologies in this perilous pandemic.

The present chapter is purely based on secondary data sources and it has written by reviewing the scientific journals, from the major sources, such as Google Scholar, Wiley Online Library, Science Direct, and Springer Link. Apart from these sources internet sources also have been used with the keyword of Corona virus pandemic, Covid-19, AI, and ML. from the search the latest information has been collected pertaining to the application AI enabled technologies in controlling the pandemic, the collected information filtered further to discover the application potential of AI to this epidemic. Thus there are ten possible ways have been identified where the AI enabled technologies functioning effectively to safeguard the public from the adverse of Covid-19. Table 1 explains the relevance of AI to control the Covid-19.

RELEVANCE OF ARTIFICIAL INTELLIGENCE IN THE MODERN HEALTHCARE

As the Covid-19 has malformed, the whole world has been experiencing a new situation called lockdown, to avoid or minimize the spread of Covid-19 as possible as, to control the infectivity, and to increase the recovered rate. Moreover, we can understand the pain of the doctors, nurses, health workers, cleaning workers, police personals, and other people who have been working for safeguarding society. Thus their sweat, blood, pain, and tears can be understood by even a common man and their efforts should also be appreciated. However, most people never realize the role of technologies in supporting Covid-19, especially, the role of AI-powered technologies have been functioning alongside human beings, to avoid the augment of covid-19. AI and its enabling technologies are contributing a lot in controlling the covid-19 (Pirouz, Shaffiee Haghshenas and Piro, 2020). The contributions made by AI and its enabling technologies are explained in the following areas.

Tracking the Spread of the Virus

AI-powered technologies have supported a lot to analyze how fast the infection cases increase and cases having the possibility to get infection. BlueDot is a Canada based institute developed one programme along with AI to predict spread of Covid -19 and its locality. That institute also has published its AI based forecast results followed by the first case diagnosed in china on 31 December 2019.This programme has treated as a well designed one that work with permutations of different cryptograms and it consider more than 1, 00,000 reports in a day from various hospices by cracking the communication fence and it alert all its clients including different government agencies, business houses, and other health care agencies (Gupta, Ghosh, Singh, and Misra, 2020). Smart glasses are the one of the outcomes of the AI-powered technologies and it is very much useful to the security guards to safeguard themselves from the infected

Table 1. Relevance of artificial intelligence in the modern healthcare

10.Other ways	1.Tracking the Pattern and Spread of the Virus	2.Reduces the Workload of Healthcare Employees	3.Controlling Spread through Contact Tracing Application
9.Sensor Enabled Self Monitoring Technologies	**Role of Artificial Intelligence in Controlling Covid-19 Pandemic**		4.Vaccine Development Through Smart Technologies
8. Decoding and Processing Images	7.Controlling Disease with Video Processing	6.Voice data support in collecting Patients details	5.Developing Response System through Chatbots

Source: Based on the Secondary Data

persons. This could be assisted the security personnel to look into the people with no physical contact, if people are looking abnormal with lofty body heat; it means it is a warning signs of the Covid-19. This smart glass technology could save the time and effort of checking every person manually. Moreover, it keeps the guards away from the risk of get in touch with of the people. This smart glass technology was in use throughout China at different public transports such as bus, train and other communal places, to test higher body temperatures without personal contact. AI-powered technologies being a critical part of integrating two technologies along with the optical vision to measure the body heat (Mufareh, 2021).

Reducing Workload of Healthcare Employees

Testing infection is one of the necessary aspects while diagnosing contaminated patients for identifying the exact reason for the contagion. Diagnosing the covid infected persons through manual tests such as blood and Swab Tests, Nasal and Tracheal aspirates and Sputum tests are ideal ways carried out worldwide. These techniques have the risk of spreading the infections from the infected person. This technique also has a limit on the number of patients confirmed in a day (Catrin, 2021). Thus it is significant to instill AI-powered technologies in hospices with an instant result. Even though the health care establishments of several countries desire to raise the tests in a day, the constraint will forever stay due to the high effort utilization in the form of manual labor, and time. By using AI-enabled technologies such as X-Ray and scanning at the present check for definite patterns such as patient's lungs and assess Covid-19 cases sooner and with no risk of virus spread (Harshita Singh, 2021).

Avoids Contact between the Infected Persons and Healthcare Employees

AI is software by using this we can develop robots with the targeted programming, and these robots can be helped us to face the outbreak. The most significant help that these AI-enabled robotics lessening contact between the contaminated and the people annoying to heal them. As robotics cannot be contaminated by the virus it can be used in healing activities, and thereby reduce infections. It has been administered in numerous hospitals to distribute foodstuff, linctus to the patients, moreover to clean and disinfect the rooms, toilets, and close surroundings often. Robots can also be used to spray cleansers on public places such as roads, parks, hospices, malls, and other common places where there is a high possibility for the crowd (Nguyen, Waurn, and Campus, 2021). Many countries have already built-in robots to check people who are in a fever and even have installed for spraying disinfectants and sanitizers and squirt gel when needed. Boston Dynamics a United States-based IT company has shaped a robotic dog that is being used in hospices. Where, the robotic dogs used to examine patients and collect health-related data, thus it reduces the contact between medical practitioners and the infected cases. In another place, Drones are used to transport medical emergency things to the people who are in quarantine (Manghnani, 2021).

Controlling the Spread of Covid-19 through Contact Tracing Applications

AI-powered Contact Tracing Applications (CTAs) are supporting a lot in controlling the spread of Covid-19. The CTAs have collected the information as the name indicates an incursion of the solitude. Characteristically, this would have for no reason been established, but this is being re-examined relating to the present situation. AI has achieved a lot through CTAs as it assists to decide the transporter of a particular mobile phone number and identifies the spot and meantime it alarms others staying nearby.

The CTAs have already been put into practice in different nations such as India, China, Italy, and Israel, and the same kind of application is in Trial in the UK. Where this application declared using Bluetooth modus operandi to identify the infected people and their place and make aware of others also in the same area (Maghdid, Asaad, Ghafoor, Sadiq, Mirjalili, and Khan, 2021,).

Developing Vaccine through Smart Technologies

Developing or preparing a vaccine is a lengthy process with all combinations and amalgamations it should design to develop an ideal medication that suits all despite the trivial variation in our genera. This process would be done with different data sources that might be cloud-based, and the computations may have more competencies than the computers. Researchers and research institutes have already begun using AI-powered supercomputers to accelerate calculations and develop different model solutions for a vaccine likely to be finalized. Many research laboratories are using various supercomputers such as Tencent, Alibaba, and Huawei (Hu, Ge, Jin, and Xiong, 2020).

Helping People through Chatbot Response Systems

Aiding the contaminated recuperate and diminish the virus contamination is an important job of the medical practitioners in the outbreak. Creating awareness among the public along with genuine information about the virus would be the best way to reduce the impact of the outbreak. The Centre for infection control and preclusion has developed a chatbot and named Clara. This chatbot has developed to direct the public to recognize signs related to the outbreak and what to suggest actions need to take. Thus, different types of Chatbots have been created, and even the World Health Organization (WHO) has its chatbot on the Whatsapp platform. Since these chatbots are designed with AI-enabled technologies, they are always smart, fast, and accurate in collecting and examining the data related to the outbreak. The responses obtained through the chatbots are based on the unique data inputs, and it is also called ML (Maghdid, Ghafoor, Sadiq, Curran, and Rabie, 2020).

Collecting and Processing Data Through Voice Data

AI plays an indispensable role in crafting a voice assistant to lend a hand to the medical practitioners' to issue the medical notes to the needy instantly because of the time limitations. 'Suki' is an application developed with the AI and ML components to understand the mode of healing and the choices of a doctor. This gadget also recognizes the background of the treatment followed by a doctor and describes their intention also. In such cases collecting and storing a patient's data is a receptive process and it is done safely with cryptographic actions to maintain its security. At present, using "Suki" is free for doctors, health care professionals, doctors, and other crucial care units until the controlling of the outbreak. "Kara" is one of the similar products to "Suki" which is purposively crafted for high-end mobile phones such as iPhone, blackberry and it is a voice-enabled technology that can direct the persons who are working for and who are affected by the outbreak. It also can be used as tone to text application, thus it saves the doctors' time to inform reports manually and it also can be used as an interface with several charting methods. In the case of telemedicine, charting directs to get perfect and regularity of data, accessible for fresh and regular medicine. At present Kara is available free of cost, and it can be accessed with proper permission from the developed organization (Varshney, 2021).

Capturing and Analyzing Data Through Video

In the recent days using videos as data at the necessary times is being a common one. Since it is simple to capture video with the digital camera, and it is available in all places. However, with the help of AI, the cameras could be activated with the visual sensors and notice irregularities as well. The same kinds of gadgets are available with the tag called "Care.ai" and it can be utilized to notice the face reactions, feelings, and it's some of the features that help to discover health issues too. These gadgets or the systems enhancing the physical readings and examining them to take decisions related to fever, allergies, discoloration, and agitations. Even though, this technique has its limitation that it has to be always on to observe the patient's situation and behavior in connection with the patient's history and other clinical details (Maghdid, Ghafoor, Sadiq, Curran, and Rabie, 2020).

Decoding and Processing Images

Images are played important role in the health sector in different ways. Images include Computed Topography, X-Rays, MRI scans, CT scan, PET scans, etc., and doctors are analyzing these images physically even now for normal cases. However, personal involvement is a threat in the present pandemic; moreover, it consumes more time as well as a human endeavor. However, the same data can be assessed by the AI-enabled gadgets it would examine the metaphors by the fraction of time, as well as it would present the reports accurately, thus it reduces the workload of the doctor either endorse otherwise make a decision subsequently. Hence, it is necessary to implement the AI-enabled gadgets in the medical field as soon as possible to collect and process thereby it can be utilized to recognize the consequences of an outbreak and to suggest precautionary to be approved and utilize (Karthikeyan, and Pandian, 2021). Behold.ai is a company that has introduced a new system called diagnostic imaging. This technology can be used to study the upper body C-Rays for patients by using the deep learning technique to generate an algorithm instead of establishing Heat Maps on the patient's upper body.

Sensor Enabled Self-Monitoring Technologies

Admitting patients into the hospital is a preliminary task of the medical staff, whether the patients infecting less or high. The abrupt increase of Covid-19 affects thousands of people every day, on the other side hospitals facing issues in admitting patients into their hospital due to the shortage of beds. Owing to this issue a new practice called Quarantine has been brought into practice, as per these quarantine patients have to separate themselves in their own houses by maintaining physical distance with others. Further, it needs to observe the patients who are in quarantine whether the health of those bettering or worsening. Due to this, a Hong Kong-based organization called Biofourmis brought some changes in its premise Biovitals Sentinel as well as Everton biosensor to ensure patients who are in house quarantine. Moreover, these gadgets can find out electro dermal, high temperature optically, and some other dimensions, followed by it collect and analyze the data by an AI-powered computer in the health center itself. At the same time as most of the medical centers are operating on AI sensors to observe patients, a digital platform called Oura ring can sense Covid-19 signs before three days they show up. This application has been designed by researchers by employing AI technology to envisage the Covid-19 outbreak and its warning signs such as high fever, continuous and rough cough, gasp problems, and drowsiness, with more precision. Moreover, this technology can be used to monitor the wellbeing of the hospice staff and doctors. This software collects biometric data from Covid-19 symptoms and identifies patterns of the start, progressing, and recovery (Neelima, Amit, and Mangamoori, 2020).

Other Ways

EKO is one of the few technologies that use AI, and it is used as an AI-enabled stethoscope to observe and identify various resonances in the body and recognize anomalies. The major benefit of this gadget is that it is wi-fi enabled one and thus it allows keep of a stretch between the physician and patients, by eradicating the possibilities of virus transmission. Further, abnormal heartbeats would be detected by EKO cardiology and monitor cardiopulmonary functions using telemedicine operations (The Economic Times, 2021).

APPLICATION OF ARTIFICIAL INTELLIGENCE IN MODERN MEDICINE

The application of AI in the modern health sector is a hot subject matter in current years. Even though there is the acumen of extreme potential in the application of AI and its enabling technologies in the contemporary medical sector, there are also qualms about the overwhelm of the human touch in such significant and human-motivated jobs. AI indicates that the use of AI and its enabling technologies, programs, and its procedures play a crucial role in the modern health sector by identifying and curing patients with utmost care at affordable cost. Moreover, several other incidental procedures also come to pass in the requirement for a patients' delegate accurately taken to attention on collecting and storing patients' data during doctor's consultation and health checks. Once it collects the data it also examining those data and produces the outcomes of the result. Thereby it applies numerous reasons of information data to obtain precise problem recognition and suggests appropriate curing techniques and treatments, and also it controls the selected technique whenever necessary (Sengupta, 2021). Divergence for engorged use of AI and its enabling technologies in the contemporary medicine is rationally planned and automated the health services frequently and thereby the jobs are completed more rapidly, and it also assists to reduce the time of a doctor, while they could be performing other errands, which cannot be automated and helps to reach more exquisite practice of human wealth. As the application of modern techniques are being occupied and helps to improve our day to life. Nowadays, there are incredible technologies, tools and robotics join hands with AI thereby they have redesigned the modern health and medicine sector by digitalizing the medical data, managing doctors' appointments online, and along with the healthcare applications installed in the smartphone, and it also helps the patients to identify the nearest clinics and health centers. Further, the AI-enabled medical evaluation systems help to analyze various health-related issues, indications, marks, lab files, etc. to build a hierarchical list of recognition and it can be used to illustrate the health and medicine indices. AI-enabled health systems are used to observe, and inspect infects of the patients accurately (Satheesh Pandian, 2020). Further, AI-powered healthcare robotics supports a lot in the surgery with required movement along with the robotic arms, and magnetized hallucination supports surgeons to carry out surgery that is impossible by manual and expertise. Thus the AI-enabled health technologies support a lot to diminish the physical involvement of the health personals in various health services, saves doctors' time, it also enables expertise service and positive service output, and thus it ensures prospect for health and medical sector, thereby it transforms the modern health sector.

IMPACT OF AI ON VARIOUS STAKEHOLDERS

On Patients

Like a self-service hotel, patient self-service is the latest health service model that ensures the option and expediency by letting patients complete the health-related activities such as appointment scheduling, hospital bill payment, entering or updating patients' details quickly and with no trouble all and also with their expediency. Patients can also be utilizing various information and communication devices such as Smartphones, tablets, and laptops to fulfill these activities at their convenient times and locations. Executing self-service health and medical programs enable hospitals to recognize various advantages such as cost reduction, patient waiting time reduction, minimizing medical errors as much as possible, make payment easy, and thereby these technologies also helps the hospitals to augment patients' satisfaction and to promote the hospitals' goodwill among the public (Bai et al., 2020). Such a wonderful self-service can be ensured in the hospitals with the help of ML and Natural Language Processing (NLP) by collecting, storing, analyzing patients health-related data, and it is also made possible to provide customized health services to the patients by accelerating health service processes to augment expediency and competence of the hospitals further. Progressively, service-providing organizations including hospitals nowadays are developing and using internet-enabled interactive platforms, along with chatbots for helping patients to complete various hospital-related services such as medication refills and simple directorial tasks. Alike to virtual health assistants (VHAs), chatbots use NLP to extract concepts and to analyze sentiments and thus a well-structured interactive can be experienced. Apart from this, image sensing is also being used in some cases to sense photos, read bar codes as well as handwritten notes. Thus the automatic interface systems enable a customized incident to the patients and it is also accessed at any time round the clock. As health service providers are trying to mounting patients' experience and satisfaction towards their services, concentrating more on the intelligent interface systems to make a distinction. By authorizing patients to do some tasks at their expediency with round-the-clock access to gain familiarity with the various functions of the chatbots, along with the health systems, the ability of the interface systems will also be representing to boost up patients' satisfaction. With patient's self-service model the health service providers can streamline the hospital operations by steering the patients to get an appointment or straight them to visit help or registration desk, according to the predefined rules, thus it facilitates the registration team to concentrate more on the select group of patients who require greater value-added services. The managerial and operational advantages of the hospital self-service model using ML and NLP ensures well-organized documentation of current and real-world scenarios as well (Li, 2020). With the help of the self-service technology model, patients' traffic in the hospitals can be reduced considerably and free healthcare staff to do their work without any disturbance. Afterward, as schedules are ended, point of service (POS) will be exposed to augment payment collection. Though hospitals integrated with various payer systems, the use of POS systems helps to speed up the payment process and more responsible for the patients. If in case of any problems arising in the collection and remittance of the payments, the ML technology will be used to remove those problems, by analyzing the payment patterns along with the interface system, thereby it will come up with the finest way to receive the payments from patients without any delay. A personal health assistant is yet another health application that leverages the experience of the patients in various ways. These personal health assistant applications collect information from the users and provide the same to the hospitals or the doctors about the intensity of diseases, various symptoms through chatbots with NLP and ML (Tim Wilson, 2020). Some types of personal health assistant applications raising questions towards the patients to build a user profile and thereby perform custom-made evaluations when the patient is not feeling well. Thus personal health assistant applications also use AI to present health-related advice based on queries raised by the patient and also provides technical support through video consultation with doctors. Further, than personal health assistants, NLP and ML are also used in various patient-oriented functions. Personal health assistant applications use optical images to confirm whether the patients have taken medicines, at the right time or not. AI plays a major role in this process for analyzing the images of both facial and medication identification and to authenticate that the medicine has been ingested.

On Clinicians

AI acts like a kit for diagnosing patients more effectively with precise treatment plans with the help of ML and NLP. There are numerous clinician-oriented applications which are using NLP and ML to collect and process the data. AI-enabled technologies are at present being used in computer-aided detection (CAD) systems to gain knowledge of how various clinical deformities become visible and it can be studied by assessing the data collected through imaging and clinic. Thus by reviewing an extremely more number of images and along with clinical data, would facilitate achieving a sufficient level of knowledge, further CAD systems are talented to use the information they have erudite to recognize areas of deformity by studying the images and produce various possible analyses for the results. CAD is the latest method that is being used largely in several imaging studies, especially in mammography to recognize areas doubtful for breast cancer for the radiologist to assess further, and high-resolution CT scans to evaluate the chest related issues by using the number of images taken during the study to spot suspicious areas which are having the possibilities for the lung cancer and thus it suggests further review from the radiologist (GGVA, 2019). Progresses in AI and its enabling technologies are expected to produce additional as well as the extraordinary potential to the solutions produced by the CAD. Over time, it would not be astonishing to see the precision of CAD technology for several images sensing studies and it surpasses that of radiologists, further along with CAD technology radiologists become the principal interpreters of various image sensing studies and radiologists only reassess the image sensing studies that go beyond a certain point of doubt of the CAD or AI technologies. Apart from the radiology application, CAD technology is also applied in dermatology to identify skin-related issues or diseases. CAD technology in the dermatology field helps to learn a lot about dermatological issues by analyzing huge numbers of images of lesions along with the dermatological-related opinions connected with them. Representing how CAD technologies are functioning in the radiology field, this CAD technology can also be helped to use the knowledge they have obtained to identify the possible dermatological lesions that are at risk for being wicked. Even though the results of these technologies are usually re-evaluated by a skin specialist, these dermatology CAD technologies can make it convenient for non-dermatologist major care doctors to screen various skin lesions (Forsee, 2020). At last, a company, further than spoken, has designed software to recognize the vocal samples to categorize the feelings for uses further than the health sector. Fascinatingly, some of the health-related researchers have established the precise relations between several patterns of voice and several diseases. At the same time as more researches need to be conducted in this field to excel the health benefits, further the initial results direct to voice analysis possibly used this method as a marker for various non-invasive sickness processes (oucks, Davenport, and Schatsky, 2018).

On Pharmaceutical Industry

The role of AI in the pharmaceutical industry is a fortunate thing, as it condenses the time and cost for discovering new drugs and developing new formulas as fast as possible. In olden times developments of pharmaceutical products were expensive and time-consuming lengthy process. Since the biological field is a multifaceted one, this AI-enabled technology inserts many layers in the drug development process within a short span with more precision. A particle that is recognized to adapt an exact step in a biochemical process and to do so efficiently, the rest of the biological process needs to be understood thoroughly. Though many formulas are reacting extremely well in the laboratories they cannot be processed further in biological setup as they have unfavourable effects. The different mix of the bio-molecular configure the number of new molecules with new possibilities to become restorative drugs is overwhelming. Further, the more tests that must be lead to high costs and lengthy as well as a slow process. AI and ML together with NLP are a tremendous technology that would facilitate to process of numerous research outputs to make the progression more competent and resourceful (Kechit, 2021). Thus the AI and its enabling technologies then decide the shortest connections among various relevant data points and thus it narrows down the number of molecules by an order of enormity. Further, the objective of drug development is to discover diminutive particles that modulate the process towards the target proteins. From the olden times, guidance has been provided from generation to generation to prepare the compounds naturally. Moreover, nature has supplied a huge number of molecules and they are facilitated to develop various modern drugs, but not in recent times, as many drugs are developed through the laboratory. And while unearthing new drug formula has a chaotic process, the modern pharmaceutical industry developing various methods and strategies to evaluate a huge number of molecules for exact desired targets (Kathleen, 2020). Yet even with contemporary techniques of high-throughput selection of molecules recognized for exact targets, and the results are frequently sub-optimal because genetic systems are multifaceted, and molecules that functioning well for transforming one pace in a process may have unfavorable relations in other branches of the biological network or the process. These concerns may not become obvious until later in the development of the drug come across several tests, and requiring more time and money for the same but results are not viable. In such cases, the modern techniques in molecular testing, called machine-vision and image sensing allow AI and enabled technologies to envisage the right number of molecules for effective results, and thus speed up the drug discovery and development process. Likewise, replications of chemical relations can be carried out to assess the efficacy of the drugs in the disease treatment (Alyssa DelPrete, 2019). The potential application of AI and its enabling technology is ensuring speedy and precise discovery of vaccines for a certain pandemic like covid-19. In such times this technology can ensure huge and immediate benefits for diseases that are spreading immediately such as Ebola or Zika, or even the rapidly transmuting HIV. While some of the drug manufacturing companies have started to use AI technology to study the drug interactions deeply, thus this technology may pave the way forward to use AI to investigate whole biological systems to observe how the drugs might influence the tissues of a patient. Through this technology requires a huge volume of data and image sensing outputs, AI technologies are the promising technology; they are helping to trim down the time as well as the cost in the drug development process by spotting the right number of molecules. Even though the brunt of ML and NLP has yet to be decided in successive stages of drug development, researchers have lots of optimism for making use of the outcome of these technologies (Laura Craft, 2017).

AI FOR DESIGNING EFFECTIVE TREATMENT PLAN AND DELIVERY

AI is contributing a lot to oncology treatment design and it is considered to be a major advantage of AI in this sector. Because treatment patterns will differ often while treating cancerous cells and it is important to consider various factors of treatment such as treatment modalities availability and the preservation of healthy hankie. As a result, this process seems to be a challenging one as well as time-consuming. However, in the field of subspecialties of oncology number of clinical tests and trials are being carried out around the globe. While understanding and assimilating all the data would be a colossal job for one oncology practice and it is not possible by a single doctor, but this job can be processed easily and precisely by computer-facilitated with ML and NLP (John Edwards, 2019). These two technologies can make this job as easy as possible by reading and understanding thousands of data and compare the same with the data of a particular patient's case, and thus a doctor can take an appropriate decision. Deciding and providing treatment is yet another complex issue and as it is a time-consuming one in oncology because treatment has to target only the cancerous cells and safely treat the area of the healthy tissue. Thus it is a difficult job, further while treating the cancerous cells spotted in the neck, and head, countless important structures are in located closeness, that too they are small spaces comparatively (Aunt Minnie.com, 2019). Charting the anatomical structures, and measuring radiation combinations at different viewpoints and beam strengths, is a time-consuming process for radiation oncologists and their employees, as they decide the right way to providing therapy. Here yet again, the ML along with NLP demonstrated medical value consistently. Further, the ML-enabled systems can process the way of treatment in less than a minute, but for the same, even the days need to spend by the manual oncology team, and it also delays the treatment process. In the cancer clinical trials, the ML-based medication plans have been compared with the plans prepared by the experts, where the ML-based medication plans have equal accuracy. Furthermore, the majority of the respondents found difficulty in distinguishing between the plans produced by experts and the ML system. In such a manner the ML-enabled systems created an accurate treatment plan.

HOW AI CAN IMPROVE OUTCOMES AND EFFICIENCY IN THE HEALTH SECTOR

From the ancient days to till today the health sector has been moving with huge volumes of data, and which have been maintained through recording and keeping the data including observation details and analyzing the same during the patient care if required. Nowadays AI-enabled systems have made these kinds of jobs including collecting, classifying, storing, retrieving, and exploring the large structured and unstructured data sets to expose veiled patterns, compare the same with past cases, and take medication decisions based on that. As mentioned earlier, ML is playing a significant role in AI-enabled health activities and it enables the quicker and more precise examination of the huge volume of data. Yet another role of AI in the health sector is health and medical proof mining and recognition of concealed tendency of the disease. AI can be applied to inspect the data for drawing the health trends of the patients or to match up with an individual patient with similar histories. Data science technologies are very much useful in examining various medical data from numerous medical records, and they can help to improve patient care during an emergency through clinical forecasting based on patterns recognized among similar cases. With the help of AI-enabled technologies patients' risks can be segregated more accurately by processing huge volumes of data with lesser resource requirements, but this facility was a tough job before the arrival of AI. In the same way, AI can be used to improve the outcomes of the pharmaceutical industry (Daniela Hernandez, 2017). AI leverages itself as an essential tool for clinicians in charting interventions and improves patient outcomes. One more area that receives significant benefits from AI is genomics. Genome examination and disease tendency forecast are keystones of accuracy health service, which is a promising move focusing towards individual's health improvement by analyzing, avoiding, and treating potential sickness through well-planned preventive techniques. AI-enabled integrated technologies ensured exact health analysis by combining the AI-powered technologies in genomics medicine with improved data compilation through electronic health records, sensors, digital wearables, and other digital devices. Thus the AL-enabled technologies not only diagnose the disease pattern but also assess the clinical information, by analyzing the data collected from a patients' biometric access, lifestyle, heredity, and current environment situation includes workplace, residence, tension, and so on. For several diseases, a patient's genomic data is used already to plan a custom-made treatment to maximize the clinical outcome. In the years to come, the accuracy of the health sector can be balanced by merging the genomic analysis with ML and AI. These technologies will ensure the suitable treatment to trim down the occurrence of certain illnesses (Nicolae et al., 2019). Thus the capacity to identify potential health risks and arbitrate with precautionary measures will alter the concept of health care. In the present disease management process, health service providers let the individuals become ill and present with symptoms, to know exactly what the disease is. But in the future, the health sector and health service providers will focus more and more to provide true and reliable health service by observing the individual health proactively, performing precautionary measures in advance, and managing people with preventive medicine. Thus the exactitude health models will have the possibility to implement using ML, and NLP. Apart from medical, AI helps to gain managerial and operational benefits, as AI will prolong to play an important role in providing a competent and gainful administration of the health sector (Cohen and Mello, 2018). Thus it enables operational effectiveness; reduce the treatment cost, data processing, speedup office automation from reception to back-end offices, and all over the place in between. Further, the systematic appraisal of medical credentials and coding hospital operations based on data analytics having the potential to raise the annual income to 80 million USD, depending upon the dimension of the health care organization.

THE FUTURE OF AI IN HEALTH CARE

The future of healthcare will depend upon AI in its operations, as it has been operating with hybrid models. With these hybrid models, health service providers can diagnose the patients accurately with less time along with less cost; these models will also guide them to charting the treatment plans, analyze and identify the health risk factors shortly, thus this technology itself is having the responsibility for the patient's care. Its result influences the health service providers to adopt this technology faster for justifying perceived risk and begin to deliver quantifiable developments in patients' outcomes and working efficiency at scale. The existing AI-enabled modern technologies and the technologies in the developmental process are leveraging themselves through ML and NLP as these technologies having their values (Atul, Ken, David, and Bill, 2019). As these technologies having the capacity to deliver potential output to the health sector, the future will be expected to obtain a synergy through the power of AI and its related technologies on patients' journeys. Though we cannot forecast the happenings in the future with the fullest accuracy, we may judge upcoming scenarios that would likely happen. Because in the upcoming days, all the patients would have access to various wearable digital devices to track different health issues right from monitoring glucose levels in the blood, heartbeat rates and rhythms, and levels of exercise over time. Thus all this monitored information will be synchronized to a centralized monitoring system installed in the hospitals. All those monitored information will be processed through ML to identify irregular or undesired change patterns. If the monitored devices found an abnormal health pattern in the patient's body, those monitoring devices will notify that information to the doctors or hospitals through messages or warning signs, and it also intimates the patients to plan an scheduled time to meet or consult with health service providers. Once the patient reaches the health center, they can check-in by themselves through voice chat-enabled biometric machines powered by the NLP to attain patients' registration data. Suppose the patient has no bill due on his hospital account, the patient need not pay at the machines or expect anyone to discuss an account balance. The doctor before checking the patient,/ will review the data sent by the digital wearable devices of the patients along with the causes why the alert was produced and a list of possible diagnoses will be produced by the monitoring systems with the help of AI capabilities. Once the doctor inspects the patient, he /she will then provide the treatment reminder (Simon Marshall, 2021).

After the treatment reminder note has been provided, the ML and NLP will convert the text in that treatment note into codified data behind the scenes, by using those codified data patients' medical records will be updated electronically, and thus it would generate appropriate billing details automatically and will send the same to the patients' insurance company for reimbursing the medical expenses. Furthermore, based on the data collected by the digital wearables as well as the electronic medical record generated by the systems, a treatment plan will be decided with the combination of ML and NLP to suggest possible changes to the patient's present treatment plan including medicine dosages and times to consume as well as diet and exercise schedule. Thus it also reveals the patients' precise clinical condition up to date. For example, a patient approaches a doctor and mentions that he feels tired and having a continuous cough in the last two months, so the doctor will dictate necessary lab tests along with a chest CT scan (Codrin Arsene, 2021). Once the lab test results come both the patient and doctor will be notified through the patient and doctor portal. Based on the results of abnormal heartbeats and chest CT scans found by the CAD it would mention the probability of the particular health issue. As a result, the patient is again impelled by the NLP-enabled chatbots to schedule and follow-up the appointment with the doctor, oncologist, and biopsy for confirming the state of the disease, and to consider the results to go for the next stage of treatment. The oncologist will check the patients' e-medical records and imaging findings before meeting the patients and will re-examine evidence-based medical treatment literature for deciding possible treatment options by using NLP and ML. If the treatment type is finalized, then the ML will be used to customize the treatment plan according to the patients' health conditions (Micah Castelo, 2020).

Both while the patient is undergoing treatment and after treatment, wearable devices will monitor the patient and again notify both the patient and provider should the AI-enabled monitoring system determine that intervention is needed. ML can then also suggest the best course of action based on the patient's clinical condition and prescriptive analytics, and monitor patient behavior in order to provide incentives for appropriate behavior. At last, data of a particular patient will be compared with the health data of other patients, and the results will be stored into the master health database. That database, with new information being added daily, is continuously being mined using NLP and ML for potential associations across a broad set of data in an effort to identify previously undiscovered causes and treatments of diseases. This situation demonstrates the possible advantages available to the patients, doctors, and other stakeholders like laboratory experts, pharmaceutical experts by increasing the use of AI throughout the medical journey the patients (analyticsindiamag.com, 2021).

Proactive oversight of the patient's health using NLP and ML to monitor data from wearable devices can mean quicker interventions and changes to treatment plans, potentially resulting in patients health state while they are coming to the treatment, and it will support doctors by making their job more easy, fast and take care of patients with affordable cost. Kiosks with NLP and ML for registration and check-in can save patients time, reduce front-desk resource costs, and increase the accuracy of information for the provider office and insurers. Using NLP and ML to codify a provider's dictated note saves the provider time because dictation is much quicker than other forms of data entry but benefits the patient, the provider, and the insurer by codifying information dictated in the visit note and generating a more accurate and complete bill to send to the insurer in a more timely fashion. Application of CAD systems into the examination of the image studies, it will help a lot to the radiologists to get better output with precision, and applying AI and ML in the treatment based on the unusual physical condition of the patients, inducing patients to make appointments means that patients can be proactively treated earlier in the process when they are less ill. The use of NLP and ML to review the literature for treatments specific to a particular patient's clinical situation helps providers and patients by making a positive outcome more likely and helps reduce costs for insurers by avoiding treatments with lower likelihoods of success. It can also benefit the pharmaceutical industry by allowing their products to be used in clinical situations where they are more likely to be successful in treating the patient. The application of NLP and ML in the public health data mining produces various benefits to various stakeholders such as patients, doctors, other healthcare service providers, and pharma industry people by discovering the diseases have not explored previously and having the possibility to the novel treatments (analyticsindiamag.com, 2021).

Patients will be monitoring during and after treatment with the digital wearable gadgets, and these gadgets will be watching patients by observing the physical condition and it will alert both the patient and doctors by the AI-powered supervising systems to decide the type of intercession is required. Meantime ML can also recommend the best course of treatment based on the patients' medical stat, analyzing prescriptive and observing patients' behavior. On the other side, patients' health data will be de-identifying with other patients' health data, and thus it will be entered into the centralized healthcare database. Such a manner database will be updated daily with new patients' data and is incessantly analyzed with the help of ML and NLP to find out the possible relations across the large set of data to discover reasons and treatments to cure the diseases. This situation demonstrates a lot of the possible positive outcomes to various stakeholders such as patients, doctors, and pharmaceutical people by augmenting the power of AI throughout the patients' medical journey (G7, 2018).

AI-enabled smart wearables induce the patients to oversees their health proactively by themselves using ML and NLP to observe and collect the data from the wearable devices, thereby it alerts the patients to go for the treatment at the earlier stage of the disease and thus it reminds the quicker intervention of the doctors either to choose or change the plan of treatment, its result patients will be checking at the initial stage of the ill and immediately will be presenting for the treatment, thereby the workload of the doctors will be reducing, and also reducing the costs for insurers. Machines powered with ML and NLP are used in the hospitals nowadays for registering patients and check-in, thus patients' time can be saved considerably on one side, on the other side it will minimize the costs of front-desk resources, and augment the correctness of data for the doctors and insurers (Geng, Daniel and Rishi 2018). ML and NLP will be used to coding the doctor's dictated notes, thus this technology banks the time of the doctor, by this way the dictation can be done much faster than different forms of data entry, meantime it also helps the

Figure 1. Patient journey
Source: Deloitte, 2021

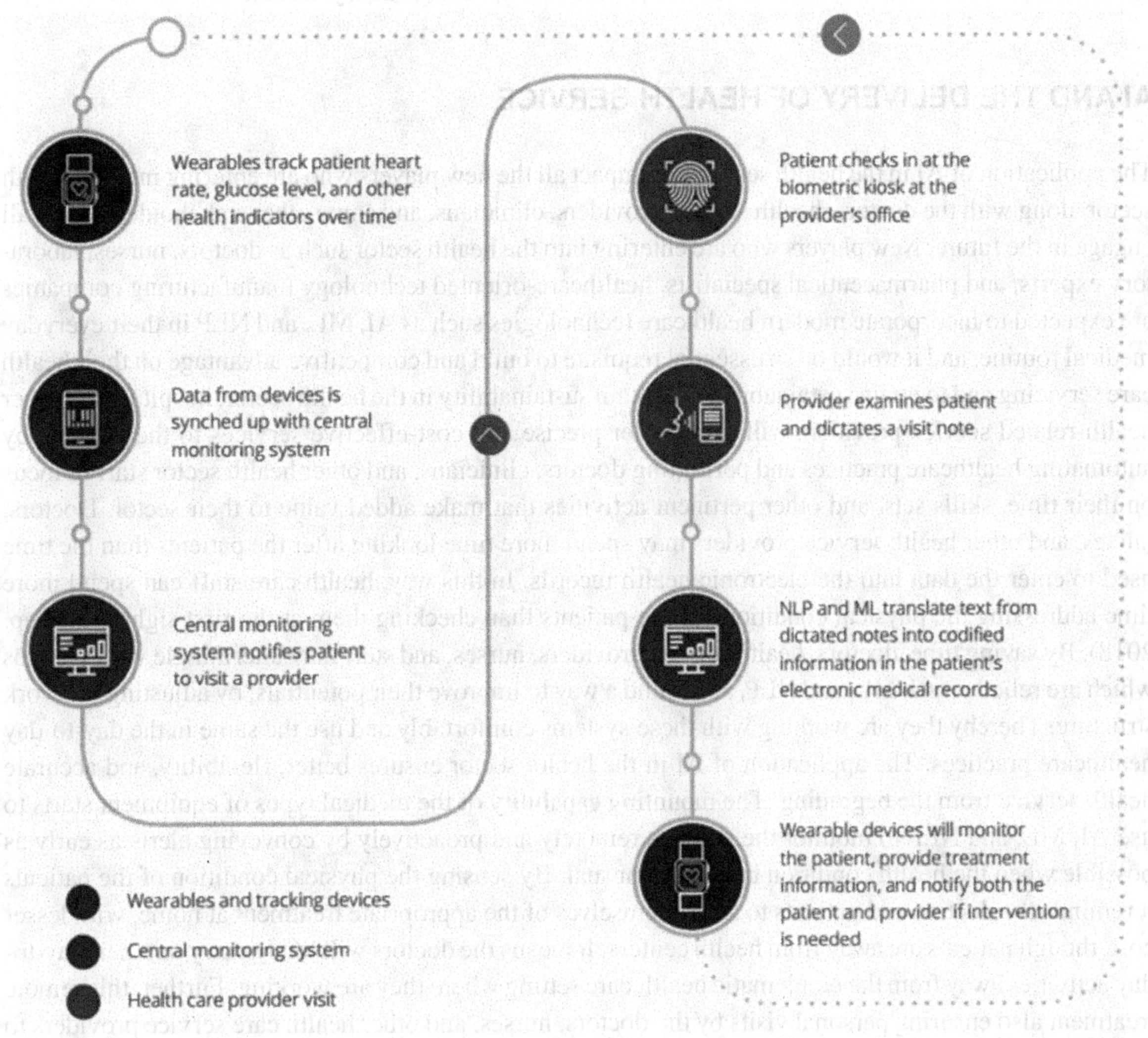

patient, doctor, and the insurance company by coding the information stated in the appointment note and producing a more precise and absolute medical bill, and the same will be sent to the insurance company in a further appropriate method. Using CAD systems in reviewing the images of the various scans, will assist radiologists to get better output and accurateness, and applying AI and ML to hold unusual health outcomes activating patients to schedule an appointment with the doctors to treat themselves as early as possible in the course while the patients are in the ill. ML and NLP will be used to re-examine the medical literature for fixing specific patterns of treatment to a patient based on their clinical condition, and thus these systems will help doctors and patients for making possible positive outcomes and assists to diminish reimbursement costs for insurers by evading treatments with lesser likelihoods. AI-enabled technologies also supporting the pharmaceutical companies by permitting the drugs and tablets to be utilized in various medical situations where they are having more possibility to treat patients successfully. Ultimately, ML and NLP help a lot to manage mass health data in a short time with high accuracy, thereby it helps patients, doctors, insurance companies, and the pharmaceutical industry by recognizing the unfamiliar relationships and ensures new possible treatments (Pandey, 2018).

AI AND THE DELIVERY OF HEALTH SERVICE

The application of AI in the health sector will impact all the new players who are entering into the health sector along with the doctors, health service providers, clinicians, and some other stakeholders who will engage in the future. New players who are entering into the health sector such as doctors, nurses, laboratory experts, and pharmaceutical specialists, healthcare-oriented technology manufacturing companies are expected to incorporate modern healthcare technologies such as AI, ML, and NLP in their everyday medical routine, and it would be an essential requisite to build and competitive advantage on their health care servicing and to attain sustainability. To attain sustainability in the health sector, hospitals and other health-related service providers will try to offer precise and cost-effective services to the patients by automating healthcare practices and permitting doctors, clinicians, and other health sector staff to focus on their time, skills sets, and other pertinent activities that make added value to their sector. Doctors, nurses, and other health service providers may spend more time looking after the patients than the time used to enter the data into the electronic health records. In this way, health care staff can spend more time addressing the physical conditions of the patients than checking them at the first sight (Sandeep, 2018). By saving time, doctors, health service providers, nurses, and staff may intermingle with systems which are relied on AI, ML, and NLP, and found a way to improve their potentials, by adjusting the work structure. Thereby they are working with these systems comfortably and use the same in the day-to-day healthcare practices. The application of AI in the health sector ensures better, flexibility, and accurate health service from the beginning. The mounting capability of the medical types of equipment starts to use AI, ML, and NLP to monitor the patients remotely and proactively by conveying alerts as early as possible when the health condition becomes unusual. By sensing the physical condition of the patients it reminds the doctors and patients to avail themselves of the appropriate treatment at home, with lesser cost, though patients are away from health centers. It means the doctors will likely carry out their day-to-day activities away from the emblematic health care setting where they are working. Further, this remote treatment also ensuring personal visits by the doctors, nurses, and other health care service providers to take care of the patients, thus it is lowering the cost of patient care on one side and also augments satisfaction (mckinsey.com, 2020). In addition, assessing where and how the health sector will be working

Figure 2. Various considerations of AI, ML, and NLP
Source: Deloitte, 2021

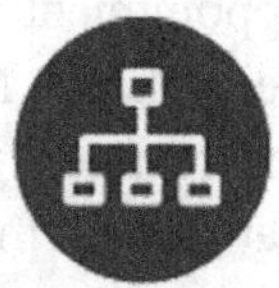

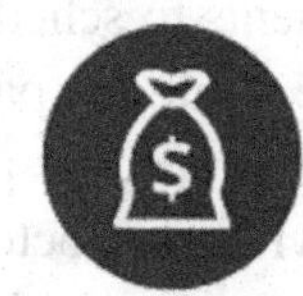

better with the application of ML and NLP will possibly shock the health sector's talents. Because, these technologies to be expected to perform better by extending the doctors' service by combining with ML and NLP, to trim down costs and saving doctors time. It is also expected that the new developments and new forms of talent models to occur in the days to come. Thus it will be changing the traditional health service from the hospital to the home environment, and it would not be astonishing to see local health care by allowing the licensed health professionals and allow them to serve as local and home extended services on behalf of the health care institutions (Sandeep, John Fox, and Maulik, 2019). Health service providers hereafter should be deemed the inevitable shifts related to NLP and ML and prepare themselves to be ready for dealing with various considerations, such as process and governance, Organizational and culture, and financial considerations (Deloitte, 2021).

Consideration of Process and Governance

The basic ideology of identifying new forms of functioning is depending upon the solid structure of the governance, process, and reliable teams. Hence every organization especially service organizations like health care centers needs to deem the development of an innovative steering commission. The commission should conduct regular conventions to discuss the things that need to be automated, modernized, and enhanced by applying the latest technology developments like AI, ML, and NLP. In this way, organizations can radically augment the output or service quality by investing capital, time, and other resources to build a solid structure of governance and process. Further, the organizations need to connect with the steering committee to innovate and recognize places where the latest digital technologies such as the Internet of Things, blockchain technology, big data can be applied to promote organizational efficiency. Cloud storage is a technology that augments the value and diminishes the cost thereby it promotes cloud-based third-party data storage structures, and ML and NLP help to build a faster, smarter, competent, and sustainable business. Thus measurable data storage can be offered by the third-party vendors that would usually be prohibitively costly, and offer a Software-as-a-Service (SaaS) move towards attaining ML and NLP resolutions that diminishes the charge and intricacy of having and keeping hardware on-site (Chelvachandran, 2020).

Consideration of Organization and Culture

While thinking about the human capital and organizational resource aspect of this revolution, organizations need to raise data analytics groups to be capable to collect data from the patients, doctors, and the public as likely to augment health care services and operations. Spawning fresh data from the patients is a tricky job for doctors due to the multifaceted and complex nature of healthcare data. On the other hand, many decisions will be made based on these data and will be used in clinical and business, it is an indispensable process to generate a culture and its related processes to endorse the formation of fresh, whole, and appropriate data from domestic sources. From the cultural point of view, health care service providing organizations should look into other businesses for motivation, as numerous companies are in a superior place to take perils coupled with modernization of business than health service providing organizations, as patients' survival would be at stake and attractive unacquainted perils are excessively risky (Tim, Brian, and Tamim, 2019).

Financial Considerations

From financial considerations, any business must be ready to do the investment in the information center sufficiently, as the IT-enabled solutions will be allowing the technologies to function as planned and fabricate the required results. Though some of the models, like SaaS, involve the development of lesser infrastructure to be built and manage by a company, and thus every data need to be analyzed thoroughly and independently.

NEW RISKS TO ADDRESS

It is time to understand that, though the technologies providing lots of benefits there are latent risks also associated with the major use of technology advancements like ML and NLP. Coding the collected data using NLP builds it easier to disseminate that data such as organizational policies and procedures throughout the organizations, as well as de-identifying the information that is disbursed in several circumstances, and these are the things that need to be industrialized to look after the privacy of the patients. Moreover, data safety against the third party or the hackers or some other unauthorized admission also requires be executing and sustaining at various levels to avoid unofficial use of the secluded individual and health care data. Though the data security issues are existing in the usage of AI, users or the service providers need to understand that AI is used in the day to day health care activities to augment the quality of service provided, increase productivity; however, all these things are indenting to provide utmost service not to reinstate healthcare and its allied activities personals (Nicholson Price, 2019). Though the AI, ML, and NLP technologies are having lots of advancement in their operations, they require some amount of human effort, without human effort it is not possible by those technologies. As far as the present situation of technologies is concerned, though the AI and its enabling technologies are suggesting suitable treatment patterns for various diseases, those treatment suggestions should be appraised suitably by the approved clinical experts to confirm the suitability of the recommendations for a particular patient's health situation. Correspondingly, doctors or health service providers should not reliant on the more use of technologies operating with the support of AI, because it may lead to the loss of medical expertise that they were skilled in training and extended through practice (Michael Walter, 2019). Though modern technologies are come up with several noteworthy paradigm shifts, the progression towards AI in the various operations will take some time to work. While there are major technological challenges that need to be addressed from the back and front ends. Moreover, the progress towards the self-service obtained by the patients indicates progress away from the status quo, changing control over some functions may create unnecessary problems for both doctors and patients. To recompense for the control greater than before by patients, effective governance policies and procedures need to be developed to make sure the sufficient number of staff and the resource are utilized properly, and effectively (Upendra, 2020).

CONCLUSION

AI is a fortunate technology that has been serving humankind a lot to deal with this pandemic. It is a future and constructive technology to recognize the Covid infections early and assists in managing the infectious. With all the new advancements and developments explained in the earlier part of the article, thus one can think about Covid-19 is an ignition for all the modernism and it makes the researchers and scientists work smarter, faster, and reliable. Thus it develops the medicinal firmness by taking decisions with well-developed algorithms. As a result this technology taking care of affected cases with the appropriate and timely monitoring. This technology also tracks the pandemic situations with various yardsticks like medicinal, biological, molecular, and epidemiological significance, and hence, it is treated as a contributive technology. Moreover, it researches the severity of the pandemic, with the available data and comes with reliable and constructive results. It also ensures world-class treatment by establishing different treatment methods and approaches for preventing disease, developing medicines, and vaccines. Exclusive of AI, the Covid-19 battle would have been harder to fight, and the potential uses of AI and its enabling technologies in the medical sector are never-ending. The further range for the advancements and developments of the healthcare industry with AI and creates an important brunt in overcoming the Covid-19 pandemic (Alloghani et al., 2018). The planet may never be similar as we know it, but it can be improved more than earlier.

REFERENCES

G7. (2018). *Charlevoix: Common Vision for the Future of Artificial Intelligence*. https://g7.gc.ca/wp-content/uploads/2018/06/FutureArtificialIntelligence.pdf

Alloghani, M., Al-Jumeily, D., Hussain, A., Aljaaf, A. J., Mustafina, J., & Petrov, E. (2018). *Healthcare Services Innovations Based on the State of the Art Technology Trend Industry 4.0* [Paper Presentation]. *11th International Conference on Developments in e-Systems Engineering (DeSE)*, Cambridge, UK. 10.1109/DeSE.2018.00016

Arsene, C. (2021). *Artificial Intelligence in Healthcare: The Future Is Amazing*. https://healthcareweekly.com/artificial-intelligence-in-healthcare/

Atul, K., Ken, A., David, S., & Fera, B. (2019). *The future of artificial intelligence in health care*. https://www.modernhealthcare.com/technology/future-artificial-intelligence-health-care

Bai, H. X., Hsieh, B., Xiong, Z., Halsey, K., Choi, J. W., Tran, T. M. L., & Liao, W. H. (2020). Performance of radiologists in differentiating COVID-19 from non-COVID-19 viral pneumonia at chest CT. *Radiology*, *296*(2), E46–E54. doi:10.1148/radiol.2020200823 PMID:32155105

Castelo, M. (2020). *The Future of Artificial Intelligence in Healthcare*. https://healthtechmagazine.net/article/2020/02/future-artificial-intelligence-healthcare

Catrin, S., Zaid, A., Niamh, O. N., Mehdi, K., & Ahmed, K. (2020). World Health Organization declares global emergency: A review of the 2019 novel corona virus (COVID-19). *International Journal of Surgery*, *76*, 71–76. doi:10.1016/j.ijsu.2020.02.034 PMID:32112977

Chelvachandran, N., Trifuljesko, S., Drobotowicz, K., Kendzierskyj, S., Jahankhani, H., & Shah, Y. (2020). Considerations for the Governance of AI and Government Legislative Frameworks. In H. Jahankhani, S. Kendzierskyj, N. Chelvachandran, & J. Ibarra (Eds.), *Cyber Defence in the Age of AI, Smart Societies and Augmented Humanity. Advanced Sciences and Technologies for Security Applications*. Springer. doi:10.1007/978-3-030-35746-7_4

Chen, S., Yang, J., Yang, W., Wang, C., & Barnighausen, T. (2020). COVID-19 Control in China during Mass Population Movements at New Year. *Lancet*, *395*(10226), 764–766. Advance online publication. doi:10.1016/S0140-6736(20)30421-9 PMID:32105609

Cohen, G., & Mello, M. (2018). HIPAA and protecting health information in the 21st century. *Journal of the American Medical Association*, *320*(3), 231–232. doi:10.1001/jama.2018.5630 PMID:29800120

Craft, L. (2017). *Emerging Applications of Ai for Health care Providers*. Gartner. https://www.gartner.com/document/3753763?ref=solrAll&refval=224860044&qid=d68fd7aaf33dc5ae74c5e8

DelPrete. (2016). *Self Service Kiosks: Improving Collections, Efficiency and Patient Experience*. American Association of Orthopedic Executives. https://www.aaoe.net/news/315967/self-service-kiosks-improving-collections-efficiency-and-patient-experience.html

Dialani, P. (2021). *How Virtual Reality Is Helping to Deal with Covid-19*. https://www.analyticsinsight.net/virtualreality-helping-deal-covid-19/

Edwards, J. (2019). *How Mobility Solutions are Increasing Patient Satisfaction in Health care*. https://healthtechmagazine.net/article/2018/05/thoughtful-healthcare-mobility-deployments-improve-patient-satisfaction

Forsee. (2020). *AI in Healthcare*. https://www.foreseemed.com/artificial-intelligence-in-healthcare

Fountaine, T., McCarthy, B., & Saleh, T. (2019). *Building the AI-Powered Organization*. Academic Press.

Geng, D., & Rishi, V. (2018). *Tricking Neural Networks: Create Your Own Adversarial Examples*. https://ml.berkeley.edu/blog/2018/01/10/adversarial-examples/

GGVS. (2019). *Importance of AI in healthcare*. https://www.gavstech.com/importance-of-ai-in-healthcare/

Gil Press. (2021). *The Future of AI in Healthcare*. https://www.forbes.com/sites/gilpress/2021/04/29/the-future-of-ai-in-healthcare/?sh=31809939163b

Gupta, R., Ghosh, A., Singh, A. K., & Misra, A. (2020, May). Clinical considerations for patients with diabetes in times of COVID-19 epidemic. *Diabetes & Metabolic Syndrome*, *14*(3), 211–212. doi:10.1016/j.dsx.2020.03.002 PMID:32172175

Hernandez, D. (2017). *How AI Is Transforming Drug Creation*. https://www.wsj.com/articles/how-ai-is-transforming-drug-creation-1498442760

Hu, Z., Ge, Q., Jin, L., & Xiong, M. (2020). *Artificial intelligence forecasting of COVID-19 in China* [Unpublished Manuscript].

Imaging Technology News. (2020). *Integrating Artificial Intelligence in Treatment Planning*. https://www.itnonline.com/article/integrating-artificial-intelligence-treatment-planning

Javaid, M., Haleem, A., Vaishya, R., Bahl, S., Suman, R., & Vaish, A. (2018). Industry 4.0 technologies and their applications in fighting COVID-19 pandemic. *Diabetes & Metabolic Syndrome*, *14*(4), 419–422. doi:10.1016/j.dsx.2020.04.032 PMID:32344370

Karthikeyan, S., & Pandian, M. S. (2021). Science and Technology in the Modern Agricultural Sector: An Overview. *Science and Technology, 7*(2).

Kathleen. (2020). *The Increasing Use Of AI In The Pharmaceutical Industry*. https://www.forbes.com/sites/cognitiveworld/2020/12/26/the-increasing-use-of-ai-in-the-pharmaceutical-industry/?sh=74a4b0cb4c01

Kechit, G. (2021). *Artificial Intelligence in Pharmaceutical Industry: 8 Exciting Applications in 2021.* https://www.upgrad.com/blog/artificial-intelligence-in-pharmaceutical-industry/

Li, L., Qin, L., Xu, Z., Yin, Y., Wang, X., Kong, B., & Xia, J. (2020). Artificial intelligence distinguishes COVID-19 from community acquired pneumonia on chest CT. *Radiology*. Advance online publication. doi:10.1148/radiol.2020200905

Loucks, J., Davenport, T., & Schatsky, D. (2018). *State of AI in the Enterprise*. https://www2.deloitte.com/content/dam/insights/us/articles/4780_State-of-AI-in-the-enterprise/AICognitiveSurvey2018_Infographic.pdf

Maghdid, Ghafoor, Sadiq, Curran, & Rabie. (2020). *A Novel AI-Enabled Framework to Diagnose Corona virus Covid 19 Using Smartphone Embedded Sensors: Design study* [Unpublished Manuscript].

Maghdid, H. S., Asaad, A. T., Ghafoor, K. Z., Sadiq, A. S., Mirjalili, S., & Khan, M. K. (2021). Diagnosing COVID-19 pneumonia from X-ray and CT images using deep learning and transfer learning algorithms. Multimodal Image Exploitation and Learning, 11734. doi:10.1117/12.2588672

Manghnani, D. (2021). *Robotics: A Layman's Guide*. https://blogs.systweak.com/robotics-a-laymans-guide/

Marshall, S. (2021). *How AI is Transforming the Future of Healthcare*. https://www.internationalsos.com/client-magazines/in-this-issue-3/how-ai-is-transforming-the-future-of-healthcare

Mckinsey.com. (2020). *Transforming healthcare with AI: The impact on the workforce and organizations*. https://www.mckinsey.com/industries/healthcare-systems-and-services/our-insights/transforming-healthcare-with-ai

Minnie, A. (2019). *AI can reduce mammography screening's workload*. https://www.auntminnie.com/index.aspx?sec=sup&sub=aic&pag=dis&ItemID=124880

Mufareh, A. (2021). *Artificial Intelligence Technology Benefits*. https://yourstory.com/mystory/artificial-intelligence-technology-benefits

Neelima, A., Amit, K. B., & Mangamoori, L. N. (2020). The role of artificial intelligence in tackling COVID-19. *Future Virology, 15*(11), 717–724. Advance online publication. doi:10.2217/fvl-2020-0130

Nguyen, T. T., Waurn, G., & Campus, P. (2021). *Artificial intelligence in the battle against corona virus (COVID-19): A survey and future research directions*. https://www.thepeninsula.org.in/2020/04/28/artificial-intelligence-in-the-battle-against-coronavirus-covid-19-a-survey-and-future-research-directions/

Nicolae, A., Morton, G., Chung, H., Loblaw, A., Jain, S., Mitchell, D., Lu, L., Helou, J., Al-Hanaqta, M., Heath, E., & Ravi, A. (2017). Evaluation of a Machine-Learning Algorithm for Treatment Planning in Prostate Low-Dose-Rate Brachytherapy. *International Journal of Radiation Oncology, Biology, Physics, 97*(4), 822–829. doi:10.1016/j.ijrobp.2016.11.036 PMID:28244419

Pandey, P. (2018). *Building a Simple Chatbot from Scratch in Python (Using NLTK).* https://medium.com/analytics-vidhya/building-a-simple-chatbot-in-python-using-nltk-7c8c8215ac6e

Pandian, M. S. (2020). Impact of new agriculture technology in prediction of modern robotic system. *Dogo Rangsang Research Journal, 10*(06), 85–94.

Pirouz, B., Shaffiee Haghshenas, S., & Piro, P. (2020). Investigating a Serious Challenge in the Sustainable Development Process: Analysis of Confirmed Cases of COVID-19 (New Type of Corona Virus) through a Binary Classification Using Artificial Intelligence and Regression Analysis. *Sustainability, 12*(6), 24–27. doi:10.3390u12062427

Price, N. (2019). *Risks and Remedies For Artificial Intelligence In Health Care.* https://www.brookings.edu/research/risks-and-remedies-for-artificial-intelligence-in-health-care/

Reddy, S. (2018). *Use of Artificial Intelligence in Healthcare Delivery, eHealth - Making Health Care Smarter.* https://www.intechopen.com/chapters/60562

Reddy, S., Fox, J., & Purohit, M. P. (2019). Artificial Intelligence-Enabled Healthcare Delivery. *Journal of the Royal Society of Medicine, 112*(1), 22–28. doi:10.1177/0141076818815510 PMID:30507284

Sengupta, R. (2021). *PM Modi to Address the Nation Again Tonight amid the Corona Virus Crisis.* https://yourstory.com/2020/03/pm-modi-address-tonight-coronavirus-crisis?utm_pageloadtype=scroll

Singh, H. (2021). *The Impact of Artificial Intelligence in Healthcare 2020.* https://blogs.systweak.com/the-impact-of-artificial-intelligence-in-healthcare/

Stefanini. (2020). *The Usage of AI in Pharma Has Been Relatively Slow; However, Unknown to Many, It Offers Immense Benefits.* https://stefanini.com/en/trends/news/a-guide-to-ai-in-the-pharmaceutical-industry

The Economic Times. (2021). *Can your Fitbit or Apple Watch detect corona virus infection early?* https://economictimes.indiatimes.com/tech/can-your-fitbit-or-apple-watch-detect-coronavirus-infection-early/tech-wearables-in-the-fight/slideshow/76319430.cms

Upendra. (2020). *Artificial Intelligence in Healthcare: Top Benefits, Risks and Challenges.* https://www.tristatetechnology.com/blog/artificial-intelligence-in-healthcare-top-benefits-risks-and-challenges/

Vaishya, R., Javaid, M., Khan, I. H., & Haleemb, A. (2020). Artificial Intelligence (AI) applications for COVID-19 pandemic. *Diabetes & Metabolic Syndrome, 14*(4), 337–339. doi:10.1016/j.dsx.2020.04.012 PMID:32305024

Varshney, R. (2021). *Coronavirus: This IIT-Delhi alumni startup develops camera to detect face masks, social distancing in crowded places.* https://yourstory.com/2020/05/coronavirus-iit-delhi-alumni-camera-face-masks-social-distancing

Walter, M. (2019). *6 Serious Risks Associated With AI in Healthcare.* https://www.aiin.healthcare/topics/diagnostics/6-risks-ai-healthcare-artificial-intelligence

Wilson, T. (2020). *No longer Science Fiction, AI and Robotics Are Transforming Healthcare.* https://www.pwc.com/gx/en/industries/healthcare/publications/ai-robotics-new-health/transforming-healthcare.html

Chapter 6
Secured Healthcare Data Analytics on the Cloud Using Blockchain-Based Techniques

Subashini B.
Department of Computer Science, Thiagarajar College, Madurai, India

ABSTRACT

Blockchain and the internet of things (IoT) are progressive technologies that are changing the world with additional special care within the healthcare system. In healthcare, IoT is a remote patient monitoring system that allows IoT devices to collect patient information such as remote monitoring, test results, pharmacy detailsm and medical insurance details, and allows doctors to provide excellent care. In order to facilitate data sharing among different hospitals and other organizations, it is necessary to secure data with caution. Blockchain is a decentralized, distributed, and an immutable digital ledger that records healthcare transactions using peer-to-peer technology in an extremely secure manner. It uses the cloud environment to store the huge amount of data on healthcare. The data generated from IoT devices uses blockchain technology to share medical information being analyzed by healthcare professionals in different hospitals in a secure manner. The objective is to benefit patient monitoring remotely and overcome the problem of information blocking.

INTRODUCTION

Today, the health sector is one of the fastest growing sectors in spite of the economic downturn. Healthcare systems are complex and the kinds of hospital systems, patient care, insurance, health care providers and legal challenges are well recognized. Research and development in the health sector should be a continuous process, as it will contribute to the improvement of the quality of life by combating various diseases and health problems. A variety of innovative computer technologies IoT, Blockchain, Machine Learning, Data Mining, Natural Language Processing (NLP), Image Processing, Cloud Computing used within the healthcare system will provide miraculous outcomes.

DOI: 10.4018/978-1-7998-9132-1.ch006

Copyright © 2022, IGI Global. Copying or distributing in print or electronic forms without written permission of IGI Global is prohibited.

Blockchain was originally introduced as a mechanism to power Bitcoin (Nakamoto, 2008), but has now evolved to the point of being referred to as a foundational technology for multiple decentralized applications (Iansiti & Lakhani, 2017). Blockchain is a relatively new database and data encryption technology that uses immutable ledgers, hash tables, and a decentralized network to verify and transfer data (Morgan P et al., 2020) (Gatteschi Vet al., 2018) (Friedewald Metal, 2020) (Ridhawi I AI et al. 2020)., Blockchain has been suggested as a way to solve critical challenges faced by healthcare, such as secured sharing of medical records and compliance with data privacy laws (Rupasinghe et al., 2019). The most interesting features in blockchain that are beneficial to healthcare applications is decentralization, privacy and security since blockchain technology may ensure for example a secure access to medical data for patients and various stakeholders such as insurance companies, hospitals, doctors, etc. (Rim Ben Fekih et al., 2020).

The Internet of Things (IoT) is a network of physical objects (or "things") that are implanted with sensors, software, and network technologies in order to connect and exchange data with other devices and systems over the Internet. Through body sensor networks and handheld devices, IoT promotes communication between doctors and patients in medical applications.

Cloud computing in health care enhances the efficiency of the industry, while lowering costs. Cloud computing facilitates and secures the sharing of health records, automates background operations, and even facilitates the creation and maintenance of healthcare data.

As a result, security must be taken into account. Blockchain is one of today's most popular study subjects, and it may be used in a variety of IoT applications (Pranav Ratta et al.2021), allowing developers to quickly deploy resources and operate from afar.

MAIN CONTRIBUTIONS

1. The opportunities, advantages and several challenges related to the use of Blockchain, IoT technologies and cloud were explored.
2. The Internet of Things (IoT), Blockchain, and cloud computing in healthcare are discussed.
3. The use of blockchain and IoT to secure medical data in the cloud was investigated.

BLOCKCHAIN TECHNOLOGY AND ASSOCIATED CONCEPTS

Blockchain is one of the leading hyped technologies of the current day with usage cases and startups showing at the rate. A Blockchain is a network of distributed software for the recording and storage of transaction records and also permit the secure transfer of properties. In a blockchain system, transaction records are stored and distributed among all network participants. Blockchain is a distributed public ledger database that is maintained by a network of verified participants or nodes (Jaoude & Saadeet al., 2019) and stores immutable blocks of data that can be shared securely without third-party intervention (Hölbl et al., 2018). Data are preserved and recorded with cryptographic signatures and use of consensus algorithms that are enacted as key enablers of its application (Mendling et al., 2018). Blockchain describes a chain of data or transactions as blocks linked or chained together by cryptographic signatures, each of

Figure 1. Blockchain structure

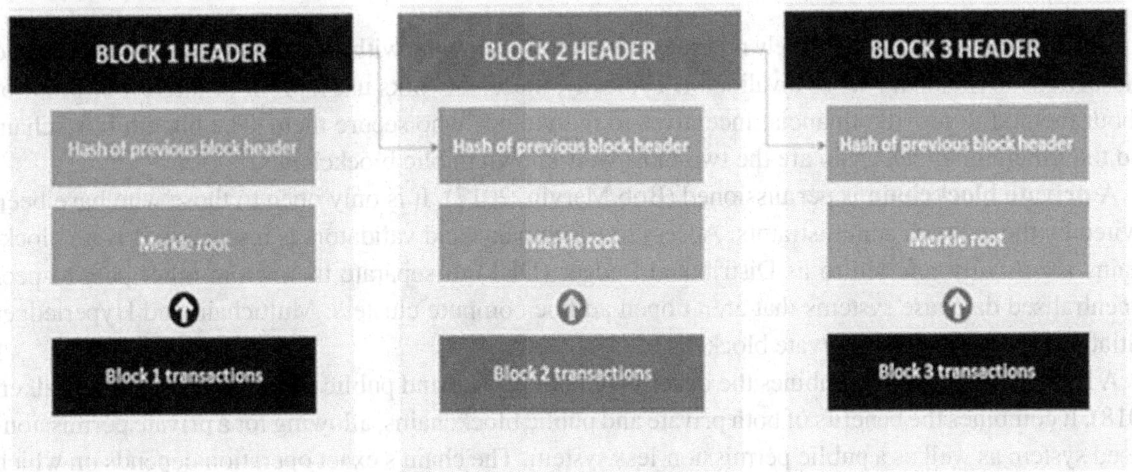

which is called a hash, stored in shared ledgers and supported by a network of connected processes called nodes. The crypto-economic realists of the blockchain protocol (consensual layer) regulate the activity rules and incentive mechanism of all network stakeholders. Blockchain has a wide range of applications and uses in the health domain. The efficient Blockchain healthcare application requires interoperability, allowing technology to keep medical data safely in a digital ledger.

Key Characteristics

Digital: Wherever all of the data on Blockchain eliminates the need for human documentation, it is digitised.

Distributed Ledger: Blockchain might be a distributed ledger in which all data is shared in indistinguishable copies. Participants verify data on an individual basis rather than as a centralised authority. Despite one of the nodes collapsing, the remaining nodes continue to function normally.

Immutability: Once entered, no one can change the data on the block chain. It also involves the system administrator as well as third parties. This allows people to demonstrate that their data is authentic and unedited.

Privacy: The value of information is encoded. Only approved Participants will have access to the information for which permissions are required.

Dynamic Consent: Allow people to provide several types of consent in accordance with different potential uses of knowledge, as well as the ability to change and revoke consent in accordance with the GDPR at any moment.

Self-Executing: The written agreement says that it supported the digitalization of written agreement relationships, which are stored in the blockchain and automate the execution of peer-to-peer transactions under user-defined conditions.

Synchronised: Every participant has access to the exact same information and status. (F. Xavier Olleros., 2016).

Types of Blockchain

A **public blockchain** has absolutely no access restrictions. Anyone with an Internet connection can send transactions to them and act as a validator. Typically, these networks use a proof of interest or proof of labour method to provide financial incentives to individuals who secure them. The bitcoin blockchain and the Ethereum block chain are the two most well-known public blockchains.

A **private blockchain** is permissioned (Bob Marvin, 2017). It is only open to those who have been invited by the network administrators. Access to participants and validators is restricted. Private blockchains are usually referred to as Distributed Ledger (DLT) to separate them from other peer-to-peer decentralised database systems that aren't open ad-hoc compute clusters. Multichain and Hyperledger initiatives are examples of private blockchain.

A **hybrid blockchain** combines the benefits of both private and public blockchains (Martin Walker, 2018). It combines the benefits of both private and public blockchains, allowing for a private permission-based system as well as a public permission-less system. The chain's exact operation depends on which parts of centralization and decentralisation are used.

A **consortium blockchain** is a semi-decentralized kind in which a blockchain network is managed by multiple organisations. This is in contrast to a private blockchain, which is controlled by a single organisation. In this type of blockchain, more than one organisation can operate as a node, exchanging information or mining. Banks, government agencies, and other institutions frequently use consortium blockchains. Energy Web Foundation, R3, and other consortium blockchains are examples. (Vitalik Buterin., 2014) (Z. Zheng 2017) (F. Xavier Olleros., 2016).

Challenges of Blockchain

There are still certain challenges that blockchain's have not yet overcome, they are Scalability, Hackers and shadow, dealing, Complex to understand and adopt, Privacy, costs and Blockchain is still a distant dream, Interoperability.

INTERNET OF THINGS AND RELATED CONCEPTS

The «thing» in the Internet of Things can be any device with any form of inbuilt sensor that can collect and transport data over a network without the need for operator intervention. Embedded technology enables them to interact with internal and external states, which aids in decision-making. All things connected to the Internet can be categorised into three categories on the Internet of Things:

1. Things that collect and transmit data.
2. Things that take action after receiving information.
3. This completes the pair.

Smart grids, smart homes, smart transportation and smart cities, health care, seismic detection, and other technologies are included.

Benefits of IoT

- Improved Customer Engagement – By automating the action, the Internet of Things improves the consumer experience.
- Technical Optimization – The Internet of Things has been a huge success in terms of advancing and upgrading technology.
- Reduced Waste – Our current data is superficial, but the Internet of Things (IoT) gives real-time data that leads to better decision-making and resource management.

Challenges in IoT

The main issues in IoT are security issues, privacy concerns, interoperability issues, it standards issues, legal issues, regulatory rights issues, emerging economic issues, developmental issues (Dubovitskaya, 2017).

CLOUD COMPUTING AND RELATED CONCEPTS

Cloud computing is the process of manipulating, configuring, and accessing physical and software assets from a distance. It provides internet infrastructure, data storage, and application development services. It provides internet infrastructure, data storage, and application development services. Behind the scenes, some services and models make cloud computing possible and available to end users. The operating models for cloud computing is as follows:

- Deployment Models
- Service Models

Deployment Models

The types of cloud access are defined by deployment models. In cloud computing, there are four different types of access.

Public Cloud

The public cloud makes systems and services available to anybody with an internet connection. Because of its openness, the public cloud may be less secure.

Private Cloud

Within a business, the private cloud offers access to systems and services. Because of its private character, it is more secure.

Community Cloud

A set of organisations can access systems and services through the community cloud.

Hybrid Cloud

The hybrid cloud is a blend of public and private clouds in which vital tasks are handled by the private cloud and non-critical tasks are handled by the public cloud.

Service Models

Service models support cloud computing. These can be divided into three types of service models:

- Infrastructure-as–a-Service (IaaS)
- Platform-as-a-Service (PaaS)
- Software-as-a-Service (SaaS)

Anything-as-a-Service (XaaS) which encompasses Network-as-a-Service, Business-as-a-Service, Identity-as-a-Service, Database-as-a-Service, and Strategy-as-a-Service, is yet another service paradigm.

The Infrastructure-as-a-Service (IaaS)

The most basic level of service is Infrastructure-as-a-Service (IaaS). The security and management mechanisms of the underlying model are passed down to each of the service models. IaaS gives users access to basic resources like physical machines, virtual machines, and virtual storage.

Platform-as-a-Service (PaaS)

PaaS provides the application runtime environment, as well as development and deployment tools.

Software-as-a-Service (SaaS)

The SaaS model allows end-users to use software applications as a service.

Challenges in Cloud Computing

Cloud computing, an emergent technology, has placed many challenges in different aspects of data and information handling. Some of the challenges include security and privacy, portability, interoperability, computing performance, reliability, cost management and containment, managing multiple clouds, performance and availability.

BLOCKCHAIN IN HEALTH DOMAIN

Blockchain technology can be tremendously useful in healthcare data group action, which is currently dispersed, with a spread of service providers. As this is a distributed network, blockchain-based systems can be useful for the integration of many intermediaries into the treatment system. Blockchain technology has the potential to reshape health care, to place the patient in the middle of the health care system, and to increase the protection, confidentiality, and capacity of health literacy. This technology could provide a whole new model for health data interchange (HIE) by creating a lot of economic, disintermediated, and secure electronic medical records. It can be applied in several areas of attention; however, all activity within the attention is not included in the transactions. Blockchain technology is based on a decentralized agreement and is currently being implemented in each public and personal context. To better understand the fundamentals of the technology as well as the potential application of blockchain with attention.

Blockchain application in focus is emerging. However, early solutions have shown the potential to reduce attention prices, contour business processes and improve access to data among diverse and numerous stakeholders working towards a typical goal.

The benefits of exploitation blockchain's, relative to ancient strategies of attention, direction systems, embody decentralised management, changeless databases for the approved user by keeping the data out from the unauthorized users with encoding the patient's personal key.

This ability to preserve data is one of the main reasons why blockchain is being used in healthcare (Kuo et al., 2019), where a large volume of data is exchanged and distributed widely (Meinert et al., 2019).

Interoperability is the use of blockchain technology to make it easier to collect vast amounts of patient data for population health efforts. The concept of immutability in a distributed transaction ledger promises architectural features that will help healthcare providers, payers, and affected patients overcome current impediments to patient health care data interoperability.

Figure 2. Blockchain cryptographic / hash security concept

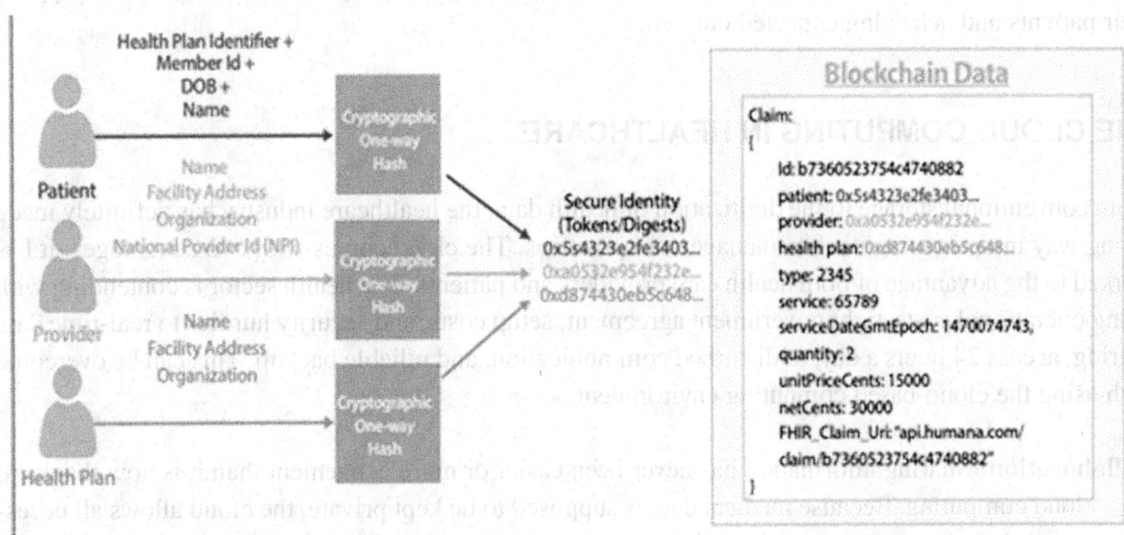

The Wall Street Journal reports that Ernst & Young is developing on a blockchain to enable businesses, governments, airlines, and others track those who have had antibody tests and may be immune to the COVID-19 pandemic in 2020. Blockchain was also used by hospitals and vendors for the essential medical equipment. Furthermore, in China, blockchain technology was employed to reduce the time it takes for health insurance payments to reach health care providers and patients. (Castellanos et al.)

IOT IN HEALTHCARE

Remote monitoring facilitated by the Internet of Things (IoT) in the health sector keeps patients safe and healthy, providing for ongoing monitoring of health conditions and empowering physicians to give high-quality care. Patient participation and satisfaction have also increased as interactions with physicians have become easier and more efficient. This has a big impact on lonely people and their families.

The frequency of health surveillance has altered as a result of wearable devices such as fitness strips and smart watches. Doctors can better monitor patient health by deploying portable devices and other IoT-enabled home monitoring equipment.

Aside from patient health monitoring, hospitals can benefit from IoT devices in a variety of ways. Defibrillators, wheelchairs, oxygen pumps, nebulizers, and other monitoring equipment are all utilised to locate real-time medical equipment using sensor-enabled IoT devices. Health insurers can use IoT-connected smart devices for a variety of purposes. For underwriting and claims operations, insurance firms may use data collected by health surveillance devices. In the pricing, underwriting, claims processing, and risk assessment procedures, IoT systems promote transparency between customers and insurers. Furthermore, if a patient arrives at the hospital via ambulance, the physicians diagnose the patient at the time of arrival and the hospital immediately begins treatment. Data generated from a variety of healthcare applications is now being analysed and used to develop cures for various diseases.

IoT helps healthcare professionals to be more observant and proactive in their communication with patients in this way. IoT device data can assist clinicians in determining the best course of therapy for their patients and achieving expected outcomes.

THE CLOUD COMPUTING IN HEALTHCARE

From conventional storage to the digitization of health data, the healthcare industry has definitely made a long way in optimizing its data management practices. The cloud comes with two advantages. It has worked to the advantage of both health care providers and patients. The health sector is contending with rising operational costs, tight government agreement, setup costs, and security hurdles to real-time data sharing, access 24 hours a day, undisturbed communication, and reliable backup. This can be overcome with using the cloud-based computing environment.

Collaboration: Sharing information has never been easier or more convenient than it is now thanks to cloud computing. Because medical data is supposed to be kept private, the cloud allows all necessary stakeholders, such as nurses, doctors, and care providers, to securely share data in real time. They can view medical reports and files at any time and from any location, in addition to sharing.

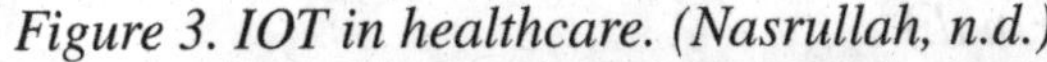

Figure 3. IOT in healthcare. (Nasrullah, n.d.)

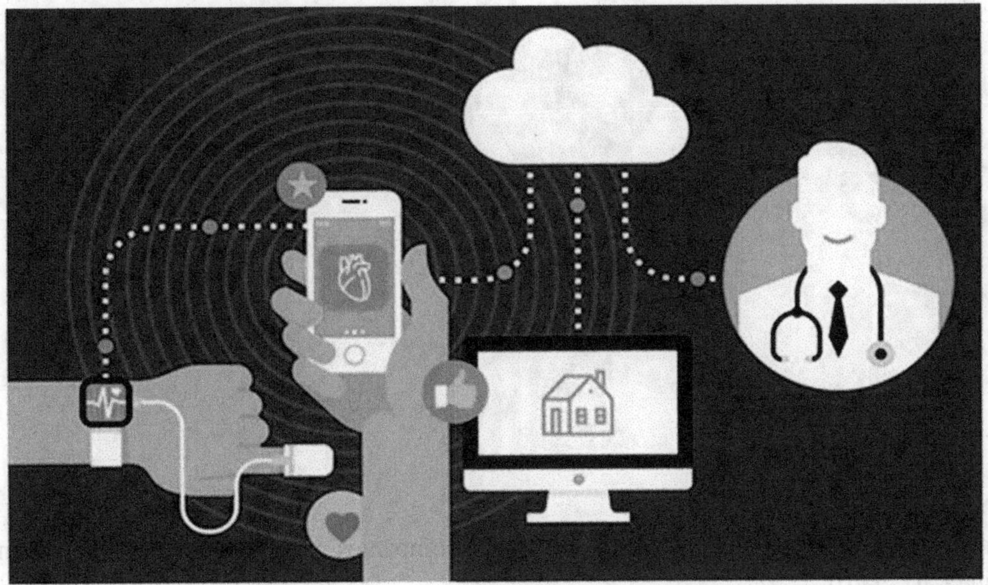

Security: Confidentiality of health information is required. Because of the large amount of data kept by this domain, it attracts malevolent actors, resulting in data and security risks.

Cost: At a low cost, the cloud can store a large amount of data.

Speed: Prior to deciding on a technology, speed is a crucial factor to consider.

Scalability and Flexibility: The healthcare industry flourishes in a dynamic environment. Electronic medical records, mobile applications, patient portals, IoT devices, and enormous data analysis are all made possible by the cloud. It provides easy scalability and flexibility, which improves the ultimate decision-making process.

Along with providing 24x7 availability, healthcare providers must substantially grow their data storage and network requirements to meet the demands of their services.

In addition to being available 24 hours a day, healthcare providers must be able to adjust to service requests in terms of data storage and network requirements.

It is critical for healthcare providers to adapt to data storage and network requirements to meet service expectations, in addition to being available 24 hours a day, seven days a week.

SECURE HEALTHCARE DATA ON CLOUD USING BLOCKCHAIN AND IOT

Health care is expected to become a trend because of changing technology and our way of life, which has resulted in changes in the health care system and increased lifespan. The confidentiality of a patient's information and preventing data theft are two key ethical concerns in the health-care system. The most intriguing features of the blockchain that are beneficial for health care applications are decentralisation, confidentiality, and security, because blockchain technology can provide secure access to health data

Figure 4. Benefits of cloud computing in healthcare (Zymr, n.d.)

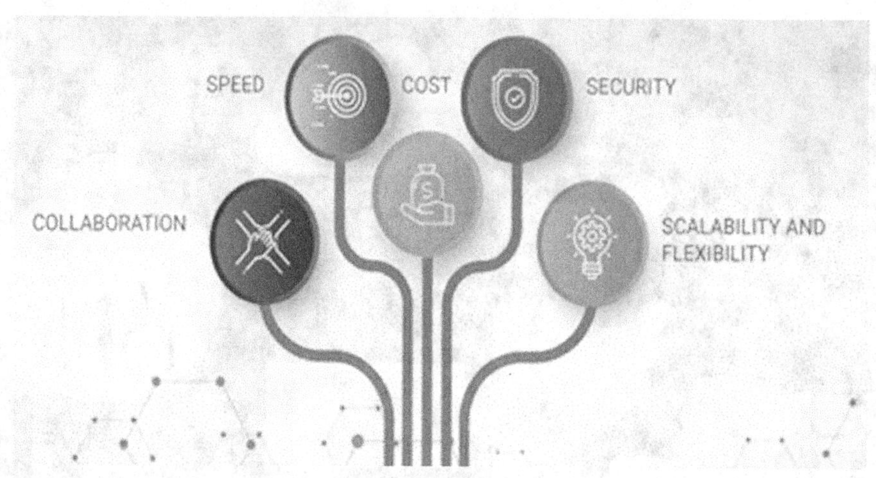

for patients and various stakeholders such as insurance companies, hospitals, doctors, and so on. (Rim Ben Fekih et al., 2020)

Remote patient monitoring includes the collecting of medical data via body sensors and IoT (Internet of Things) devices in order to remotely monitor patient status. Blockchain has a wide range of applications and uses in the field of health care. It's essential for storing, exchanging, and retrieving data generated by IoT devices. To make the secure transmission of patient health records and to govern the pharmaceutical supply chain, ledger technology is deployed. The patient's medical information, including past and present diseases, treatments, and medical family history, will be stored on the blockchain.

Remote patient monitoring includes the collecting of medical data via body sensors and IoT (Internet of Things) devices in order to remotely monitor patient status. In the field of health care, blockchain has a wide range of applications and uses. It is critical for the storage, exchange, and retrieval of data collected remotely via IoT devices. Ledger technology is used to ease the secure transfer of patient health records and to control the pharmaceutical supply chain. The blockchain will contain the patient's medical information, including past and present ailments, treatments, and medical family history. Medical records will not be lost or altered because they will be permanent, portable, and accessible. The patient will have access to the information. This information is only accessible to permitted users, such as healthcare providers and insurance companies. Patients have access to all stored information. The healthcare provider or insurance company will send a request, along with the contents of the information to consult. Patients' personal information will be kept confidential, and they will be the sole owners of it. This avoids the theft of a patient's medical identity. As a result, the Block chain can be used to address security issues in an IoT system.

The cloud provides on-demand computing by deploying, accessing, and utilising networked information, applications, and resources using the most up-to-date technology. In the health-care industry, cloud computing is increasingly becoming a must. It aids the healthcare system by allowing medical providers to share patient information concerning emergency cases in real time. Cloud solutions, service providers, and carriers all have enhanced security and protection mechanisms in place. Healthcare organisations should be assured that they are safeguarded against the loss of control over some critical patient information.

Figure 5. Integration of IOT, blockchain and cloud computing in healthcare

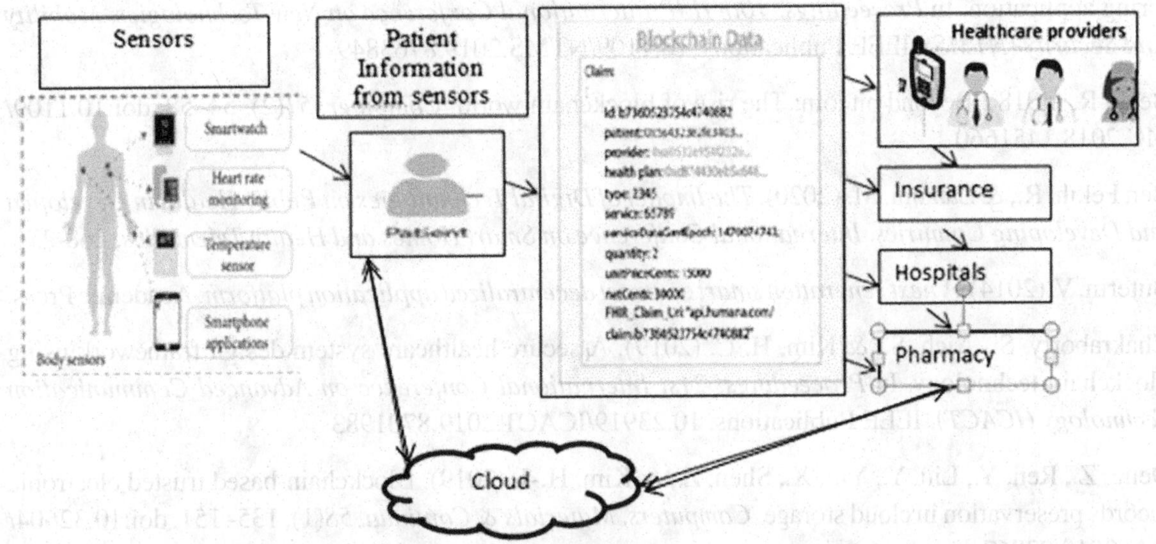

CONCLUSION AND FUTURE ENHANCEMENT

Blockchain is a fairly replacing capability that will be on the rise in the coming years. The promise of Blockchain in the healthcare industry is enticing enough to create a technical framework for the creation of blockchain-based healthcare apps. The Blockchain technology must be of higher quality, with the network's latency being reduced by utilising completely different algorithms and a wide range of secure settings for the storage and distribution of touch-and-go data. In the future, blockchain technology combined with other developing technologies such as AI, big data, cloud computing, and IoT computing will provide really effective medical help and blockchain healthcare solutions. With the development of technology tools to allow the sharing of patient data and improve health-care procedures, the trade is seeking for secure and clear ways to conduct business so that they may maintain complete confidence inside the systems and provide their patients with consistent care. The data created by IoT devices employs Blockchain technology to securely communicate medical data from the cloud environment, which is being analysed by healthcare professionals in various hospitals.

REFERENCES

Akhtar, M. M., & Rizvi, D. R. (2021). Traceability and detection of counterfeit medicines in pharmaceutical supply chain using blockchain-based architectures. In *Sustainable and Energy Efficient Computing Paradigms For Society* (pp.1–31). Springer. doi:10.1007/978-3-030-51070-1_1

Alonsa, G. S., Arambarri, J., Lopez Coronado, M., & de la Toree Diez, I. (2019). Proposing new blockchain challenges in e-health. *Journal of Medical Systems*, *43*(64).

Attaia, O. (2019). An IoT-blockchain architecture based on hyperledger framework for healthcare monitoring application. In *Proceedings: 10th IFIP International Conference on New Technologies, Mobility And Security (NTMS)*. IEEE Publications. 10.1109/NTMS.2019.8763849

Beck, R. (2018). Beyond bitcoin: The rise of blockchain world. *Computer, 51*(2), 54–58. doi:10.1109/MC.2018.1451660

Ben Fekih, R., & Lahami, M. (2020). *The Impact of Digital Technologies on Public Health in Developed and Developing Countries. International Conference on Smart Homes and Health Telematics*, 268-276.

Buterin, V. (2014). *A next generation smart contract decentralized application platform*. Academic Press.

Chakraborty, S., Aich, S., & Kim, H. C. (2019). A secure healthcare system design framework using blockchain technology. In *Proceedings: 21st International Conference on Advanced Communication Technology (ICACT)*. IEEE Publications. 10.23919/ICACT.2019.8701983

Deng, Z., Ren, Y., Liu, Y., Yin, X., Shen, Z., & Kim, H.-J. (2019). Blockchain-based trusted electronic records preservation in cloud storage. *Computers, Materials & Continua, 58*(1), 135–151. doi:10.32604/cmc.2019.02967

Dubovitskaya, A., Xu, Z., Ryn, S., Schumacher, M., & Wang, F. (2017). Secure and trustable electronic medical records sgaring using blockchain. *AMIA Annual Symposium Proceedings*, 650-659.

Fernández-Caramés, T. M., & Fraga-Lamas, P. (2018). A review on the use of blockchain for the internet of things. *IEEE Access: Practical Innovations, Open Solutions, 6*, 32979–33001. doi:10.1109/ACCESS.2018.2842685

Friedewald, M., Önen, M., Lievens, E., Krenn, S., & Fricker, S. (2020). Distributed ledger for provenance tracking of artificial intelligence assets. *IFIP Advances in Information and Communication Technology*. Advance online publication. doi:10.1007/978-3-030-42504-3

Gatteschi, V., Lamberti, F., Demartini, C., Pranteda, C., & Santamaria, V. (2018). Blockchain and smart contracts for insurance: Is the technology mature enough? *Future Internet, 10*(2), 20. doi:10.3390/fi10020020

Gokhale, P., Bhat, O., & Bhat, S. (2018). Introduction to IOT. *International Advanced Research Journal in Science, Engineering and Technology*, *5*(1), 41–44.

Haq, I., & Esuka, O. M. (2018). Blockchain technology in pharmaceutical industry to prevent counterfeit drugs. *International Journal of Computers and Applications, 975*, 8887.

Hemalatha, P. (2021). Monitoring and securing the healthcare data harnessing IOT and blockchain technology. *Turkish Journal of Computer and Mathematics Education, 12*(2), 2554–2561.

Hoy, M. B. (2017). An introduction to the blockchain and its implications for libraries and medicine. *Medical Reference Services Quarterly, 36*(3), 273–279. doi:10.1080/02763869.2017.1332261 PMID:28714815

Iansiti, M., & Lakhani, K. R. (2017). The truth about blockchain. *Harvard Business Review, 95*(1), 118–127.

Jamali, M. A. J. (2020). *IoT architecture towards the internet of things*. Springer. doi:10.1007/978-3-030-18468-1

Jamil, F., Ahmad, S., Iqbal, N., & Kim, D.-H. (2020). Towards a remote monitoring of patient vital signs based on IoT-based blockchain integrity management platforms in smart hospitals. *Sensors (Basel), 20*(8), 2195. doi:10.339020082195 PMID:32294989

Jamil, F., Hang, L., Kim, K., & Kim, D. (2019). A novel medical blockchain model for drug supply chain integrity management in a smart hospital. *Electronics (Basel), 8*(5), 505. doi:10.3390/electronics8050505

Jiang, S., Cao, J., Wu, H., Yang, Y., Ma, M., & He, J. (2018). A blockchain-based platform for healthcare information exchange. *IEEE International Conference on Smart Computing*, 49-56. 10.1109/SMART-COMP.2018.00073

Jin, H., Luo, Y., Li, P., & Mathew, J. (2019). A review of secure and privacy-preserving medical data sharing. *IEEE Access: Practical Innovations, Open Solutions, 7*, 61656–61669. doi:10.1109/ACCESS.2019.2916503

Kizza, J. M. (2017). Internet of things (IoT): Growth, challenges, and security. In *Guide to Computer Network Security* (pp. 517–531). Springer. doi:10.1007/978-3-319-55606-2_24

Kumar, N. M., & Mallick, P. K. (2018). Blockchain technology for security issues and challenges in IoT. *Procedia Computer Science, 132*, 1815–1823. doi:10.1016/j.procs.2018.05.140

Kumar, T. (2018). Blockchain utilization in healthcare: Key requirements and challenges. In *Proceedings: IEEE 20th International Conference on E-Health Networking, Applications and Services (Healthcom)*. IEEE Publications. 10.1109/HealthCom.2018.8531136

Li, H., Zhu, L., Shen, M., Gao, F., Tao, X., & Liu, S. (2018). Blockchain Based Data Preservation System for Medical Data. *Journal of Medical Systems, 42*(8), 141. doi:10.100710916-018-0997-3 PMID:29956058

Linn, L. A., & Koo, M. B. (2016). Blockchain for health data and its potential use in health IT and health care related research. Proceedings of the ONC/NIST use of Blockchain for Healthcare and Research Workshop.

Mazlan, A. A., Mohd Daud, S., Mohd Sam, S., Abas, H., Rasid, S. Z. A., & Yusof, M. F. (2020). Scalability challenges in healthcare blockchain system-a systematic review. *IEEE Access: Practical Innovations, Open Solutions, 8*, 23663–23673. doi:10.1109/ACCESS.2020.2969230

Morgan, P. (2020). Blockchain technology: Principles and applications in medical imaging. *Journal of Digital Imaging, 33*(3), 726–734. doi:10.100710278-019-00310-3 PMID:31898037

Nakamoto, S. (2008). *Bitcoin: A peer to peer electronic cash system*. Academic Press.

Nasrullah, P. (n.d.). *Peerbits*. Retrieved from https://www.peerbits.com/blog/internet-of-things-healthcare-applications-benefits-and-challenges.html

O'herrin, J. K., Fost, N., & Kudsk, K. A. (2004). Health Insurance Portability Accountability Act (HIPAA) regulations: Effect on medical record research. *Annals of Surgery, 239*(6), 772–778. doi:10.1097/01.sla.0000128307.98274.dc PMID:15166956

Rathee, P. (2020). Introduction to blockchain and IoT. *Studies in Big Data*, 1–14.

Raval, S. (2016). *Decentralized applications: Harnessing Bitcoin's Blockchain technology*. O'Reilly Media, Inc.

Ray, P. P., Dash, D., Salah, K., & Kumar, N. (2020). Blockchain for IoT-based healthcare: Background, consensus, platforms, and use cases. *IEEE Systems Journal*.

Reyna, A., Martín, C., Chen, J., Soler, E., & Diaz, M. (2018). On blockchain and its integration with IoT. Challenges and opportunities. *Future Generation Computer Systems*, *88*, 173–190. doi:10.1016/j.future.2018.05.046

Ridhawi, I., Aloqaily, M., & Jararweh, Y. (2020). *An incentive-based mechanism for volunteer computing using blockchain*. Academic Press.

Roehrs, A., Da Costa, C. A., & Da Rosa Righi, R. (2017). OmniPHR: A distributed architecture model to integrate personal health records. *Journal of Biomedical Informatics*, *71*, 70–81. doi:10.1016/j.jbi.2017.05.012 PMID:28545835

Rupasinghe, T., Burstein, F., Rudolph, C., & Strange, S. (2019). Towards a blockchain based fall prediction model for aged care. *Proceedings of the Australasian Computer Science Week Multiconference*, 1–10, 10.1145/3290688.3290736

Stagnaro, C. (2017). *White paper: Innovative blockchain uses in health care*. Freed Associates.

Wang, J., Chen, W., Wang, L., Ren, Y., & Simon Sherratt, R. (2020). Blockchain-based data storage mechanism for industrial internet of things. *Intelligent Automation & Soft Computing*, *26*(5), 1157–1172. doi:10.32604/iasc.2020.012174

Wang, Q., Zhu, F., Ji, S., & Ren, Y. (2020). Secure provenance of electronic records based on blockchain. *Computers, Materials & Continua*, *65*(2), 1753–1769. doi:10.32604/cmc.2020.07366

Wood, G. (2014). *Ethereum: A secure decentralized generalized transaction ledger*. Academic Press.

Xavier Olleros, F. (2016). Blockchain technology: Principles and applications. *Research Handbook on Digital Transformations*, 225.

Xia, Q., Sifah, E. B., Asamoah, K. O., Gao, J., Du, X., & Guizani, M. (2017). MeDShare: Trust-less medical data sharing among cloud service providers via blockchain. *IEEE Access: Practical Innovations, Open Solutions*, *5*, 14757–14767. doi:10.1109/ACCESS.2017.2730843

Yue, X., Wing, H., Jin, D., Li, M., & Jiang, W. (2016). Healthcare data gateways: Found healthcare intelligence on blockchain with novel privacy risk control. *Journal of Medical Systems*, *40*(10), 218. doi:10.100710916-016-0574-6 PMID:27565509

Zhang, A., & Lin, X. (2018). Towards secure and privacy-preserving data sharing in e-health systems via consortium blockchain. *Journal of Medical Systems*, *42*(8), 140. doi:10.100710916-018-0995-5 PMID:29956061

Zhang, P., White, J., Schmidt, D. C., Lenz, G., & Rosenbloom, S. T. (2018). FHIRChain: Applying blockchain to securely and scalably share clinical data. *Computational and Structural Biotechnology Journal, 16*, 267–278. doi:10.1016/j.csbj.2018.07.004 PMID:30108685

Z. Zheng, S. Xie, H. Dai, X. Chen, & H. Wang (Eds.). (2017). Big data (bigdata congress) *IEEE International Congress on 2017*. IEEE Publications.

Zhou, L., Wang, L., & Sun, Y. (2018). MIStore: A blockchain-based medical insurance storage system. *Journal of Medical Systems, 42*(8), 149. doi:10.100710916-018-0996-4 PMID:29968202

Zymr. (n.d.). Retrieved from https://www.zymr.com/5-key-benefits-of-cloud-computing-in-healthcare-industry/

Chapter 7
IoT Security Issues, Challenges, Threats, and Solutions in Healthcare Applications

Sudhakar Hallur
KLS Gogte Institute of Technlogy, India

Roopa Kulkarni
Dayanand Sagar Academy of Technology and Management, India

Prashant Patavardhan
RV Institute of Technology and Management, Bengaluru, India

Vishweshkumar Aithal
KLS Gogte Institute of Technology, India

ABSTRACT

A majority of the applications now go wireless involving IoT as a technology to communicate to their respective destination. IoT is considered as a future of internet. The internet of things integration and efficient communication of the patient health monitoring parameters is the need of the hour in this pandemic. This chapter discusses the three-layer architecture involving hardware communication protocols supporting a layer of healthcare services and applications. Also, the data-guarantee, security and integrity issues, threats risks, and solutions involving deployment of efficient privacy, control, integration methods to confront various prominent and erroneous data manipulation techniques, malicious, and a series of cyber-attacks are proposed. The deployment of various efficient privacy and security protocols in IoT networks is of extreme need to ensure the confidentiality, access-control, authentication, and integrity of the health data transferred and to guarantee the availability of the services to the user at any point of time.

DOI: 10.4018/978-1-7998-9132-1.ch007

Copyright © 2022, IGI Global. Copying or distributing in print or electronic forms without written permission of IGI Global is prohibited.

INTRODUCTION

Healthcare with inclusion of IoT is the need of the hour during this pandemic as a result of social-distancing between the people. Also, combining the Healthcare using IoT with successful communication would result in the fastest growth of one of the aspects of medico-engineering infrastructure. The main objective of combining is to provide mere rapid, successful and in-time management of the patient health taking into consideration, the various health parameters of the patient. Combining healthcare applications with IoT also arises a need for security. The security mitigation is to pre- serve privacy, confidentiality, ensuring the security of the data of the patient, infrastructures, data and medical devices of the IoT and to guarantee the availability of the services offered by an IoT Medico-Engineered ecosystem. Thus, the mitigation, countermeasures, portability, compatibility and data-guarantee need to be achieved and enhanced to support the existing IoT based medical applications.

Also, the IoT industry with the inclusion of healthcare is expected to be into boom by about approximately $10billion by the year 2024 end. Also, parallelly wireless 5G network is also developing at a faster pace. The combination of these two technologies to combine it for utilization with IoT and healthcare would be a definite lead front improvement.

IoT gadgets and their organizations should be joined with different advancements to help medical services offices change in a significant way. 5G will give the super low idleness paces and versatility that the IoT in the medical care industry needs. Thusly, artificial intelligence driven arrangements will sort out the information lakes assembled from an assortment of gadgets. Huge Information methodologies will utilize such simulated intelligence calculations to investigate information progressively and settle on basic wellbeing choices. Virtualization will assist with lessening or dispose of old framework in clinics.

Advancing the pace in the medico-engineering division just as a transmission dependent on routine wireless technology using Internet of Things would empower the accomplishment of the objectives of utilization of wireless communication. Various challenges involve in integration of IoT devices and component sources and transmitting the health data vehicle from adjusting the precision and transmitting using certain protocols to indicate complete utilization of the medical infrastructure and wireless technology to improve the performance of the system most efficiently.

One of the significant angles is that maturing of the populace brought about new difficulties for the general public and medical services systems. Assisted Way of life that relies upon Internet of Things (IoT) gives help to the handicapped individuals and supports their essential everyday life exercises. Moderateness and Openness and the use of IoT begins altering medical care administrations.

Some of the challenges include the intermitted power disruption of the transmitted signals, data security and privacy in real time, integration of the IoT end devices and protocols, data overload and accuracy and cost.

BACKGROUND

In clear words, the Internet of Things (IoT) is the arrangement of interconnected gadgets/tasks consented to all the organization components, for example, equipment, programming, availability of the organization, and some other required electronic/PC implies that eventually makes them responsive by supporting in information quarrel and assortment. In the event that we talk a touch more about IoT, it is past to an idea that fosters the in general engineering foundation which at last permits the incorporation and the viable trade of the information between the individual out of luck and the specialist organizations. The utilization of the IoT idea makes the reachability to the patients very valuable, which at last assistance to give them huge consideration so they can escape this illness. (Wang et al., 2020)

Dealing with the heterogeneous assets that get that information is a region that requests more consideration. The design introduced centers around the utilization of virtual assets as an administration idea and recognizes various methodologies in the exhibition assessment tense figuring gadgets. Utilizing the IoT convention CoAP, virtual assets are uncovered in the edge organization. An assessment of a Go CoAP virtual asset is introduced(Samaniego & Deters, 2016). IoT zeroing in on empowering innovations, conventions, and application issues, and feature security as one of the primary difficulties that should be tended to in IoT (Al-Fuqaha et al., 2015). A center around the cutting edge of IoT security dangers and weaknesses, offering a scientific categorization of dangers and examining conceivable cyberattacks(Alaba et al., 2017).

Survey eight IoT structures monetarily accessible, bringing up the security components of the individual architectures(Ammar et al., 2018). Investigation of open difficulties on IoT security, introducing a scientific categorization of safety issues, zeroing in on blockchain-based arrangements(Khan & Salah, 2018). A guide of safety in the IoT is presented through a fundamental and intellectual methodology. By intellectual, the creators imply that their methodology gives intricate and dynamical connections between measure, individuals, innovation and association, to give the adaptability for the framework to have the option to dissect various circumstances(Sfar et al., 2018). A review center around data security the executives structures for IoT(Irshad, 2016) and in (Nguyen et al., 2015) the creators examine about security issues in IoT considering their attributes concerning the application layer, network layer, and discernment layer. At last, in (Zhao & Ge, 2013) the creators examine the appropriateness and constraints of existing IP-based Internet security conventions, just as different kinds of safety conventions utilized in remote sensor organizations.

A complete report on security issues in IoT organizations. Different security prerequisites like validation, trustworthiness, secrecy was discussed(Shehab, 2018). Dynamic situating strategies have been utilized for concealing data in the further layer of the picture channels with the assistance a common mystery key(Bairagi et al., 2016).A procedure to get any kind of pictures particularly clinical pictures. To begin with, the AES encryption method was applied on the initial segment(Anwar et al., 2015). The clinical applications can be ordered into remote checking, analytic help, therapy support, clinical data, instruction and mindfulness(Elhoseny et al., 2018). Likewise, talked about the security methods that utilized for taking care of the security issues of medical care frameworks particularly crossover security techniques(Yehia et al., 2015).A clinical uprightness check framework to work on the security of clinical picture. The proposed framework primarily decayed into two phases: assurance and check. (Sreekutty & Baiju, 2017).A technique that concentrates on the clinical picture quality corruption when concealing information in the recurrence space. The mystery plaintext was encoded utilizing RC4 encryption before the implanting system.(Khalil, 2017)

IOT ARCHITECTURE

The design of IoT comprises of a few layers as shown in Figure 1, beginning from the edge innovation layer at the base to the application layer at the top. The two lower layers add to information catching, while the two higher layers are liable for information use in applications.

Figure 1. Layered structure of IoT

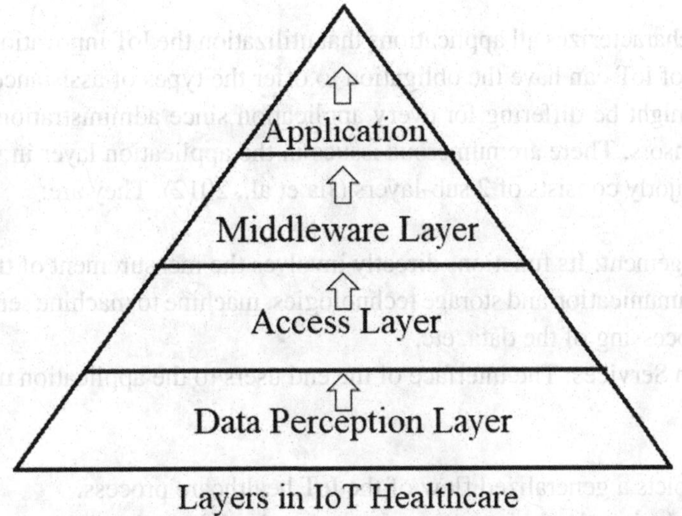

[The layered design in the IoT architecture depicts the flow of data from the point of origination to the point it reaches the user. The data flow in the diagram is bottom to top]

1. Data Perception Layer:

This is a hardware component layer that consists of various hardware components that relatively act as sensors such as Wireless Sensor Networks, Radio frequency identification components, storage devices, data processing devices, etc. to direct the information towards communication so that the information can be easily processed and broadcasted easily via various miniature trans-reception devices.(Hussain et al., 2009)

2. Access Layer:

This layer is mainly responsible for handling the data, transmission, rerouting of the messages, publication and subscription of various messages related to the intended application. The data transfer then occurs from access layer to the next layer. i.e. middleware layer where the transmission of the data takes places using the wireless communication technologies such as WiMax, WAN, WIFI, Ethernet, etc. (Atzori et al., 2010; Santucci, 2009)

3. Middleware Layer:

A software platform that provides flexibility to the users and also a simple flow functionality to the applications. The various functions that are being performed by this layer include device management and discovery, information segregation and filtering, data combining, recent and historical data analysis, access to the data control by various layers and devices and data recognition.

4. Application Layer:

Application layer characterizes all applications that utilization the IoT innovation or in which IoT has sent. The utilizations of IoT can have the obligation to offer the types of assistance to the applications. The administrations might be differing for every application since administrations rely upon the data that is gathered by sensors. There are numerous issues in the application layer in which security is the central question. It majorly consists of 2 sub-layers.(Jia et al., 2012). They are:

a. Data Management: Its functions directly involves the measurement of the Quality of service (QoS), communication and storage technologies, machine to machine services and processing and pre-processing of the data, etc.
b. Application Services: The interface of the end users to the application utilization is done via this layer.

Figure 2 below depicts a generalized flow of the IoT healthcare process.
(The process flow depicts the various components involved from the capture and monitoring of the victim's bodily parameters using sensors to its efficient and secure transmission via channels, its storage and usage.)

Figure 2. Generalized IoT-healthcare process flow

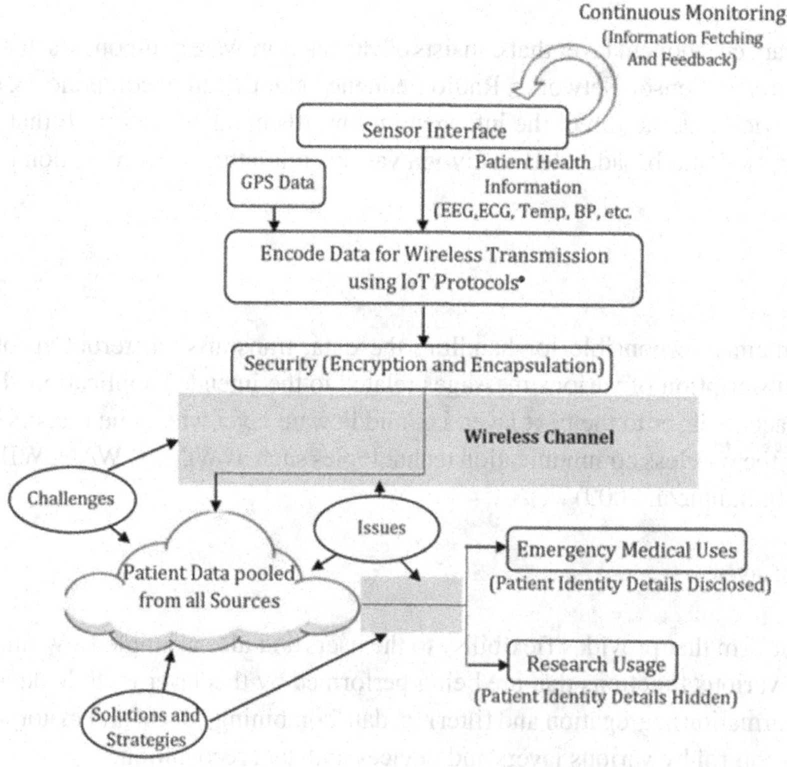

IOT PROTOCOLS FOR HEALTHCARE

In this section, three of the few standardized IoT application layer protocols used for message passing (related to healthcare or patient monitoring data) have been discussed as follows:

1. Hypertext Transfer Protocol (HTTP)

The HTTP is an application-level convention for conveyed, collective, hypermedia data frameworks. The HTTP is a nonexclusive and stateless, convention which can be utilized for some undertakings past its utilization for hypertext, for example, name workers and circulated object the executive's frameworks, through augmentation of its solicitation techniques, mistake codes and header. An element of HTTP is the composing and arrangement of information portrayal, permitting frameworks to be constructed autonomously of the information being moved. The HTTP convention is a solicitation/reaction convention. A customer sends a solicitation to the worker as a solicitation strategy, URI, and convention adaptation, trailed by a Multipurpose Internet Mail Extensions (MIME)- like message containing demand modifiers, customer data, and conceivable body content over an association with a worker. The worker reacts with a status line, including the message's convention adaptation and a triumph or blunder code, trailed by a MIME-like message containing worker data.

2. Constrained Application Protocol (CoAP)

CoAP is an application convention used to furnish compelled conditions with HTTP (for example demand/reaction) web move systems. CoAP has been given an inherent enrollment component which makes the convention likewise fitting to bar/sub applications. One of the primary plan objectives of CoAP was to limit the message overhead and oblige the parcel fracture.(De Caro et al., 2013)

3. Message Query Telemetry Transport (MQTT)

It is a lightweight convention suitable for gadgets with limited handling and memory abilities, to send information over low data transmission organizations. MQTT characterizes three Quality of Service (QoS) levels for message conveyance. With QoS 0, messages are conveyed all things considered once (MQTT is just about as reliable as TCP); with QoS 1, messages are conveyed essentially once through affirmations with QoS 2, messages are conveyed precisely once. MQTT dependent on the bar/sub model, where numerous customers can construct an association with agents.(De Caro et al., 2013)

4. Open Data Protocol (ODATA)

The Open Data Protocol, frequently condensed OData, is an open convention that permits making and devouring queryable APIs following the REST standards. It is normalized by OASIS and is very helpful in the transmission of medical data of the patients reliably from the source to the destination and the questions can be made in an information base like way. (OData, 2015) (OData - the Best Way to REST, n.d.)

5. Zigbee

A good example for master-slave combination is Zigbee which is also a good example for near-distance communication. The data received from the slave node is communicated to the master node which sometimes fails due to long placement of the receiver. So, in order to assist the communication, a LoraWAN protocol is used in place. During correspondence, such as exact area discovery by ZigBee terminal when it goes through ZigBee switch region. At the point when detected information of patients are contrasted and manual perusing, maximum matches occurred.(Vineetha et al., 2020) (Hiraguri et al., 2015)

6. Sigfox/LoRa

Reduced cost, extended battery life and range of radio communication under low power WAN are the extensive benefits offered by these protocols for transmission of any data. These protocols are frequently used to transmit medical patient data if used in closed perimeter area.(Vineetha et al., 2020) (Hiraguri et al., 2015)

IOT COMPONENTS

Remote advancements like RFID, ZigBee, and so forth assume a critical part in giving End to End IoT correspondences by making utilizing of the radio frequencies (Jaswal et al., 2017). The vast majority of the significant RFID parts like labels, perusers, sensors, network frameworks, and so forth are connected as stickers on the items to be detected. The IoT components may have inbuilt force (dynamic) or may depend for power on some regular asset, for example, sun oriented, and so on (detached). These sensors joined to objects work together inside themselves to make an organization which will be going by a pioneer chose on various imperatives. These sensors are called as hubs. The RFID labels might be recognized as dynamic (having installed power supply) and uninvolved (no locally available force supply). The sensors have a pivotal job in man-made reasoning, e-medical care and removing ecological information like temperatures, quakes, mechanical dangers, safeguard frameworks, and so on The primary part of IoT will be IoT middleware, making out of sub-layers which lie in the midst of the application level and specialized level layers. The middleware is deteriorated into different basic parts that follows an assistance arranged methodology allowing the utilization of any equipment just as programming.

CHARACTERISTICS NEEDED BY IOT FOR HEALTH MONITORING PURPOSES

There are a few characteristic features that need to be possessed by the IoT devices for the transfer of data in healthcare infrastructure. Some of them are listed below: (Verma et al., 2021)

1. Large Heterogenous device attachment capacity

Millions of gadgets will be required to construct a huge IoT framework, and every one of these gadgets should likewise be altogether different from one another. The majority of the IoT gadgets are assorted relies on the information and yield format of specifics and the correspondence conventions. So, to make a solid IoT framework, between gadget correspondence, interoperable gadgets, and examination of the information from all different gadgets is a major challenge.

2. High Reliability

Proper and accurate information delivery is the main purpose of usage of IoT. This is a highly expected feature at every layer so as to deliver uninterrupted and non-erroneous data from source to the destination.

3. Real Time Data Transfer

These gadgets send ongoing information to the base station (BS), which can additionally be utilized in various applications and that too with a base deferral. Under sufficient force availability, remote transmissions from sensors can be planned at ordinary time stretches to keep up with real-time information procurement

4. Safeguard data flows

Various methods are used to transfer the data through different layers from the source to destination. Thus, there is a high risk of data breach. Safeguarding the data is the primary feature.

5. Ability to Configure Application

Sensors get obsolete occasionally, and there are odds of breakdown, so it is smarter to arrange them from time to time as indicated by the application.

6. Device Level Monitoring and Traffic Management

Observing all actuates of associated gadgets and overseeing all traffic or we can say appropriate steering ought to be there

7. Cost-Effectiveness

The more devices are added, the more cost will increase. So, there is a need for efficient system that supports more devices on less interfaces.

HEALTHCARE APPLICATIONS

1. Scope and Role of Healthcare Applications in the Pandemic

In the present COVID-19 circumstance, there is a prerequisite to recognize the high-hazard patient, the death rate for various gatherings, following the spread of the infection, and appropriate observing of the medical services system.(Chen et al., 2020) Present day, IoT-empowered gadgets are valuable for managing a patient's internal heat level and advising something very similar to the specialist during any unusual circumstance. The savvy IoT-based wearable gadgets are helpful in giving checking during various medicines. This innovation can assist with giving progression to handle the COVID-19 pandemic. The IoT-empowered gadgets have the capacity for distant observing in a medical services framework, in this way protecting the patient solid and with the help of this innovation, the patient cooperation with the specialist becomes compelling and reasonable during the COVID-19 pandemic. It forestalls clinic re-affirmation and diminishes the length of stay of a patient in the clinic. The treatment results of COVID-19 patients are additionally improved adequately by continue to track of a patient's wellbeing. (Materia et al., 2020)

The utilization of versatile innovation and gadgets has been discovered to be fruitful in the medical care setting. The expression "versatile Health" (mHealth) has been utilized to portray any medical services practice that is upheld by cell phones. For example, a mHealth application may help medical services experts in treating clinical infections and instructing patients on self-checking of the sickness just as supporting therapy adherence. The utilization of mHealth applications has made medical services and wellbeing data effectively accessible. Furthermore, the utilization of mHealth applications at the client's comfort additionally assists with decreasing the recurrence of superfluous emergency clinic visits by stable patients, consequently lessening the versatility of patients who are immunocompromised to high-hazard regions. (Were et al., 2019)

The execution of key highlights in mHealth that can help in conclusion or side effect announcing has extraordinary potential in the administration of contaminations. Also, the joining of pertinent epidemiological information and geological data of communicable illness pervasiveness in a locale will permit the following of cases, which can be utilized as a viable apparatus to control the spread of contamination. It is more successful to convey wellbeing related data through mHealth applications, as data can be traded quickly and refreshed powerfully. Versatile applications can conceivably forestall the event of a specific sickness, as traded messages through a portable application can advance correspondence, stockpiling of data, and message conveyance that drives clients to make sound way of life changes

2. IoT Devices in Healthcare

There are a lot many healthcare devices or sensors that needs to be integrated with the main systems in order to process and analyse the data and arrive at a conclusion with respect to the patient's health. Some of the health acquisition devices in IoT are as given below:

a. Smartwatches:

Wearables sold at shopper gadgets stores accompany a sensor and internet association. Some of them can even screen your pulse, control diabetes, help in discourse treatment, help in further developing stance, and identify seizures.

b. Smart Glucose Monitoring System:

These gadgets can screen blood glucose levels and send the information to a committed cell phone application. Patients with diabetes can utilize these gadgets to follow their glucose levels and even send this information to a medical services office.

c. Brain Sensors / EEG Sensors:

These minuscule sensors are embedded inside the noggin to assist with braining specialists monitor extreme cerebrum wounds and keep away from additional dreadful growing. They measure tension on the mind and can break down without help from anyone else in the body minus any additional clinical impedance. Also, these sensors assist in determining the seizures prior to their occurrence and intimate the same beforehand.(Hallur et al., 2018) There are some sensors called as mood-enhancers which are special head-mounted sensor devices that affect the mental status of the patient by transmitting lesser power and intensity signals to the brain. This control and co-ordination of the sensors can be done via IoT by operating from a remote place.

d. Ingestible Tots:

There are some sensors which are ingested via a patient's entry to extract the images inside of the body. These sensors capture the images of the interior of the organs of the body and transmit the same wirelessly so as to be displayed on a monitor or a smartphone screen. This helps in analysing the medical condition of the patient. Also, endorsed drug is gulped with a minuscule swallowable clinical sensor that conveys a little message to a wearable recipient on the patient, which, thusly, sends information to a committed cell phone application. This sensor can assist specialists with guaranteeing patients take their medicine consistently.

e. Diabetes Monitoring Tools:

There are some of the sensors such as m-IoT which monitors the patient's glucose level by taking the pictures of the finger tip of the patient. This is accompanied by the laser beam to extract the pictorial data from the patient's finger tip's blood stream from inside. Also, optical sensors such as infrared LED and photodiodes in the infrared layer band can help with the detection of patient's diabetic condition. (Pradhan et al., 2021)

f. Temperature Monitoring Tools:

A small 3D printed ear-placeable temperature monitoring electrode is used in case of wirelessly monitoring the patient's temperature. This sensor tracks the body temperature from the tympanic membrane using a sensor making use of Infrared light. The extracted temperature is stored in the database which is then wirelessly transmitted to the destination to a nearby/far station so as to monitor it distantly on a web page and provide feedback.(Pradhan et al., 2021)

g. Hypertension Monitoring Tools:

Cuffs around the patient's arm and pumping till the bulb fills up to the maximum and the reduction in the mercury level indicates the BP of the patient. Bu now-a-days automated pumping to the cuffs around the arm occurs and automated monitoring, storing and transmission of the readings is done.

h. Pulse Oximeter:

The headway in the beat oximetry that comes from the reconciliation of IoT-based innovation has shown expected application in the medical care industry. A noninvasive tissue oximeter estimates the blood oxygen immersion level, alongside pulse, and heartbeat boundaries.

i. Asthma Monitor:

A respiratory monitor which records a respiratory rate of the patient's inhaled and exhaled air and setting a threshold to indicate the criticality of the patient's respiratory status.

3. Applications of Health IoT to monitor certain body parameters

COVID19 has had a highly devastating effect on the majority of the world's population. As indicated that it spreads through air-medium, it becomes very much necessary to safeguard the health of the health-monitoring officials such as doctors, nurses, etc. and also of the adjacent patients and family members of the patients in case of non-availability of beds and home-quarantine. No near accommodation or close monitoring of the patient's health is possible in case of COVID affected patient. So, some of the bodily parameters that can be measured remotely using IoT data transmission and reception are listed below:

a. EEG Monitoring

It becomes very much difficult to monitor the patient's oxygen level during the critical Covid times. The person affected with COVID need to be monitored for his brain activities if he is very critically ill. Extracting the EEG signal from the victim's brain via EEG electrodes of various kinds, aggregating the information and then transmitting it to the remote stations where the doctors can analyze the information by decoding the info and respond appropriately.

b. ECG Monitoring

Electrocardiogram (ECG) addresses the electrical movement of the heart because of the depolarization and repolarization of atria and ventricles. An ECG gives data about the essential rhythms of the heart muscles and goes about as a marker for different cardiovascular irregularities. The utilization of IoT innovation has discovered possible application in the early discovery of heart anomalies through ECG observing. IoT-based ECG checking framework is made out of a remote information obtaining framework and a getting processor that utilized a hunt computerization technique that was utilized to distinguish cardiovascular anomaly continuously. A bio-potential chip is utilized to catch great quality information which can be communicated through Bluetooth or any IoT viable convention. The recorded information can be then sent to the end-clients where the recorded ECG information could be pictured utilizing a versatile application.(Pradhan et al., 2021)

c. Glucose Monitoring

In cases of the COVID affected patients who have been affected by diabetes, glucose-monitoring is a must. Thus, a non-invasive, convenient, comfortable and safe wearable gadget named m-IoT to monitor glucose wirelessly can be used in real-time. (Pradhan et al., 2021)

d. Temperature Monitoring

A primary symptom in COVID affected patient is fever and so monitoring the patient's temperature becomes most critical. Monitoring the adjustment of temperature after some time assists the specialists with making derivations about the patient's ailment. The ordinary method of estimating temperature is utilizing a temperature thermometer that is either appended to the mouth, ear, or rectum which can be awkward to the patients. So, a remote wearable sensor should be utilized to screen the patient's temperature distantly.(Pradhan et al., 2021)

e. Hypertension Monitoring

A compulsory procedure in any patient's diagnostic is Blood Pressure monitoring. In case of COVID patients monitoring becomes highly critical as it indicates the speed of patient's blood circulation to all the parts of the human body especially to the lungs and the three-way blood circulation system of the heart.

f. Oxygen Saturation Monitoring

Monitoring the oxygen level is one of the most critical requirements in case of a COVID patient as the patient mainly suffers from the deficit of oxygen to all the parts of his body since the mainly affected organs in case of COVID are lungs which are the main sources of oxygen exchangers in human body. The oxygen level in the patient's body is measured using the Pulse Oximeter. Pulse oximetry is the noninvasive estimation of oxygen immersion and can be utilized as a fundamental boundary in medical care investigation. The noninvasive strategy takes out the issues identified with the regular methodology and gives ongoing observing.(Pradhan et al., 2021) Integrating the oximeter with IoT monitors, stores and transmits the data via IoT integrated technologies on a long range or via WIFI on a shorter range.

g. Asthma Monitoring

A side effect of COVID is asthma. Asthma is a persistent disease that can influence the respiratory routes and may cause trouble in breathing. In asthma, the respiratory routes recoil because of the expanding of the air section. This follows numerous medical problems, for example, wheezing, hacking, chest agony, and windedness. The inhaler or nebulizer one of the sole lifelines right now. Recent technology advancement has incorporated a respiratory sensor which measures the inhaled and exhaled air by the patient, stores the data and transmits it via a IoT-integrated transmitter.(Pradhan et al., 2021) A wearable asthma sensor, can decide the manifestations of an asthma assault ahead of time, which permits the proprietor to take preventive measures on schedule. A vibration sign and a message cautioning about a danger are sent to the person linked with the patient. Among different highlights, the gadget has an inhaler utilization tracker. Such respiratory disorder monitoring is very helpful in cases on the patients affected with Covid'19. The sensors sense the oxygen level in the blood using oximeter along with the sensing of the breathing pattern of the patient and transmit it over IoT.

h. Mental State Monitoring

Deprivation of the oxygen level of the patients directly affects the blood circulation to the brain of the patient by shutting down the parts of the brain and abnormally functioning of the brain. This can be monitored by measuring the brain signals using the EEG electrodes, storing the values in the database and then explicitly transmitting it to display it on a webpage or on any software.

i. Medication Management

Prescription adherence is a typical issue in the medical care industry. Nonadherence to the medicine timetable may build the antagonistic unexpected issues in patients. Prescription nonadherence is generally found in old individuals as they foster clinical conditions like psychological decay, dementia, etc as the age advances. Henceforth, it is hard for them to stringently follow the medicines of specialists. A keen clinical box was fostered that can help individuals to remember their drug. The case has three plates where every plate contains the medication for three unique occasions (morning, evening, and evening). The framework likewise gauges a portion of the indispensable health parameters (blood glucose level, blood oxygen level, temperature, ECG, etc). Every one of the recorded information are then shipped off the cloud worker. A portable application was utilized to build up correspondence between the two end-clients. The recorded data can be gotten to by specialists and patients utilizing the versatile application. (Pradhan et al., 2021)

4. IoT Mobile/Desktop Applications for Health Monitoring

There are a lot many applications developed by companies that monitor the health data by extracting the body health parameters using various sensors. Some of the health applications are as listed below:

a. Google Fit

It is a wellbeing follow application. It is the lone arrangement of application programming interfaces (API) that consolidate information from various gadgets and applications. Programming interface is a processing edge that characterizes trades of information between various programming. Google fit uses sensors of a client's cell phones to observe our actual wellness conduct for a case running, strolling, cycling, and some more. According to the client's wellness objective, they estimated against a broad perspective on their wellness level. (Selvaraj & Sundaravaradhan, 2020)

b. Noom Walk

Noom Walk is like a pedometer as it checks steps all over the course of the day. It doesn't utilize GPS innovation, so the application utilizes less battery and subsequent to checking ventures for 24 h, Noom Walk utilizes around the equivalent battery life as a GPS-empowered application only for few moments. (Selvaraj & Sundaravaradhan, 2020)

c. MI Fit

MI Fit is another application that monitors the health of an individual based on the steps taken throughout the day. The MI Fit also monitors the patients pulse rate, heart rate, sleep cycles and weight. It consolidates the information obtained and transmits it to the user via Bluetooth or the information can also be shared to other individuals via IoT protocols.

d. Finger Print Thermometer

It is a sensor-based application that takes a client's finger to identify internal heat level and pressing factor. It perceives the finger which we push on the showcase board. These sensors can allow clients to simply put their finger on the screen and perceive the print, instead of on a catch. Irregular organizations of a crossover nanostructure remain on super long silver nanofibers, and fine silver nanowires are utilized to create clear, adaptable terminals of this performing multiple tasks sensor cluster. (Selvaraj & Sundaravaradhan, 2020)

e. On Track Diabetes

This API associates with Dexcom-glucometer to follow the degree of glucose. An individual can likewise give related data dependent on advances, practice levels, suppers, and so on. (Selvaraj & Sundaravaradhan, 2020)

f. Instant Heart Rate

Fundamentally, this application and innovation are very comparative to the innovation which is being utilized in Heart rate checking. For example, some predefined calculations and programming are utilized in this. The principle nature of this application is to gauge pulse right away or in a small amount of a second.(Selvaraj & Sundaravaradhan, 2020)

CHALLENGES

IoT gadgets are significant for wellbeing applications. IoT gadgets gather quantifiable and analyzable medical care information to work with the work medical care applications. Hence, security of IoT medical care applications is significant for medical care frameworks. IoT gadgets are undermined by numerous security weaknesses. Some of them are:

1. Cost

Cost is certainly one of the key difficulties confronted with IoT execution. This innovation driven arrangement isn't yet moderate to the average person! Most individuals living across the globe are stressed over the expanding costs in the medical services area and things are extreme particularly in created nations. IoT in medical services is as yet a promising thought however an exorbitant issue. This can just contribute towards better medical services once the partners associated with it make it financially savvy for the general population. Assuming IoT stays a costly model, just the rich individuals will actually want to manage the cost of its offices later on.

2. Data Overload and Accuracy

Information collection is troublesome because of the utilization of various correspondence conventions and norms. Be that as it may, IoT gadgets actually record a huge load of information. The information gathered by IoT gadgets are used to acquire essential experiences. Nonetheless, the measure of information is gigantic to such an extent that getting bits of knowledge from it are turning out to be very hard for specialists which, eventually influences the nature of dynamic.

3. Massive Inputs of Generated Data

Having a huge number of gadgets in a solitary medical care office and all of them seriously sending data from far off areas — all continuously — will create tremendous measures of information. The information produced from IoT in medical services will probably cause stockpiling necessities to develop a lot higher, from Terabytes to Petabytes. Whenever utilized appropriately, computer-based intelligence driven calculations and cloud can assist with sorting out and coordinate this information, however this methodology needs an ideal opportunity to develop.

4. Existing Software Infrastructure is Obsolete

IT frameworks in numerous clinics are outdated. They won't consider legitimate mix of IoT gadgets. Subsequently, medical care offices should patch up their IT cycles and utilize new, more current programming. They will likewise have to exploit virtualization, and super quick remote and portable organizations like Progressed LTE or 5G.

5. Integration: Multiple Devices and Protocols

Integration of different gadgets likewise causes obstruction in the execution of IoT in the healthcare sector. The justification this obstruction is that gadget makers haven't arrived at an agreement in regards to correspondence conventions and standard. Along these lines, regardless of whether the assortment of gadgets are associated, the distinction in their correspondence convention confuses and blocks the interaction of information conglomeration. This non-consistency of the associated gadget's conventions hinders the entire interaction and diminishes the extent of adaptability of IoT in medical services.

6. Privacy(Buttyan & Hubaux, 2007)

Privacy can be defined as the data needed from few components and properties as below:

a. No Traceability: Making it hard for a foe to recognize that similar subject played out a given arrangement of activities.
b. No observability: Hiding or disguising the fact that an information was passed from a sender to a receiver.

c. No linkability: Not disclosing the relationship information between anything. Ex: objects, patients, etc.
d. Anonymity: Not disclosing the data such as what action was performed by whom. Ex: Who performed the surgery.
e. False – Anonymity: Usage of false identifiers instead of true identifiers.

Medical services information are gathered from IoT gadgets. These gadgets assemble information by far off access systems which make them challenge about protection and security. Information gathered by the sensor is communicated to the information base or cover over web. In expansion, IoT gadgets interface web and speak with one another from the Internet. Security weaknesses on Internet and IoT gadgets are undermined wellbeing information. Moreover, medical services information are gathered from various wellbeing units. Wellbeing information is shared by different wellbeing units. Each unit should give protection of information. Since medical care information incorporates fundamental critical data. Thus, security of information should be ensured.(Thilakanathan et al., 2013)

7. Trust

Information assortment trust is not kidding issue due to enormous volumes of information are gathered from gadgets. Large information is utilized by IoT wellbeing application inferable from make right choice about patients and work on nature of medical care. Also, IoT medical care administrations incorporate information interaction, investigation and mining. Assailants could be harmed large information with make harm or vindictive contribution of IoT gadgets. Subsequently, specialists concentrate about difficulties of trust the executives in IoT. Trust the executives in IoT should carry out network layer and application layer. (Abomhara & Køien, 2014)

8. Data Manipulation

Information is significant IoT medical care applications. Information is utilized all means of medical care frameworks. Hence, assaults are against to information security and protection. Assaults are taking information, information control and harming information. Wellbeing information is significant and touchy information. Information is utilized numerous ways in the IoT. These are IoT gadgets, the web, the cloud, the machine.(Bing et al., 2011) They take information when information is created furthermore, shipped by IoT gadgets. Aggressor's control or on the other hand change information to divert casualties what aggressors need.

9. Reliable Connectivity

Organization disappointments aren't adequate in gadgets that require continuous admittance to information, as numerous clinical gadgets do. Keeping up with availability is particularly difficult in cell phones like wearables, which travel anyplace the patient does, across lines and inclusion zones. Cell availability is frequently the best answer for IoT organizations that cover a huge topographical region. With an open meandering, non-controlled SIM card, IoT gadgets can naturally switch among organizations and stay associated with the most grounded accessible sign. The quantity of organizations that might be gotten to relies upon the SIM supplier's wandering connections and the area of arrangements.

10. Scalable Platforms

For medical services IoT to succeed, it should be upheld by and consistently incorporate into the more prominent medical care framework. Patients, specialists and other approved experts should have the option to utilize the gadgets, screen their status as well as investigate them distantly. This requires a versatile, adaptable and easy to understand IoT stage that can adjust to explicit use cases, ideally with a strong help group to help with arrangement plan and assist with guaranteeing a smooth joining.

11. Incompatible Architecture:

The devices that communicate with each other often need to be on the same platform for the data encoding and decoding or transmission or reception purposes. Incompatible hardware or software may lead erroneous analysis of the medical data of the patient which might result in wrong diagnosis of the patient.(Noura et al., 2019)

12. Limited Resource Availability

The IoT gadgets often work on battery power leading to limited processing power, memory and online power. This limited power resource makes the communication and implementation of the designated protocol more difficult since they are compute intensive.(Noura et al., 2019)

13. Power Consumption and Energy Optimization

The majority of the HIoT gadgets run on battery. When a sensor is put on, the substitution of the battery isn't simple. Consequently, a powerful battery was utilized to power such a framework. Nonetheless, right now, specialists overall are attempting to plan medical services gadgets that can create power for themselves. One such potential arrangement might be the mix of the IoT framework with environmentally friendly power frameworks. These frameworks can help in reducing the worldwide energy emergency somewhat.(Pradhan et al., 2021)

Sensors are critical gadgets for medical services frameworks. Quantifiable and analyzable medical services information are assembled effectively with the improvement of sensor innovation. Lately, wearable gadgets are very mainstream for medical services frameworks. Wearable gadgets could gather numerous medical services information without upsetting patients. Nonetheless, energy burning-through is significant issue for wearable gadgets. Since wearable gadgets are little and they are utilized to gather information structure individuals' body. They gather medical services information from body persistently. Battery isn't sufficient to gather and send wellbeing information to medical services applications. Also, battery of wearable gadgets is important to be continually charge. These are not kidding issues for IoT gadgets in medical services frameworks (Decuir, 2015)

14. Standardization

In the medical services industry, an enormous number of sellers are fabricating a shifting scope of items. The greater part of these items guarantees to keep standard guidelines and conventions in the plan cycle. Notwithstanding, there is an absence of legitimacy. Henceforth, the development of a devoted gathering is required that can normalize these HIoT gadgets dependent on the correspondence conventions, information collection, and entryway interfaces. The approval and normalization of electronic clinical records (EMRs) recorded by the HIoT gadgets are likewise to be thought about widely. This can be accomplished when different associations and normalization bodies like Information Technology and Innovation Foundation (IETF), the European Telecommunications Standards Institute (ETSI), the Internet Protocol for Smart Objects (IPSO), etc can team up with the scientists to frame working gatherings for the normalization of the gadgets. (Pradhan et al., 2021)

15. Identification

Medical care experts manage numerous patients and parental figures simultaneously. Also, when a patient arrangement with different medical problems, he associates with numerous specialists. Consequently, it is critical to trade the character of the patient, parental figure, and specialists among one another during a solitary treatment cycle to stay away from disarray and keep up with the smooth working of the medical care framework.(Pradhan et al., 2021)

16. Self-Configuration

The IoT gadgets should give more capacity to the clients by including the element like manual setup. This will empower the clients to change the framework boundaries as indicated by the application interest and furthermore with the adjustment of the natural conditions.(Pradhan et al., 2021)

17. Continuous Monitoring

Numerous medical care circumstances request long haul checking of the patient during therapy as on account of ongoing illnesses, heart infections, and so forth. In such circumstances, the IoT gadget should have the option to perform ongoing observing effectively.(Pradhan et al., 2021)

18. Exploration of New Diseases

With the quick development in portable innovation, new medical care applications are added with spending days. However, an enormous number of versatile applications are accessible for medical services applications, the sorts of infections for which these applications were planned are as yet restricted. Thus, there is a need to incorporate more sicknesses that were either disregarded or got lacking thought before. This will amount to the variety of the HIoT applications.(Pradhan et al., 2021)

19. Environmental Impact

The improvement of a HIoT framework requires the incorporation of different biomedical sensors with semiconductor-rich gadgets. The assembling and manufacture generally require the utilization of earth metal and other poisonous synthetic compounds. This may establish an unfavourable impact on the climate. Consequently, an appropriate administrative body should be made to control and manage the assembling of the sensors. Further, more examination should be committed to making sensors utilizing biodegradable materials.(Pradhan et al., 2021)

20. Physical assaults

Most of IoT gadgets are little and remotely associated, for example, obliged asset hubs. Hence, secure the put away delicate information in IoT gadgets furthermore, give secure capacity devices with regards to IoT. In addition, since it is normal that a larger number of information would be on the way than in conventional models, there is an expanded danger of acknowledgment of assaults and getting non-approved admittance to information being communicated characterize a foundational approach for IoT security.(Djenna & Saïdouni, 2018) (Hussain et al., 2009)

21. Bodily Injury:

On the off chance that an IoT gadget doesn't work as arranged, innovation organizations could be responsible for coming about wounds, or even the passing, of a client or patient. Organizations who produce IoT innovation ought to comprehend their openness to real injury hazard because of inadequate plan, an assembling imperfection, item abuse or an inability to caution buyers about a potential peril identified with the utilization of the item.

For instance, if a specialist recommends a pill with a swallowable chip to check consistence for a patient with a memory impedance, and a blemish keeps the transmitter from sending consistence information to the doctor, the specialist may not get alarms that the patient isn't taking the drug. In case the patient's condition deteriorates and the patient requirements costly medical procedure, the patient may sue the organization that made the associated pill for inability to send consistence information in an ideal style.

22. Technology Errors and Omissions:

The IoT innovation may neglect to fill in as proposed because of a blunder, exclusion or careless demonstration in the plan of the innovation. In the event that the buyer supports monetary misfortunes, like lost benefits or business interruption, they may record a risk guarantee. Safeguard expenses alone might be disastrous to an innovation business. For instance, if a wellbeing safety net provider offers an impetus to clients utilizing a wellness tracker, and a mistake in the following programming exaggerates the quantity of steps, then, at that point the organization may give a bigger number of limits than it ought to. The insurance agency may credit the monetary misfortune to inaccurate advance considers an aftereffect of outer wellness tracker control.

SOLUTIONS TO RISKS AND THREATS

General Solutions

Every security danger and dangers present issue to the further advancement of IoT medical care. To accelerate the cycle of the IoT, each security hazard, dangers and provokes should be given an answer for defeat with (Hallur et al., 2020). A portion of the answers for difficulties and dangers are recorded beneath:

1. Authentication Issues:

It uses a customer configurable epitome part, for instance, application layer show called the Intelligent Service Security Application Protocol which joins encryption with validation, cross-stage correspondences, and mark to ad lib the correspondence between the applications and things. The Datagram Transport Layer Security (DTLS) utilized with cryptographic calculation RSA guarantees information privacy, trustworthiness, low bundle delay, energy productivity, and low memory load. The Key Management System (KMS) is utilized. Another arrangement proposed for the security issues incorporates a verification convention that utilizes a straightforward encryption calculation dependent on a boolean XOR activity which makes the work simpler of ensuring the information of the patient.

2. False Online Storage Devices

Medical data need to be very carefully stored on to a very true storage cloud online. There are false clouds that imitate of being true and leaking the confidential data. This bogus redirection of information can be forestalled by at first checking the information parcels IP address to objective at the hour of information extraction and sending and afterward looking at it at the hour of putting away on the cloud. This might be finished by separating the information parcels dependent on IP-address and the arranged Port of objective.

3. Interoperability

The interworking with respect to data transfer from one medical institution to another medical institution during the shifting of the patient needs high interoperability among the clouds in order the data is not lost or corrupted. Normal guidelines and calculations for correspondence models, principles for plan and engineering should be characterized to interface the diverse IoT gadgets to the cloud. Additionally, this issue can be settled by infusing them into the middleware of the gadget cloud at runtime.

4. Allotment of Resources

The asset distribution issue can be overwhelmed by conveying an example parcel from each recently added hub to demonstrate the hub needs the assets to measure or concentrate the information.

5. Centralization and Decentralization

In light of the aggressor model applied to both unified and decentralized IoT engineering models, principle challenges are contemplated and proper arrangements might be applied to send security instruments. To defeat the issue of the information handling at just one spot, decentralization of the cloud assets and preparing CPU's might be finished by the client area, information characters, network thickness, and so forth. The decentralized engineering essentially can manage the information which can be prepared and put away autonomously. A brought together design might be an answer for the information that is reliant upon itself. Ex: Multimedia, Medical, Defence information.

FUTURE SCOPE

With the progression of time and the presentation of IoT wellbeing checking instruments, the decision of recuperating at home will turn into a practical choice. With the coordination of constant observing and different modules, patients basically won't should be in a medical clinic bed to be treated. The expansion of wearable innovation assists with making mending at home a chance as well as a likelihood. Wearable gadgets can follow a patient's condition while alarming their doctor on account of any irregularities. This advantageous solution integration will have the highest impact on the patient coordination with the medical field

CONCLUSION

With the advent of IoT integration into medical field to co-ordinate the patient health monitoring remotely, there are some of the drawbacks that needs to be overcomed. Though most of the advantages are in place, there might occur some mishap if any of the IoT components fail to coordinate. These non-coordination and drawbacks can be overcome by improvements or enhancements in the existing IoT infrastructure and architecture which may someday lead to independent health monitoring and peace of mind of the patients.

Case Study: Myocardial Infarction Detection using Sensor Technology during Covid-19 pandemic (Hallur & Bajantri, 2018)

Deaths caused due to myocardial infraction as a side effect of COVID-19 have become a major concern. Most of such deaths are caused due to the non-availability of medical assistance in time of need. This section describes a technology that explores a solution to such problems using wireless communications via IoT which includes an enabled RFID (Radio Frequency Identification) frontier in which the victim's actual location is tracked for providing the necessary medical services. This section also describes the interworking of wireless communications systems and miniature sensors such as RFID passive Tags, whose function is to capture the signals and wirelessly transmit all the data such as person's vital body-function signal data and GPS data to the nearest ground station. Thus, both the sets of data and the medical status and the location of the patient will then be wirelessly transmitted to the ground station from where patient's medical conditions are remotely monitored, thus providing emergency rescue units with the person's exact location. The Algorithm for processing the patient location, health status and rescue is also being discussed.

Sensors Used: ECG Sensors, RFID Sensors, Location Sensors (GPS), EEG Sensors, Pulse Oximetry sensor, etc.

The Myocardial Infarction Alert Unit consists of the following components:

1. RFID Tag implanted into the human body.
2. RFID Reader placed in any tracking object/cellular/mobile phone.
3. ECG Sensors Placed onto the victim's chest to monitor the heartbeat.
4. EEG Sensors placed on to the victim's scalp to monitor the mental status.

5. Pulse Oximeter placed onto the thumb of the patient.
6. Global Positioning Satellite System (GPS) for tracking purpose.
7. Location & Tracking Base Station Unit.
8. Ambulances / Mobile Rescue Units.

Process

Any sensors incorporated onto the body of the victim such as RFID, ECG, EEG, Pulse Oximetry initially captures the signals from victim's body in an analog form, which then needs to be converted to discrete form whose algorithm and pseudocode is as shown in Figure 3.

(An algorithm to briefly depict the steps of the process flow from capturing the victim's health signals to its transmission and processing. A pseudocode of the same is written in C language)

The receiver (such as RFID receiver) in the nearby electronics device such as laptop or a mobile phone continuously need to monitor the received bits from the sensors embedded onto the human body. The monitoring of the pulse oximetry and the respiratory system measurement become extremely important in case of COVID19 infection. The receiver continuously commands the sensors to send the data in the form of the voltages via the gateway. The bits are being monitored with respect to the threshold being

Figure 3. Process algorithm and pseudocode

Algorithm:

Step 1: Acquire the analog signals from the pulses originated from the human heart/brain/thumb.

Step 2: Generate a series of samples from the analog signals acquired with respect to the RFID Tag frequency/sampling frequency

Step 3: Assign integral values to the samples generated.

Step 4: Compare each and every sample value with the average voltage level of the human heart.

Step 5: If the compared value lies within the range of the averaged voltage level value of the heart, assign value as BIT=LOW else assign BIT=HIGH.

Step 6: Generate the bit sequence by comparing each and every individual pulse to the average value.

Pseudocode:

```
int main()
{Int analog_value = 0, a1,b1,c1=0;
a1 = Int adc (int analog_value);
b1 = Int avg (int a1);
c1 = int bit_assign (b1,a1);}

Int avg (int a)
{Intprev_avg, n;
prev_avg = ((prev_avg + a) / n);
n++;
return (prev_avg);}

Int adc (int b)
{int Temp=0;
b = (b&0xFFFFFF00);
b|=(1 << 24);
while((b&0x80000000)==0)
{Temp = b;
Temp = (Temp>>8) & 0x00FF;
Return(Temp);
}}

Int bit_assign (int b1, int a1)
{Int BIT=0;
BOOL LOW=0,HIGH=1;
if (a1 < = b1) : BIT = LOW ? BIT = HIGH;
return (BIT); }
```

Figure 4. Algorithm and pseudocode for pulse value count

Algorithm for Sensing High/Low Pulse Rate:	Pseudocode for Sensing High/Low Pulse Rate:

Step 1: The RFID tag continuously senses the body for determining the Heart Pulses and sends to the receiver upon the command.
Step 2: The bits obtained from the tag are compared every time to check whether a BIT=LOW or a BIT=HIGH has occurred.
Step 3: If consecutive five BIT=LOW is observed in the sequence, the tracking and locating base station is alerted. Else the counter is reset to 0.
	/*Piece of Code for detecting a Weak Pulse */
	ALERT ()
	{ if (bit==LOW)
	{ counter++; }
	else
	{counter=0 ;}
	if(counter==5)
	{ Alert Locating &Tracking System");
	counter=0; } }

set. A counter is set to monitor the number of pulses high and low. High indicates the person is not critical and Low indicates the person is critical. One such scenario that monitors the victim's pulse rate is as shown in the Figure 4 below.

(The counter is responsible for counting the number of bits that are assigned with value 1 and value 0. This depicts the patient's condition whether healthy or not.)

Location and Tracking gets a unique RFID ALERT message by means of an electronics device receiver nearby victim with features like Auto-sending, Auto- Resending and Auto Messaging. These administrations are given by the Cellular Network Service Provider via Data Services. Thus, the Locating and Tracking Station quickly communicates an ALERT message back to the Mobile Rescue Unit and sends a solicitation to Global Positioning System for the specific area of the Radio Frequency Identification Reader implanted inside the Cellular Phone. The Locating &Tracking Station sends an ALERT message along with the location data via IoT protocols to the Mobile Rescue Unit to alarm the Doctors/Rescue group in the Mobile Rescue Unit showing a potential Heart Failure. The Global Positioning System mean-while finds the specific area of the Victim and guides the Mobile Rescue Unit to the objective on schedule and gives quick clinical help to the Victim.

REFERENCES

Abomhara, M., & Køien, G. M. (2014). Security and privacy in the Internet of Things: Current status and open issues. *2014 International Conference on Privacy and Security in Mobile Systems (PRISMS)*, 1-8. 10.1109/PRISMS.2014.6970594

Al-Fuqaha, M., Guizani, M., Mohammadi, M., Aledhari, M., & Ayyash, M. (2015). Internet of Things: A Survey on Enabling Technologies, Protocols, and Applications. *IEEE Communications Surveys and Tutorials*, *17*(4), 2347–2376. doi:10.1109/COMST.2015.2444095

Alaba, F. A., Othman, M., Hashem, I. A. T., & Alotaibi, F. (2017). Internet of things security: A survey. *Journal of Network and Computer Applications*, *88*, 10–28. doi:10.1016/j.jnca.2017.04.002

Ammar, M., Russello, G., & Crispo, B. (2018). Internet of things: A survey on the security of IoT frameworks. *J. Inf. Security Appl.*, *38*, 8–27. doi:10.1016/j.jisa.2017.11.002

Anwar, Ghany, & El Mahdy. (2015). Improving the security of images transmission. *Int. J. Bio-Med. Inform. e-Health, 3*(4), 7-13.

Atzori, L., Iera, A., & Morabito, G. (2010). The Internet of Things: A survey. *Computer Networks, 54*(15), 2787-2805. doi:10.1016/j.comnet.2010.05.010

Bairagi, Khondoker, & Islam. (2016). An efficient steganographic approach for protecting communication in the Internet of Things (IoT) critical infrastructures. *Information Security Journal: A Global Perspective, 25*(4-6), 197-212. doi:10.1080/19393555.2016.1206640

Bing, C., Yuebo, D., Bo, J., Xiang, Z., & Lijuan, Z. (2011). The RFID-based electronic identity security platform of the Internet of Things. *2011 International Conference on Mechatronic Science, Electric Engineering and Computer (MEC)*, 246-249. 10.1109/MEC.2011.6025447

Buttyan, L., & Hubaux, J. P. (2007). *Security and cooperation in wireless networks: Thwarting malicious and selfish behavior in the age of ubiquitous computing*. Cambridge University Press. doi:10.1017/CBO9780511815102

Chen, C., Jyan, H., Chien, S., Jen, H., Hsu, C., Lee, P., Lee, C.-F., Yang, Y.-T., Chen, M.-Y., Chen, L.-S., Chen, H.-H., & Chan, C.-C. (2020, May 5). Containing COVID-19 among 627,386 persons in contact with the Diamond Princess cruise ship passengers who disembarked in Taiwan: Big data analytics. *Journal of Medical Internet Research, 22*(5), e19540. doi:10.2196/19540 PMID:32353827

De Caro, N., Colitti, W., Steenhaut, K., Mangino, G., & Reali, G. (2013). Comparison of two lightweight protocols for smartphone-based sensing. *2013 IEEE 20th Symposium on Communications and Vehicular Technology in the Benelux (SCVT),* 1-6. 10.1109/SCVT.2013.6735994

Decuir, J. (2015). The Story of the Internet of Things: Issues in utility, connectivity, and security. *IEEE Consumer Electronics Magazine*, *4*(4), 54–61. doi:10.1109/MCE.2015.2463292

Djenna, D. & Saïdouni, E. (2018). Cyber Attacks Classification in IoT-Based-Healthcare Infrastructure. *2018 2nd Cyber Security in Networking Conference (CSNet),* 1-4. 10.1109/CSNET.2018.8602974

Elhoseny, Salama, & Riad. (2018). A machine learning model for improving healthcare services on cloud computing environment. Measurement, 119, 117-128. doi:10.1016/j.measurement.2018.01.022

Hallur & Bajantri. (2018). Myocardial Infraction Alert System using RFID Technology. *International Journal of Innovative Science and Research Technology, 3*(6), 45-49.

Hallur, S., Kulkarni, R., & Patavardhan, P. (2020). *Introduction, Security Challenges, and Threats in IoT, Internet of Things: Integration and Security Challenges.* CRC Press. doi:10.1201/9781003032441

Hallur, S. N., Torse, D. A., Aithal, V. K., & Santaji, S. S. (2018). Epilepsy Detection by Processing of EEG signals using LabVIEW Simulation. *2018 International Conference on Electrical, Electronics, Communication, Computer, and Optimization Techniques (ICEECCOT)*, 1101-1106. 10.1109/ICEECCOT43722.2018.9001570

Hiraguri, T., Aoyagi, M., Morino, Y., Akimoto, T., Nishimori, K., & Hiraguri, T. (2015). Proposal of ZigBee systems for the provision of location information and transmission of sensor data in medical welfare. *E-Health Telecommunication Systems and Networks*, *4*(3), 45–55. doi:10.4236/etsn.2015.43005

Hussain, S., Schaffner, S., & Moseychuck, D. (2009). Applications of Wireless Sensor Networks and RFID in a Smart Home Environment. In *Proceedings of the 2009 Seventh Annual Communication Networks and Services Research Conference (CNSR '09)*. IEEE Computer Society. 10.1109/CNSR.2009.32

Irshad, M. (2016). A Systematic Review of Information Security Frameworks in the Internet of Things (IoT). *2016 IEEE 18th International Conference on High Performance Computing and Communications*, 1270-1275. 10.1109/HPCC-SmartCity-DSS.2016.0180

Jaswal, K., Choudhury, T., Chhokar, R. L., & Singh, S. R. (2017). Securing the Internet of Things: A proposed framework. *2017 International Conference on Computing, Communication and Automation (ICCCA)*, 1277-1281. 10.1109/CCAA.2017.8230015

Jia, X., Feng, Q., Fan, T., & Lei, Q. (2012). RFID technology and its applications in Internet of Things (IoT). *2012 2nd International Conference on Consumer Electronics, Communications and Networks (CECNet)*, 1282-1285. 10.1109/CECNet.2012.6201508

Khalil, M. I. (2017). Medical image steganography: Study of medical image quality degradation when embedding data in the frequency domain. *Int. J. Comput. Netw. Inf. Secur.*, *9*(2), 22–28. doi:10.5815/ijcnis.2017.02.03

Khan, M. A., & Salah, K. (2018). IoT security: Review, blockchain solutions, and open challenges. *Future Generation Computer Systems*, *82*, 395–411. doi:10.1016/j.future.2017.11.022

Materia, F. T., Faasse, K., & Smyth, J. M. (2020, May 25). Understanding and preventing health concerns about emerging mobile health technologies. *JMIR mHealth and uHealth*, *8*(5), e14375. doi:10.2196/14375 PMID:32449688

Nguyen, K. T., Laurent, M., & Oualha, N. (2015). Survey on secure communication protocols for the internet of things. *Ad Hoc Networks*, *32*, 17–31. doi:10.1016/j.adhoc.2015.01.006

Noura, M., Atiquzzaman, M., & Gaedke, M. (2019). Interoperability in Internet of Things: Taxonomies and Open Challenges. *Mobile Networks and Applications*, *24*(3), 796–809. doi:10.100711036-018-1089-9

OData. (2015). *Libraries*. Retrieved January 14, 2016, from OData - the Best Way to REST: https://www.odata.org/libraries/

OData - the Best Way to REST. (n.d.). Retrieved January 14, 2016, from OData - the Best Way to REST: https://www.odata.org/

Pradhan, Bhattacharyya, & Pal. (2021). IoT-Based Applications in Healthcare Devices. *Journal of Healthcare Engineering*. doi:10.1155/2021/6632599

Samaniego, M., & Deters, R. (2016). Management and Internet of Things. *The 13th International Conference on Mobile Systems and Pervasive Computing (MobiSPC 2016)*, *94*, 137 – 143. 10.1016/j.procs.2016.08.022

Santucci, G. (2009, January). Internet of things–when your fridge orders your groceries. In *International Conference on Future Trends of the Internet* (*Vol. 28*). Academic Press.

Selvaraj, S., & Sundaravaradhan, S. (2020). Challenges and opportunities in IoT healthcare systems: A systematic review. *SN Appl. Sci.*, *2*(1), 139. doi:10.100742452-019-1925-y

Sfar, R., Natalizio, E., Challal, Y., & Chtourou, Z. (2018). A roadmap for security challenges in the internet of things. *Digital Commun. Netw.*, *4*(2), 118–137. doi:10.1016/j.dcan.2017.04.003

Shehab. (2018). Secure and Robust Fragile Watermarking Scheme for Medical Images. *IEEE Access, 6*, 10269-10278. . doi:10.1109/ACCESS.2018.2799240

Sreekutty, M. S., & Baiju, P. S. (2017). Security enhancement in image steganography for medical integrity verification system. *2017 International Conference on Circuit, Power and Computing Technologies (ICCPCT)*, 1-5. 10.1109/ICCPCT.2017.8074197

Thilakanathan, D., Calvo, R., Chen, S., & Nepal, S. (2013). Secure and Controlled Sharing of Data in Distributed Computing. *2013 IEEE 16th International Conference on Computational Science and Engineering*, 825-832. 10.1109/CSE.2013.125

Verma, N., Singh, S., & Prasad, D. (2021). A Review on existing IoT Architecture and Communication Protocols used in Healthcare Monitoring System. *J. Inst. Eng. India Ser. B*. doi:10.1007/s40031-021-00632-3

Vineetha, Misra, & Kishore. (2020). A real time IoT based patient health monitoring system using machine learning algorithms. *European Journal of Molecular & Clinical Medicine, 7*(4), 2912-2925.

Wang, Y., Hu, M., Li, Q., Zhang, X., Zhai, G., & Yao, N. (2020). *Abnormal respiratory patterns classifier may contribute to large-scale screening of people infected with COVID-19 in an accurate and unobtrusive manner.* ArXiv, abs/2002.05534.

Were, M. C., Sinha, C., & Catalani, C. (2019, August 1). A systematic approach to equity assessment for digital health interventions: Case example of mobile personal health records. *Journal of the American Medical Informatics Association*, *26*(8-9), 884–890. doi:10.1093/jamia/ocz071 PMID:31188438

Yehia, L., Khedr, A., & Darwish, A. (2015). Hybrid security techniques for Internet of Things healthcare applications. *Adv. Internet Things, 5*, 21-25. https:// doi:10.4236/ait.2015.53004

Zhao, K., & Ge, L. (2013). A Survey on the Internet of Things Security. *2013 Ninth International Conference on Computational Intelligence and Security*, 663-667. 10.1109/CIS.2013.145

KEY TERMS AND DEFINITIONS

Application (API): A graphical user interface or a software that helps user to interact with it for some purpose or outcome. Usually, a mobile or computer application.

COVID-19: COVID-19 is a disease caused by a new strain of coronavirus. 'CO' stands for corona, 'VI' for virus, and 'D' for disease.

Monitoring: A continuous review of a review of a process from time to time.

Omissions: A skip of a step in the process of achieving an outcome.
Regulation: Moderating any parameter or bringing it to a predefined level.
Resource: A source/input for some task, which provides an outcome.
Threats: A blockage or a disruptive process to some productive task that may lead to hampering of the expected outcome.

Chapter 8
Edge Analytics With Machine Learning Technique for Medical IoT Applications

Jeya Mala D.
https://orcid.org/0000-0002-2100-8218
Jain University, Bangalore, India

Pradeep Reynold A.
GEMS Polytechnic College, India

ABSTRACT

Edge analytics are tools and algorithms that are deployed in the internal storage of IoT devices or IoT gateways that collect, process, and analyze the data locally rather than transmitting it to the cloud for analysis. Edge analytics is applied in a wide range of applications in which immediate decision making is required. In the case of general IoT data analytics on the cloud, the data need to be collected from the IoT devices and to be sent to the cloud for further processing and decision making. In life-critical applications such as healthcare, the time taken to send the data to the cloud and then getting back the processed data to take decisions will not be acceptable. Hence, in these kinds of MIoT applications, it is essential to have analytics to be done on the edge in order to avoid such delays. Hence, this chapter is providing an abstract view on the application of machine learning in MIoT so that the data analytics provides fruitful results to the stakeholders.

INTRODUCTION

The Internet of Things (IoT) is a collection of interrelated devices which maybe machines, electrical appliances, electronic gadgets, computer systems, smartphones, and objects with sensors, animals with RFID cards, and even people with wearable devices which are equipped with the ability to send and/or receive data over a network in an automated way. An IoT platform can connect everyday things that are embedded with electronics, software, and sensors to the internet enabling them to collect and exchange

DOI: 10.4018/978-1-7998-9132-1.ch008

Copyright © 2022, IGI Global. Copying or distributing in print or electronic forms without written permission of IGI Global is prohibited.

data. The term 'thing' in IoT refers to any device that can automatically collect and transmit data over a network or internet using any kind of sensors (Whitepaper, 2018 by Dataflair Team).

Edge analytics is an approach used for the collection and processing of data at the devices such as sensors, network switches, or other devices instead of waiting for the data to be sent back to a centralized data store (Whitepaper, 2018 by Microfocus). This processing part will be accomplished through automated analytical computation as it's generated by these devices. This can decrease latency in the decision-making process on connected devices. By placing the analytics algorithms to sensors and network devices alleviates the processing strain on enterprise data management and analytics systems. This helps even as the number of connected devices being deployed by organizations is increasing and the amount of data being generated and collected also increases.

Hence, to address this most important and crucial problem of collecting the voluminous amount of medical data, preprocess them and decision making based on them is the need of the hour, The application of Machine Learning techniques could be the right choice for providing an efficient solution to this stated problem. In this chapter, the application of a Machine Learning technique in IoT based edge analytics is going to be discussed by simulating the Medical IoT environment using IBM Watson Studio and showing the result.

INTRODUCTION TO INTERNET OF THINGS (IOT)

The term 'Internet of Things" was first used by Kevin Ashton who is a co-founder of the Auto-ID center at MIT in the year 1999 in a presentation he made to Proctor & Gamble to get the need for RFID in tracking and monitoring. Also, in the same year Neil Gershenfeld, MIT professor has mentioned the interconnection of the devices in his book "When Things Start To Think".

From these views, the IoT has evolved using the convergence of various technologies such as Wireless, MEMS, Micro Services, and the Internet. This has enabled the unstructured machine-generated data in the form of Operational Technology to be converged with software development in the form of Information Technology for further processing of these data to get the insights of such operations and further decision making.

Even though the term IoT has come during 1999, the concept of connected devices over the embedded internet has been used during the 1970s.

Then the communication between Machine to Machine (M2M) has made the machines being connected using a network with data being stored in the cloud to collect and manage the data without user interaction This M2M currently offers the interconnection of smart devices that connects applications and people also to establish a smart communication gateway.

This chapter is further divided into the following sections: IoT Architecture; Edge Analytics; Why Edge Analytics is important?; IoT testing; Machine Learning Approaches; Application of ML in MIoT with a case study application implemented in IBM Watson Studio and finally the conclusion.

IOT ANALYTICS

Before going to the detailed discussion on IoT Analytics, let us first know about the entire process involved in it. The data collected by the sensors from the things that are smartphones, production machinery, electronic appliances will be securely communicated using the Internet of Things platform. As per the whitepaper given by Dataflair (2018), this IoT platform is acting as the backbone in IoT Analytics, as it collects and combines data from multiple devices and other platforms connected through the internet. This platform then applies analytics to take decision making and further processing and transfer of data.

IoT Analytics offers a futuristic dimension to the smart application areas such as medical and health-care applications in which the devices are connected through the IoT platform.

Data collection from IoT devices is really a big challenge as the devices are independent in nature and hence collection, aggregation, classification, and making decisions are extremely difficult. Hence, nowadays the IoT platforms provide a way to send the sensor collected data to the cloud or the clusters or a centralized data store or a data warehouse for data analytics.

As the amount of data collected from these sensors will be voluminous in nature, and this collection termed as big data, collecting and storing them into the cloud for further processing is the current area of development in IoT Analytics.

This is applicable in any of the IoT architectures, in which as soon as the sensors collect and store data, these data should be processed to provide some useful outcomes to do a decision making process. Hence, the data collected and stored in the cloud or any local storage devices will then be taken for analysis to take further actions over it.

But when the IoT platform is expanded to include more sensors then collecting data and sending data to the cloud or any other storage medium for further processing will be a cumbersome task as many of the times all the data collected from the sensors need not be valuable and need not contribute any of the decision making processes. In these kinds of situations simply storing all the collected data without validating them will not be an advisable one and also some important actions or decisions need to be taken immediately after the sensor collects the data instead of waiting for storing and retrieving data from the storage media.

If we try to compress the data to minimize the storage issue, the computation overhead involved in compressing the data will be another issue or problem. Even if we have added more IoT gateways to handle this voluminous amount of data by the way of the distribution of process overhead into these gateways, once again we will face the problem of assembling the data for further processing, issue of scaling, etc. will happen. Hence, we need an alternate solution to take resolve all the stated problems. From the literature study, it has been observed that Edge Analytics is an alternate way to handle these kinds of problems.

EDGE ANALYTICS

In the referential architecture discussed earlier, the IoT devices at the bottom have one or more sensors, switches, actuators, or a combination of all these. When these devices are constantly generating streams of data, the amount of data will be significantly high and hence, a need to store these data to a highly scalable storage system is highly necessary to access this data later to take decision making by applying analytics to them.

In real-time systems, the processing of data and decision making should be done at the device itself and not sending and retrieving back the data to and from the cloud. In these situations, real time analytics namely Edge Analytics is required (Dan Liu et.al. 2019).

Edge analytics is an approach to data collection and analysis in which an automated analytical computation is performed on data at a sensor, network switch, or other devices instead of waiting for the data to be sent back to a centralized data store (Truong, Hong-Linh, 2018).

Nowadays due to Industry 4.0 based industrial evolution, Edge analytics is applied in industries that have limited resources in terms of bandwidth, Wi-Fi, etc. But this chapter shows how it can also be applied for applications in which immediate decision making is essential once the data collection is done.

Some of the survey results given in an industrial whitepaper given by Microfocus (2018) have also indicated that data from the sensors and other forms of data collection are becoming more and more ubiquitous across all walks of life; For example, a single Airbus A350 generates 2.5 TB of data per day. Cisco estimates that 507.5 Zettabytes of data will be generated in 2019 alone, A typical solution will be having interim processing is increasingly relevant for handling this staggering volume of data, and edge analytics offer a cost-effective, relatively efficient solution. About Forty percent of IoT data in 2019 is expected to be processed through edge analytics, and this number will surely grow with IoT.

Edge analytics is performed by either tools or algorithms that sit on or close to IoT devices to collect process and analyze data at the source rather than sending that data back to the cloud for analysis. This streamlines the data analysis process by performing it in real-time and to ensure as much useful information is garnered from the device as possible (Xiaomin Xu et.al. 2017).

A typical real-time example is a Traffic Management system. A light sensor at a traffic light can be built with intelligent monitoring for traffic management. Real-time feedback within the device itself ensures immediate and appropriate use of the data it is gathering, circumventing the need to send the data elsewhere for outside consideration.

There are several advantages we can get due to this Edge Analytics (Vivian Zhang, 2017). By pushing analytics algorithms to sensors and network devices alleviates the processing strain on enterprise data management and analytics systems, even as the number of connected devices being deployed by organizations and the amount of data being generated and collected increases.

There are several edge analytics tools developed by many different organizations. A typical example is the IBM Edge IoT Analytics application which pushes the processing application modules to the IoT gateways which are now called Edge Gateways will only store the results of the analysis. The analysis part is done at the IoT device itself thus avoids sending all the information to the cloud or any other storage medium. If any further computationally high overhead processes need to be done, the essential processed data sent to the cloud is then taken for analysis using Bluemix service. This helps in visualizing the results and any other outcomes to the end-users (Andrea Reale, 2017).

In many organizations, streaming data from manufacturing machines, industrial equipment, pipelines and other remote devices connected to the IoT creates a massive glut of operational data, which can be difficult -- and expensive -- to manage.

By running the data through an analytics algorithm as it's created, at the edge of a corporate network, companies can set parameters on what information is worth sending to a cloud or on-premises data store for later use.

MACHINE LEARNING IN EDGE ANALYTICS FOR IOT TESTING

Nowadays, several industries and businesses are applying Machine Learning (ML) techniques for data analytics and intelligent decision making to increase their productivity and efficiency. Based on an industrial whitepaper (2018) given by Thinkxtream, IoT Edge Analytics & Machine Learning for Real-time Device Control", the ML is a powerful analytical tool for the voluminous amount of data which is normally termed as big data.

In an IoT based application development, a similar scenario exists. As the data from the sensors of IoT devices are voluminous as they are collected every millisecond or second or minute as per the requirement, there is a need to process this collected data using ML to make intelligent decisions for further processing. From the IoT architecture, the data collected from the sensors are stored in the cloud through the IoT gateways. This stored data is then processed and analyzed for further visualization, reporting, or decision making.

However, as the data collected by the sensors is from the real time environment, dynamic processing at the edge of the IoT device i.e. at the gateway to take intelligent decisions immediately at that point itself will definitely increase the efficiency of the decision-making process.

Also, the turnaround time of storing in the cloud and then take the data for processing and then applying some ML algorithms to derive some decisions out of them will really be an overhead. And that too, when it is coming on the End-user application testing, storing this real-time data into the cloud and then selecting the relevant data to act as test cases to validate the various use case scenarios will become a cumbersome process as the amount of data will be voluminous (White paper, 2018 on IoT Edge Analytics & Machine Learning for Real-time Device Control).

Hence, this chapter proposes a novel framework to apply ML algorithms at the edge of the IoT device to do End-user application testing to validate the use case scenarios based on the behavioral analysis at the edge itself.

As the ML algorithms placed at the edge can filter most of the noisy data collected by the sensors and take only the relevant data to be analyzed by the edge and by the cloud will be stored for decision making. As these algorithms have intelligence, they can easily be applied to test the use case scenario at that point of time.

This can be achieved in two ways: (I) Keep the limited ML algorithms at the edge as the IoT devices have only limited processing capabilities and evaluate the test results (ii) Keep local IoT networks and have the analytics and decision making algorithms using ML on this edge networks to achieve higher-level decision making to evaluate the test results.

PROPOSED IOT OPERATIONS FRAMEWORK USING MACHINE LEARNING ON THE EDGE

The proposed framework for IoT operations using ML algorithms on the edge of the IoT devices is shown in Figure. 1.

CASE STUDY – A REAL TIME HEALTHCARE APPLICATION IMPLEMENTATION OF EDGE ANALYTICS IN IBM WATSON STUDIO

This case study is to monitor a patient's pulse, temperature and temperature to find whether the person's health is good or critical. This application is an IoT based application which is developed using IBM Watson IOT platform.

Figure 1. Proposed framework using machine learning on the edge

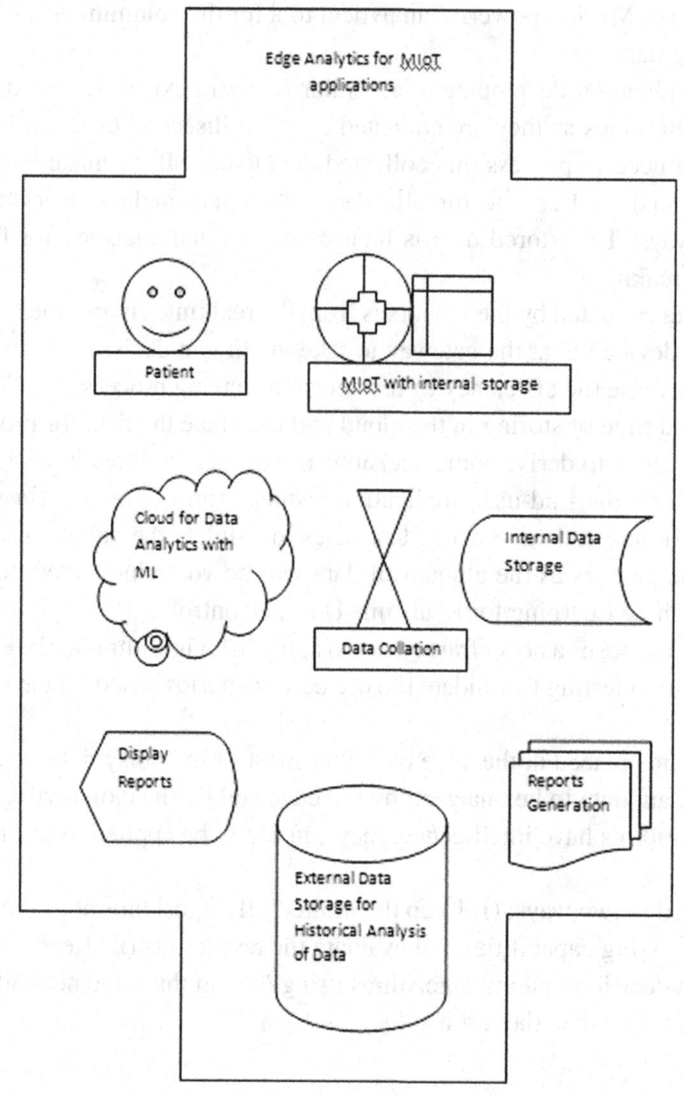

The test data are generated using the IoT platform and the sample is showed in Figure 2:
The sample test data generated are shown below:


```
{"pulse":132,"temperature":62,"heartrate":88}
{"pulse":102,"temperature":130,"heartrate":18}
{"pulse":43,"temperature":128,"heartrate":50}
{"pulse":79,"temperature":66,"heartrate":107}
{"pulse":118,"temperature":65,"heartrate":72}
{"pulse":89,"temperature":59,"heartrate":27}
{"pulse":32,"temperature":121,"heartrate":186}
{"pulse":6,"temperature":96,"heartrate":153}
```

Figure 2. Patient's medical data generated using IBM Watson IoT platform

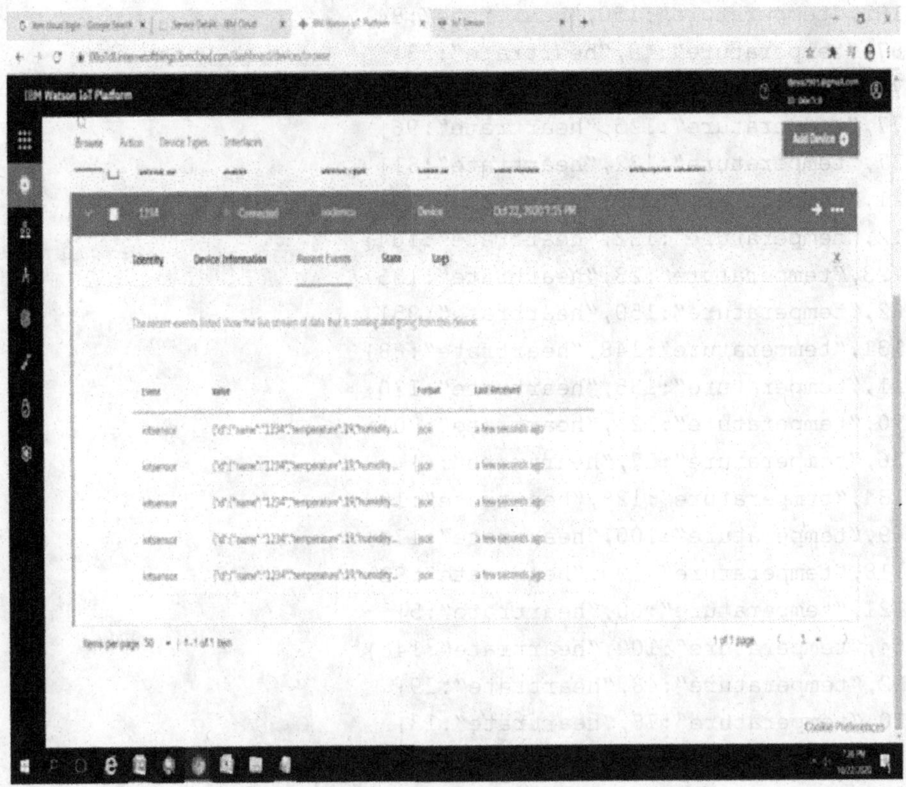

{"pulse":101,"temperature":113,"heartrate":190}
{"pulse":47,"temperature":66,"heartrate":48}
{"pulse":39,"temperature":99,"heartrate":84}
{"pulse":56,"temperature":84,"heartrate":67}
{"pulse":105,"temperature":33,"heartrate":111}
{"pulse":119,"temperature":62,"heartrate":126}
{"pulse":38,"temperature":69,"heartrate":188}
{"pulse":10,"temperature":125,"heartrate":25}
{"pulse":107,"temperature":101,"heartrate":26}
{"pulse":120,"temperature":122,"heartrate":49}
{"pulse":11,"temperature":134,"heartrate":6}
{"pulse":27,"temperature":116,"heartrate":199}
{"pulse":56,"temperature":122,"heartrate":156}
{"pulse":45,"temperature":23,"heartrate":38}
{"pulse":139,"temperature":89,"heartrate":181}
{"pulse":50,"temperature":89,"heartrate":4}
{"pulse":105,"temperature":49,"heartrate":36}
{"pulse":68,"temperature":113,"heartrate":185}
{"pulse":106,"temperature":85,"heartrate":91}

```
{"pulse":119,"temperature":133,"heartrate":154}
{"pulse":103,"temperature":150,"heartrate":84}
{"pulse":87,"temperature":49,"heartrate":33}
{"pulse":71,"temperature":58,"heartrate":70}
{"pulse":77,"temperature":125,"heartrate":96}
{"pulse":37,"temperature":132,"heartrate":81}
{"pulse":21,"temperature":138,"heartrate":20}
{"pulse":12,"temperature":122,"heartrate":104}
{"pulse":123,"temperature":23,"heartrate":155}
{"pulse":62,"temperature":150,"heartrate":95}
{"pulse":131,"temperature":148,"heartrate":88}
{"pulse":11,"temperature":135,"heartrate":120}
{"pulse":70,"temperature":126,"heartrate":70}
{"pulse":36,"temperature":57,"heartrate":4}
{"pulse":134,"temperature":128,"heartrate":184}
{"pulse":69,"temperature":100,"heartrate":179}
{"pulse":118,"temperature":100,"heartrate":92}
{"pulse":121,"temperature":60,"heartrate":5}
{"pulse":64,"temperature":100,"heartrate":148}
{"pulse":32,"temperature":48,"heartrate":29}
{"pulse":10,"temperature":78,"heartrate":13}
{"pulse":140,"temperature":108,"heartrate":92}
{"pulse":95,"temperature":111,"heartrate":80}
{"pulse":93,"temperature":46,"heartrate":187}
{"pulse":107,"temperature":84,"heartrate":100}
{"pulse":18,"temperature":56,"heartrate":117}
{"pulse":0,"temperature":23,"heartrate":40}
{"pulse":49,"temperature":135,"heartrate":100}
{"pulse":8,"temperature":119,"heartrate":140}
{"pulse":23,"temperature":72,"heartrate":147}
{"pulse":118,"temperature":133,"heartrate":63}
{"pulse":129,"temperature":35,"heartrate":181}
{"pulse":12,"temperature":136,"heartrate":113}
{"pulse":68,"temperature":25,"heartrate":198}
{"pulse":38,"temperature":87,"heartrate":58}
{"pulse":103,"temperature":128,"heartrate":199}
{"pulse":71,"temperature":142,"heartrate":28}
{"pulse":28,"temperature":72,"heartrate":21}
{"pulse":113,"temperature":44,"heartrate":18}
{"pulse":87,"temperature":100,"heartrate":28}
{"pulse":35,"temperature":35,"heartrate":143}
{"pulse":115,"temperature":53,"heartrate":35}
{"pulse":85,"temperature":84,"heartrate":187}
{"pulse":134,"temperature":36,"heartrate":94}
```

{"pulse":101,"temperature":61,"heartrate":117}
{"pulse":102,"temperature":146,"heartrate":134}
{"pulse":72,"temperature":50,"heartrate":162}
{"pulse":74,"temperature":33,"heartrate":197}
{"pulse":104,"temperature":115,"heartrate":64}
{"pulse":57,"temperature":123,"heartrate":34}
{"pulse":137,"temperature":54,"heartrate":89}
{"pulse":89,"temperature":38,"heartrate":28}
{"pulse":92,"temperature":40,"heartrate":60}
{"pulse":127,"temperature":71,"heartrate":54}
{"pulse":148,"temperature":92,"heartrate":186}
{"pulse":61,"temperature":141,"heartrate":116}
{"pulse":97,"temperature":135,"heartrate":14}
{"pulse":119,"temperature":75,"heartrate":77}
{"pulse":10,"temperature":32,"heartrate":86}
{"pulse":70,"temperature":87,"heartrate":154}
{"pulse":72,"temperature":148,"heartrate":57}
{"pulse":18,"temperature":114,"heartrate":183}
{"pulse":78,"temperature":24,"heartrate":162}
{"pulse":49,"temperature":133,"heartrate":25}
{"pulse":3,"temperature":21,"heartrate":88}
{"pulse":1,"temperature":145,"heartrate":51}
{"pulse":135,"temperature":62,"heartrate":87}
{"pulse":75,"temperature":111,"heartrate":22}
{"pulse":57,"temperature":68,"heartrate":180}

As the data generated is voluminous, the ML algorithm is proposed which will filter the data based on the similarity based measure.

Data Analytics using the ML based approach is given below:

id"42812c30f7a6a79ee6d9cf6ba090aca0"
{
 "id": "42812c30f7a6a79ee6d9cf6ba090aca0",
 "key": "42812c30f7a6a79ee6d9cf6ba090aca0",
 "value": {
  "rev": "1-3b6566160612e27aa22fb61e51654be3"
 },
 "doc": {
  "_id": "42812c30f7a6a79ee6d9cf6ba090aca0",
  "_rev": "1-3b6566160612e27aa22fb61e51654be3",
 "pulse": 124,
 "temperature": 32,
 "heartrate": 98
 }

```
id"42812c30f7a6a79ee6d9cf6ba0909d92"
{
 "id": "42812c30f7a6a79ee6d9cf6ba0909d92",
 "key": "42812c30f7a6a79ee6d9cf6ba0909d92",
 "value": {
  "rev": "1-8b7f2a52c10107df77f03ad43857082b"
 },
 "doc": {
  "_id": "42812c30f7a6a79ee6d9cf6ba0909d92",
  "_rev": "1-8b7f2a52c10107df77f03ad43857082b",
  "pulse": 123,
  "temperature": 72,
  "heartrate": 61
 }
}
```


EXPECTED ADVANTAGES AND CHALLENGES IN APPLYING ML IN EDGE ANALYTICS

Even though there are several advantages in placing the ML algorithms in the processing element at the edge of the IoT device, it has its own downsides. The cost incurred in deploying such algorithms on the edge will be viewed as huge. If the processing part is high in ML algorithms to make intelligent decisions, it may be impossible to deploy the software on the edge as it has only limited capability. The deployment, operating, and maintaining such computationally intensive algorithms has its own risks. There may be the problems of security breaches occurring while sending the processed data to and from the edge to the local or cloud storage for further processing.

Taking into consideration all these flip sides, the researchers are currently working on providing a more efficient and effective solution for End-user application testing on the Edge using ML algorithms.

Any ML algorithm can be applied to achieve this End-user application testing and in this work, an SVM classifier has been used to classify the sensor data into different groups and then filtered the sensor data as test cases relevant to test the particular scenario. Through an intelligent decision-making process, only the relevant test cases are identified and used to test the application. This reduces the time is taken and the number of test cases needed to test the application. Due to the reduction of test cases, the processing at the edge with limited capability has also been achieved.

CONCLUSION

The Internet of Things (IoT) is a connected set of various devices with processing capabilities to acquire, analyze, and leverage data collected from these devices. All the devices used in the IoT application are termed as assets and they could be industrial machines, generators, robots, building components, temperature monitoring systems, etc. In these kinds of applications, the data collected by the sensors will be the raw or unprocessed data and so, they should be processed to get some solutions out of them. Hence, a cloud or a local storage based repositories have been proposed by several researchers and nowadays several of the industries are going ahead with such cloud-based data processing and decision making to achieve IoT based industrial automation.

When such voluminous amounts of data collected from the sensors are simply stored in the cloud and then later to take any decisions taking them back using some processing components will be the right technique only for those applications that need later processing or only for data visualization or reporting. But in the case of critical applications in which the devices need to take immediate decision making based on the data collected from the sensors, the data needs to be processed at the edge. In these kinds of situations, Edge Computing comes into the picture.

In Edge Computing, the necessary processing elements are placed on the device itself as it has some limited internal storage and processing capacity. Even by placing some external storage medium as part of the entire system could also help in achieving this edge computing.

When some decisions to be taken from the past data along with the current data, the system needs intelligent data processing which is called data analytics and so, when it is done at the edge it is termed as edge analytics. This has also emerged as a very important area of research and several software industries have come up with interesting solutions to achieve it.

Hence, in this chapter, a novel framework to achieve ML based edge analytics is proposed. The case study taken is a real-time one and has been analyzed for the quick decision making process.

REFERENCES

Data Flair. (2019a). *IoT Tutorial for Beginners | What is Internet of Things?* Dataflair Team. https://data-flair.training/blogs/iot-tutorial

Data Flair. (2019b). *IoT Analytics – 3 Major Uses Cases of Internet of Things Analytics*. https://data-flair.training/blogs/iot-analytics

Data Flair. (2019c). *IoT Analytics at the Edge Vertica Brings Analytics to Where the "Things" are*. https://www.microfocus.com/media/white-paper/iot_analytics_at_the_edge_wp.pdf

Fremantle, P. (2016). *White paper, A Reference Architecture for the Internet of Things*. https://wso2.com/whitepapers/a-reference-architecture-for-the-internet-of- things/

Liu, D., Yan, Z., & Wenxiu, D. M. A. (2019). *A Survey on Secure Data Analytics in Edge Computing*. *IEEE Internet of Things Journal*. doi:10.1109/JIOT.2019.2897619

Reale, A. (2017). *A guide to Edge IoT analytics*. White paper. https://www.ibm.com/blogs/internet-of-things/edge-iot-analytics/

Thinxtream's White Paper. (2018). *IoT Edge Analytics & Machine Learning for Real-time Device Control*. https://www.thinxtream.com/whitepapers/thinxtream-iot-edge-analytics-machine-learning-real-time-device-control-wp-003.pdf

Truong, H-L. (2018). *Enabling Edge Analytics of IoT Data: The Case of LoRaWAN*. doi:10.1109/GIOTS.2018.8534429

Xu, X., Huang, S., Feagan, L., Chen, Y., Qiu, Y., & Wa, Y. (2017). EAaaS: Edge Analytics as a Service. *IEEE International Conference on Web Services (ICWS)*. 10.1109/ICWS.2017.130

Zhang, V. (2017). *The pros and cons of IoT edge analytics, White paper*. https://internetofthingsagenda.techtarget.com/blog/IoT-Agenda/The-pros-and-cons-of-IoT-edge-analytics

Chapter 9
AI-Based IoT Analytics on the Cloud for Diabetic Data Management System

S. V. K. R. Rajeswari
SRM Institute of Science and Technology, India

Vijayakumar Ponnusamy
SRM Institute of Science and Technology, India

ABSTRACT

It is very evident by looking at the current technological advancements that the interrelation and association of artificial intelligence (AI) and IoT in the Cloud have transformed the way healthcare has been working. AI and Cloud-empowered IoT boosts operational efficiency enhanced risk management. This combination creates products and services by enhancing the existing products while increasing scalability. To reduce costs, data analytics on the Cloud is much preferred in the current formation of technologies. This chapter focuses on the integration of different AI techniques in Cloud datasets for IoT data analytics. Analyzing, predicting, and making decisions by comparing the current data with historical data. The theory of AI-based IoT analytics will be much investigated with a healthcare application. Different approaches to implementing data analytics on the Cloud for a diabetic management system will be explored (human body). Finally, future trends and possible areas of research are also discussed.

INTRODUCTION

The future of the world is in Artificial Intelligence(AI). Its merge with the Internet of Things(IoT) and Cloud is an added advantage. Due to the monumental advancement in technology,they have found their application in health care, eCommerce, tourism, education, customer care etc. The data analytics performed are stored in the cloud. This helps in managing large amounts of data for storing and accessing it. Integrating AI, IoT, Cloud computing will assist in the development of smarter applications, networks

DOI: 10.4018/978-1-7998-9132-1.ch009

Copyright © 2022, IGI Global. Copying or distributing in print or electronic forms without written permission of IGI Global is prohibited.

and data systems.The primacy of this amalgamation is that greater productivity with the highest quality, safety, reliability and manufacturing units can beachieved(Goel et al., 2020).

With the advancement in the emergence of AI in IoT and the Cloud from the last decade, the technology has improved operational efficiency, increasing profitability, asset reliability and availability, decision support, process safety, and abnormal situation management(Goel et al., 2020).The independent technologies that contribute towards the future of data analytics in the cloud with AI and IoT will be further discussed in the succeeding sections.

The strength of the chapter lies in

- Discussing the trending technologies, i.e., AI, IoT and Cloud.
- Tri-union of technologies.
- Integration of data analytics with the cloud.
- Analysis of data analytics with real-time diabetic management dataset.

Artificial Intelligence

Artificial Intelligence is a well-investigated expression for today's smart generation of electronics and communication.The varied applications of AI range from fraud detection,predictive marketing,machine monitoring and inventory management(Linthicum,2017). Before the emergence of the cloud, there were many open source and proprietary computing techniques in AI. Cost-effectiveness and in-house talent to use the technology were the drawbacks when AI first hit the market in 1985(Linthicum,2017). To handle the heavy load in web servers, the Quality of Services (QoS) was achieved using client end-to-end(Jianbin&Cheng 2006).There was no emergence of the cloud.To communicate between client and server model with synchronous and asynchronous messages, a multilayer queuing network was proposed(Ramesh&Perros2000).How did the emergence of the cloud change the way AI was working?

The answer to the question raised above can be justified with the following advantages.

1. Compared with traditional computing methods such as local computing or client-server model,cloud computing has the advantage of being economical.This is the power of cloud computing(Linthicum,2017).
2. Data storage has become economical in cloud computing(Linthicum,2017).
3. APIs and SDKs are provided by cloud computing that would allow embedding AI indirect functionality applications.
4. Seamless data processing in AI on the cloud has advancement in data updating, management and consumption.

It is very evident by following the advantages that AI has much potential for smarter applications. Figure 1 represents the integration of AI and the cloud. Smart gadgets can be mobile, computers or any monitoring devices that integrate with the cloud. AI powers the cloud in self-managing with respect to the applications that have been implemented.

Figure 1. Integration of AI and cloud

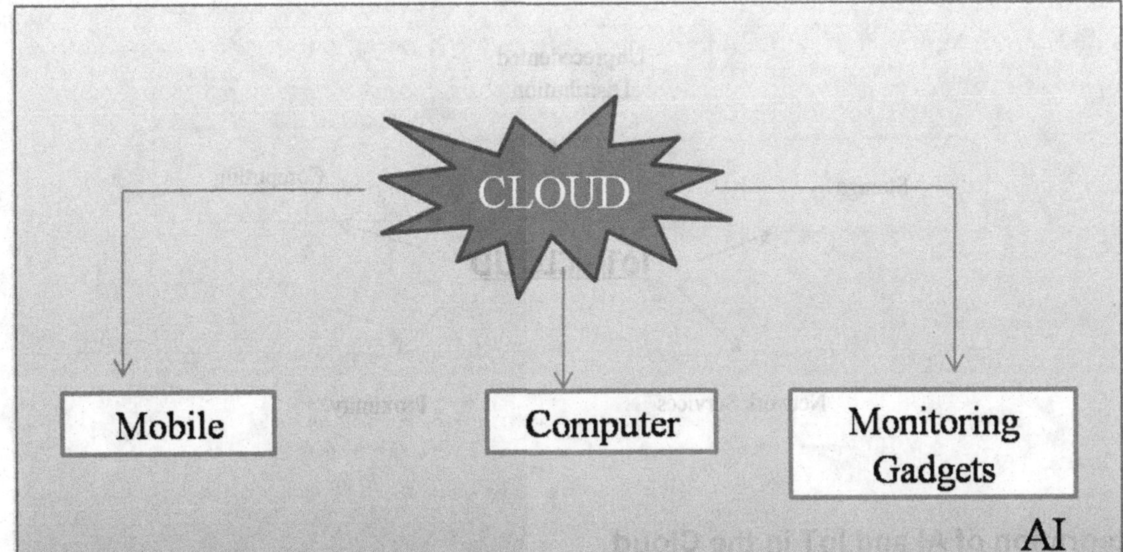

Internet of Things

The publicizing of new technologies with integration on the cloud has created a stir in the Internet of Things(IoT).This blend of technologies makes the IoT system intelligent(Gill et al., 2019).IoT is not restricted to a single device. It is the combination of sensors that can sense the parameters from the physical world. These sensors are powered to transfer the information using Wi-Fi /BLE module. Many times IoT devices have many sources to gather information. Hencethe huge amount of data collected through these sensors need a secure storage place. The main purpose for storing the data is to utilize the data for processing,analyzing and providing beneficial insights to the end-users(Barcelo etal.,2016). The next generation smart world can be achieved by smarter IoT and cloud-enabled applications. The smart world applications include smart city, smart healthcare,smart agriculture (Kamruzzaman, 2020; Peng et.al, 2019, Ayaz, 2019).

The IoT cloud network is formed due to device layer virtualization and a highly distributed network computing platform.The benefits of blending IoT and cloud are depicted in figure.2.Computing, storage,network services with unprecedented distribution and proximity to the end-user are the advantages of IoT combined with the cloud. The services in the cloud also include server management, analytics, intelligence and databases (Barcelo etal.,2016).

Figure 2. Advantages of IoT and cloud

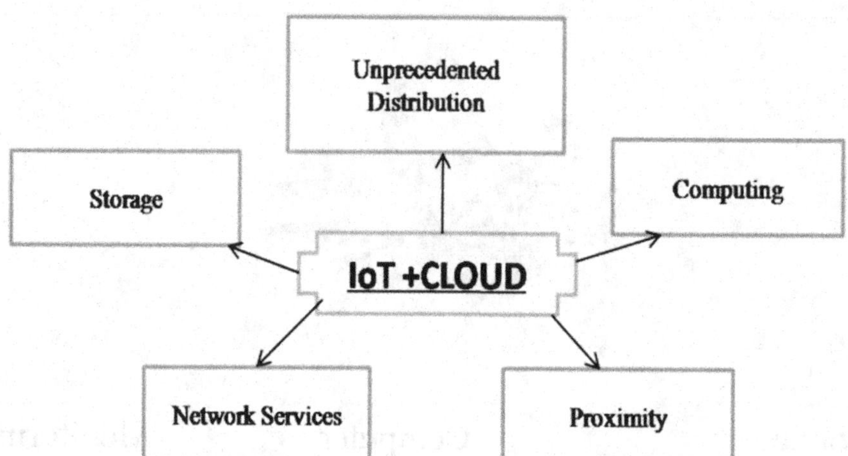

Integration of AI and IoT in the Cloud

One of the most promising fields when integrating AI and IoT in the cloud is a wearable platform. A wearable can vary from smart glasses, smartwatches, smart shirts,smart shoes,smart city,smart energy, smart agriculture(Barcelo et al.,2016.,Ayaz et al., 2019., Mahdavinejad 2018 etal.). Current studies and research on the composition of AI, IoT and cloud will be much explored in this section.

The union of three technologies, i.e., AI, IoT and Cloud, have raised the market from USD 7,740.0Million in 2019 to USD 52,190.0 Million by 2027 with a CAGR of 26% (Reports.,2021).The sensing pursuit takes place in IoT devices.The IoT device comprises sensors.These sensors can be placed at different places. The information gathered from different sensors is sent to the cloud through Wi-Fi or Bluetooth module. Data analytics using AI are implemented in the cloud. Prediction, detection,diagnosis and filtered results are sent to the end-users for real-time insight. Extensive research has resulted in smart applications making AI and IoT with cloud more smarter for the future world.The vitality of this tri-union is described below.

These applications vary from:

1. Smart healthcare application: There was a time when a patient had to carry health records and the doctors had to take time to analyze the health record every time the patient visited. With the emergence of AI, this challenge has been overcome while saving a lot of time. A smart healthcare application is proposed in (Kamruzzaman, 2020), where an AI-assisted system processes patients' data, provides emergency services, detects complicated patterns, and early detects serious diseases. qScout-EMR, InMotion ARM are few applications of smart healthcare(Kamruzzaman., 2020).
2. Smart city application: AI finds its extensive application in the smart city. Multi-access of many devices has been derived using AI (Peng etal., 2019).There is a challenge of signal processing and multiple accessing for the heterogeneous network when multiple devices try to interact. This issue has been solved by implementing AI flexible scheduling method under channel multiple access(CFMA).Low complexity with high-performance gain has been achieved(Peng et al., 2019).
3. Natural language processing: Conversation is an important part of human life. With the busy schedules that humans are running into, conversational agents are one of the promising applications of

Figure 3. Tri-union of IoT, cloud and artificial intelligence

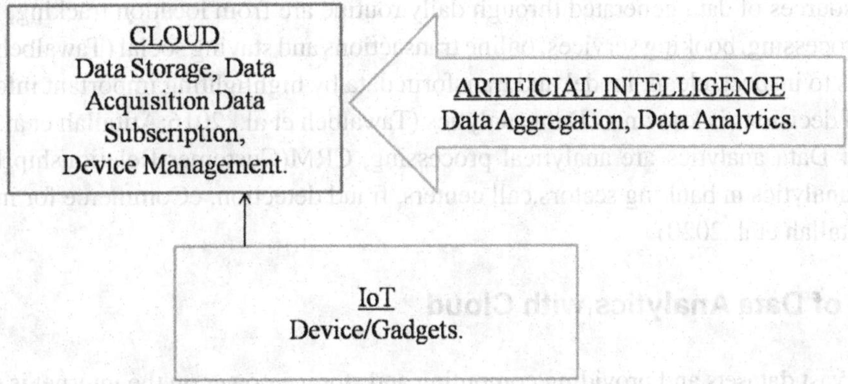

AI. Conversational agents find their importance in health care, customer care, eCommerce and education. Chatbots, Siri of Apple, Alexa by Amazon are few examples of conversational agents. These conversations range from placing an order, requesting or informing an order etc.(Kulkarni et al., 2019).

4. Smart Telecom: Telecom is an industry that is very less spoken. Handling better traffic classification, accurate network fault prediction, time optimization, heightened customer services are the fields that can be enhanced. By integrating AI in the telecom industry, MGA-MENA (Middle-east company),a study has determined how it can overcome the existing challenges and increase operational services, better products and efficiency(Gill et al., 2019).
5. Smart Agriculture: Agriculture itself is a sphere of services. The service varies right from irrigation, fungicides, fertilization, soil monitoring, diseases and bug monitoring, crop health monitoring (Ayaz et al.,2019).A farm area network is an area of crop forecasting to predict yield and production. Monitoring the crop right from fertilizing the soil, height of the crop, size of the fruit etc., helps in planning for better yield and planning for the future in case of crop rotation etc. (Ayaz et al.,2019).

For all of the above-discussed applications,different sensors aligning with the requirement are implemented in the IoT devices.The monitoring environment varies right from the human body for health care application, pollution,traffic and population for smart city application. Message and voice automation and communication for NLP, networking and fault management in signals for telecommunication application and farm area network for smart agriculture.

DATA ANALYTICS IN CLOUD

Rise of Data Analytics

Every day the four-letter word 'Data' in the form of emails, financialtransactions, webpages, audio files,structured data, unstructured data-id produced by a human. According to a report generated in 2020,The more astonishing outcome is that an everyday person generates 2.5quintillion bytes of data broken into 1.7 megabytes in a second. It is also expected to rise in the coming years (Education.,2020). The different sources of data generated through daily routine are from location tracking, time management, image processing, booking services, online transactions and staying social (Tawalbeh et .al., 2016).

The process to inspect, clean, model and transform data by highlighting important information such as insights and decisions is known as Data analytics (Tawalbeh et al., 2016;Atitallah et al.,2020). Other applications of Data analytics are analytical processing, CRM(Customer Relationship Management) management, analytics in banking sectors,call centers, fraud detection, eCommerce for inspecting web traffic etc.(Atitallah etal.,2020).

Integration of Data Analytics with Cloud

Collecting the vast datasets and providing computing and storage power on the internet is accomplished by Cloud services, also known as cloud computing. It is implemented as SOA(Service Oriented Architecture).One of the major advantages of integrating data analytics in the cloud is the ability to run millions of commands per second by removing complexities in the hardware and software for maintenance,installation and scalability at the tips(Mahmud etal.,2016).Smart technologies that integrate with the cloud are proven to be playing a vital role in reducing the cost and time of computation when implemented with the cloud (Mahmud etal.,2016).The idea of implementing cloud computing with data analytics remains to provide centralized database management and computing system (Goel etal.,2020). The amount of data collected, which can be in the form of reports, dashboards and business specification applications, is often huge for a centralized system.The information extracted is divided into four types. Figure.4.shows different types of Data analytics(Goel et al. 2020,Mujawar etal.,2015,Atitallah etal.,2020) .

1. Descriptive Data Analytics-This is the first step of performing data analysis. The objective of descriptive data analytics is to evaluate, classify and categorizethe data. This is achieved by fast-performing algorithms. The data realized is converted in the form of histograms, charts and graphs(Goel et.al 2020,Mujawar et.al.,2015,Atitallah etal.,2020).
2. Diagnostic Data Analytics-The main objective of diagnostic data analytics is to discover a reason of an event happened. It can be further described as data discovery, data mining.It helps in determining correlations between data (Goel etal.,2020).
3. Predictive Data, Analytics-The main objective of predictive data analytics is to predict the past raw data and make predictions for the future.It involves business intelligence techniques.Another advantage of this analysis is to examine the data(Goel et.al 2020,Mujawar et.al.,2015,Atitallah et.al.,2020) .
4. Prescriptive Data Analytics-Prescriptive analysis is done before making any decisions. It uses actionable data and a feedback system to track the output based on the action taken. It helps in analyzing the data to provide real-time information(Goel et.al 2020,Mujawar et.al.,2015,Atitallah et.al.,2020)

At each phase of data analytics,there rises complexity, need for more information (Goel et.al.,2020). When data is acquired from IoT devices, data analytics are performed.Depending on the application, detection, prediction, decision-making are analyzed. The integration of data analytics with the cloud when acquiring data from IoT devices is much discussed below.

Figure 4. Types of data analytics

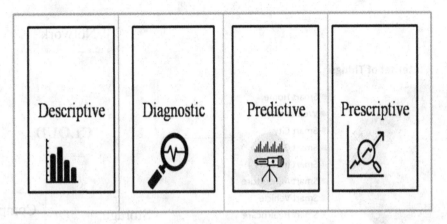

Approaches of Data Analytics in the Cloud while Integrating AI and IoT(Smart Applications)

Data analytics is humongous. IoT devices consist of sensors,actuators. The data generated from IoT are extremely huge.The transport of data from IoT to wireless technologies ranges from Bluetooth,Zigbee,Wi-Fi,LoRa and mobile technologies, i.e., GPRS/2G,eMTC,NB-IoT and other fixed technologies like PLC,optical access and Ethernet (Munoz etal.,2018). Figure.5 depicts the different applications while integrating IoT with the cloud. Different approaches of data analytics in various applications with the integration of IoT will throw light on existing technological aspects and choices. Following are the different IoT applications and their communication method for data aggregation and data analytics from the current state of the art:

1. Smart Home: Smart homes are a very common application of IoT.The most commonly used sensors for home management are gas sensors,temperature sensors,motion sensors.Often the transfer of data from these sensors to the cloud layer needs a service for dispute management. In (A.,2020) an algorithm is proposed for emergency notification systems and performance awareness as well. The cloud state also provides current relocation for achieving enormous resource usage while assigning tasks by IoT is enormous.
2. Wearables:Wearables are a substantial innovation in today's era of life. When wearables meet IoT, the enormous amount of data produced are stored in the cloud.Thecloud usage is to store data and use it for preventive measures, alerts and immediate actions. A wearable to measure the Covid-19 signs in quarantined patients are detailed in(Al Bassam et.al.,2021).The cloud in this application is used to support infrastructure,applications and teams. A firewall application is built in order to protect the data for privacy by making the system secure and reliable for a wearable application.
3. Smart City: When integrating IoT and cloud, an eco-friendly energy management system is very essential. It helps in saving the computational cost. Various technologies are implemented for utilizing energy efficiency. The solution to the service distribution problem is achieved in(Barcelo et.al., 2016) by proposing an optimization framework. It is achieved by optimally placing the service

Figure 5. Integrating IoT with cloud

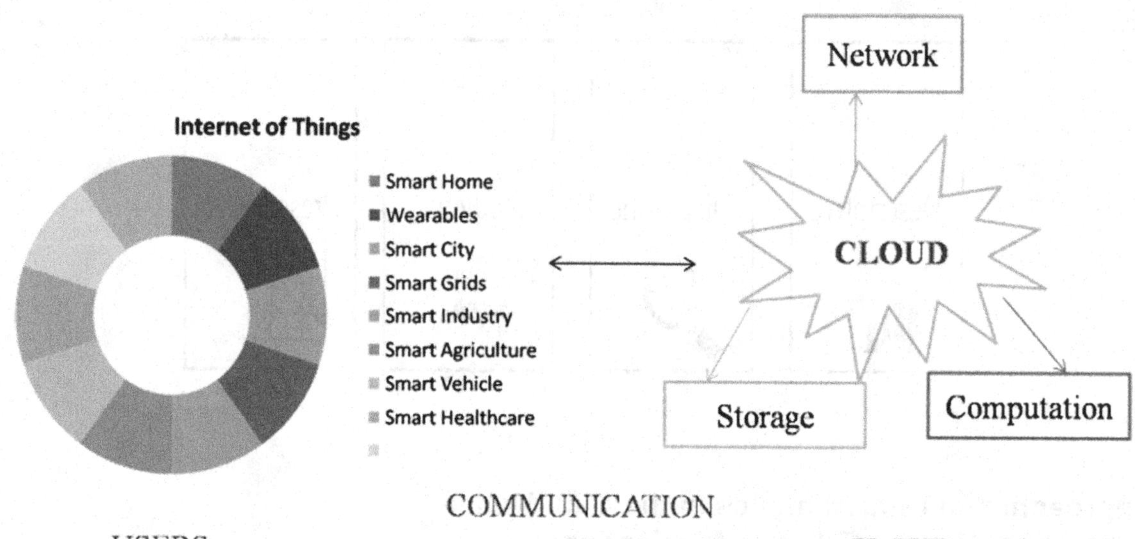

functions and routing the network flows while considering heterogeneous capacities, efficiencies of sensing, computing and transport resources in IoT-Cloud infrastructure(Barcelo et.al., 2016).

4. Smart Grids: Smart grids play a key role in IoT systems. It is a method from generating data to points of consumption. The data generated by the smart grid mainly includes about network status. Virtualization technologies are implemented in(Meloni et.al.,2018) that decouples the data coming from physical devices.
5. Smart Industry: Storing a large amount of data is a challenge by IoT in the cloud. To encounter this problem, an algorithm is implemented (Raja Singh et.al.,2020)that alters the data acquired efficiently by event data logging with pre and post-values. Mechanical parameters are monitored for pre and post-values with a high sampling rate.By enhancing the system performance and accuracy of the measurement,storage space is made limited.This decreases the cost needed to save the data.
6. Smart Vehicle: Proper communication is important while sending and receiving data from different IoT vehicular devices to the cloud. Smart computing is implemented in(Deebak et.al 2020).It proposes aframework that makes the system location independent and the communication between the devices is made smarter by better decision making and reliable computation—all these channels towards reducing the cost of the system and channels towards communication fairness.
7. Smart Agriculture: Real-time information gathering has also found its application and benefit in agriculture. Similarly, smart agriculture is helping farmers with human labor optimization by increasing the quantity and quality of the products by implementing the predicting algorithms found in data analytics.An irrigation system is a major contributorto agriculture. Continuous monitoring and controlling of agriculture are of greater importance. For meeting the same in irrigation, in(Dobrescu et.al.,2019)real-time context-aware system is developed to control and monitor irrigation systems.
8. Smart Healthcare: Remote patient monitoring, effective disease management,error reduction and reduction in costs are a few of the advantages which took IoT in healthcare the storm. While these are the most prominent fields of research in healthcare, determining health shocks in underprivi-

leged countries also serves a greater advantage. Predicting health shocks help in providing better insight for the government sectors to determine policies for general practitioners. Context-aware on health shocks are developed by socio-economic,cultural and geographic conditions that would impact an individual's health status (Mahmud et.al.,2016).More insights on data analytics will be continued further section.

HEALTHCARE DATA ANALYTICS

Data analytics forms the core of healthcare. It helps in making predictions, detection and monitoring of the patient. Among other applications, the most important application that serves humankind is healthcare. In health care applications, IoT in health care has become a boon for futuristic service.Further healthcare and data analytics associated with it will be discussed.

Exploring Healthcare Data Analytics

The data acquired from the sensors in IoT transfer the raw information to another layer for data processing that includes analysis of the data, making decisions, detection and prediction of disease. It depends on the nature of the data and the purpose of acquiring it; hence, different data analytics approaches are further described in Table 1.

Ambient assisted living (AAL) is a potential-filled boon for humankind, especially for the elderly. It is a blend of individual technology with solution and service.Data is store in IBM Bluemix with MQTT(Bianchi et.al.,2019,Bassoli et.al.,2017) .To enter the log of sleeping postures, offline big data analytics is implemented in (García-Magariño et.al.,2018).The customizable deployment method is achieved by integrating cloud and edge together (Aloi et.al.,2021).This approach, by increasing scalability, flexibility and interoperability, reduces the system costs.

A collective study that comprises of different studies in medicine has been explored in (Sadoughi et.al., 2020).Neurology, cardiology,psychology and psychiatry are the most explored fields of IoT in medicine. The data is collected in an excel sheet and then decisions are made. A new method that breaks the traditional work of the cloud is discussed in(Latif et.al.,2020).IoT-based cloud application Rx-expert system is discussed.It has the advantage of closing the feedback loop of communication from doctor to patient and from patient to doctor. Cloud storage with big data analytics is performed. To present configuration, deployment, monitoring and controlling the tasks for cloud resources, orchestration is used for resource description,policies rules and resource description in (Abdul Minaam et.al.,2018).

The approach of integrating fog and cloud-like in (Aloi et.al.,2021)is discussed in(Moghadas et.al.,2020,Abdel-Basset et.al.,2019).This approach is much faster in terms of latencies and delays. This implementation is very beneficial where continuous monitoring is very necessary,monitoring arrhythmia(Moghadas et.al.,2020) and type-2 diabetes(Abdel-Basset et.al.,2019).Covid-19 symptom management is channeled on the app directly in (Paganelli et.al.,2021), which clearly indicates that the technology to be used depends a lot on the nature of the disease and the purpose of monitoring.

IoT-based smart rehabilitation system is advantageous for activity monitoring in hospitals and rehabilitation centers. The IoT system that acquires the information is sent to the cloud. In (Hanet.al.,2020), instead of transferring information to the cloud directly, the processing layer is divided into three layers. Active CPS which is responsible for the interconnection between itself and other nodes,whereas the

Table 1. Approaches to different data analytics and diseases

Healthcare scenario	Ref	Description	Inference
Assisted Living	Bianchi et.al.,2019, Bassoli et.al.,2017, García-Magariño et.al.,2018, Aloi et.al.,2021	Human activity recognition. Ambient assisted living. Active assisted living. Ambient assisted living.	Activity recognition by implementing IoT is explored in this scenario. Different approaches to store data are discussed.
Medication intake Smart pharmaceuticals	Sadoughi et.al., 2020, Latif et.al.,2020, Abdul Minaam et.al.,2018	IoT in medicine. Medicine dispensing system. Smart pillbox.	Smart pharmaceutical devices are a new era of technological devices. Different approaches to store and process the data are discussed.
Monitoring Health	Paganelli et.al.,2021, Moghadas et.al.,2020, Abdel-Basset et.al.,2019	Remote monitoring of Covid-19 . Monitoring cardiac arrhythmia. Type-2 diabetes monitoring.	Remote health monitoring is a crucial part of health care. In this scenario, cloud and edge computing are integrated to provide better performance.
Rehabilitation	Hanet.al.,2020, Bianchi et.al.,2019	Cancer rehabilitation. Activity monitoring to record abnormal behaviors.	Use cases of rehabilitation are considered. The model acquires data and for storing and processing [39]implements three different layers on cloud and IBM Bluemix cloud services by [40].
Wearable technology	Wu et.al.,2020, Forooghifar et.al.,2019, Chen et.al.,2020, Sciarrone et.al.,2021.	Body temperature,PPG,ECG monitoring. Epilepsy monitoring. Chronic kidney disease prediction. Neurological disorder monitoring.	Wearable technology is presented in this literature. The model consists of a sensor patch that acquires the physiological data and sends it to the cloud. In every wearable technology mentioned, the data is stored and different frameworks have been applied for reducing energy consumption and overall cost reduction.

middleware layer is implemented for integration of data collected and, finally, the cloud to process data from middleware. Hence the data is processed in individual layers. Unlike in(Hanet.al.,2020),data is sent to IBM bluemix cloud services through MQTT protocol with QoS equal to 2.This method ensures reliability to the transmission process. For recording abnormal behavior through this process is not continuous, due to the flexibility that is offered by the cloud and the advantage of the reduction in the number of devices for data acquisition, the cloud is implemented(Bianchi et.al.,2019).

Wearable technology is the most promising trend in today's era. Though the size and shape of wearable differ with respect to the requirement,the amalgamation of IoT with cloud remains the same.Physiological parameters such as PPG and ECG with body temperature are monitored in(Wu et.al.,2020).The data acquired are transferred to the cloud for storage and further decision-making(Wu et.al.,2020,Forooghifar et.al.,2019,Chen et.al.,2020,Sciarrone et.al.,2021). The sensor patches are configured in different operative modes to reduce energy consumption. The complex machine learning computations for energy consumption are distributed among cloud, edge and fog in(Forooghifar et.al.,2019).

DATA ANALYTICS INDIABETIC MANAGEMENT SYSTEM

Different approaches in data analytics for different disease scenarios are explored in the former section. Diabetes is one of the leading diseases in the world; according to statistics, over 700 million adults will be affected by it by the year 2045(Diabetes.,2020).The number of leading deaths is related to diabetes. With diabetes, curing of life-threatening diseases makes the condition worse. Diabetes changes the structure of the cell. Due to high blood pressure, red blood cells destroy the erythrocyte membrane, which leads to oxygen binding disorders. These contribute towards the modification in the cell that makes the body sensitive to various diseases(Szablewski & Sulima, 2017).

Exploring Diabetic Management System

AI in healthcare enables to convert the descriptive raw data into insights and with the behavior and correlations,predictive data analysis is performed.Predictive data analysis also helps in forecasting information of the diseases. Prescriptive data analysis implements methods of handling the upcoming event depending on the predictive data analysis. With the information gathered through descriptive, predictive and prescriptive data analysis, customized medicare and therapy can be provided(Musacchio et.al.,2020). Table 2 provides an insight into different data analytics and their use-cases from different kinds of literature.

Descriptive data analysis discusses about the event that happened that includes the Hospital Information System(HIS).HIS depicts the information about the number of patients joined, outpatients records, and the no of patients discharged with respect to time period .This data is helpful in analyzing the overall analysis of a system.SQL is implemented for extracting the HIS data in(Bakar et.al.,2020).The information extracted were demographics, history, details of the visit, previous prescription and active medication. The data acquired give an insight into Type-2 diabetes management systems(T2DM).Using the State Version tool and Stata Software v12, data analytics are performed.The information acquired through descriptive analysis showed 7.5% of prevalence in T2DM in outpatient department (OPD) setting,patients who continued the treatment were found out to be 61.1%. The number of patients who received glycemic targets was 18%(Bakar et.al.,2020).

The dataset considered in(Kumar et.al.,2015) was plasma glucose concentration, serum insulin, diastolic blood pressure, diabetes pedigree, Body mass index(BMI), age, and the number of times pregnant.When the dataset is received, the map-reduce function is applied in Hadoop. Pattern matching and predictive matching are done and the results are distributed to various servers that would predict the happening of eye diseases, kidney diseases, heart strokes (Bakar et.al.,2020).

Many times the requirement to continuously monitor glucose arises for diabetic management. An IoT-based CGM is proposed in (Fernández-Caramés et.al.,2018).Fog computing is implemented, which collects and processes the data. It sends the data to a remote server and to the blockchain encrypted. For transaction privacy and validation, a federated blockchain is implemented.It stores the data and provides access to the public in a private way(Fernández-Caramés et.al.,2018).Prescriptive data analytics is needed for predicting futuristic diagnostics in diabetic management.Dataset from EMR is considered. k-nearest neighbor is implemented on the dataset. The improvement of 0.44%(4.8mmol/mol)HbA_{1C} outcome is achieved (Bertsimas et.al.,2016).

Predictive data analytics are proposed in (Ara .,2017).The dataset consists of the glucose levels of patients. Azure machine learning along with Azure SQL database produce predictive algorithm on

Table 2. Data analytics in the diabetic management system

Ref	Description	Inference
Bakar et.al.,2020	Descriptive data analytics of type-2 diabetes mellitus is proposed by using a patient information system.	Using Structured Query Language (SQL),data is collected and descriptive data analytics are performed.
Kumar et.al.,2015	Predictive data analytics for diabetic management is proposed.	Hadoop/Map Reduce data analytics method is implemented for predicting diabetes prevalence and complications.
Fernández-Caramés et.al.,2018	Diagnosis data analytics for diabetic management using fog computing and blockchain is proposed.	An IoT-based continuous glucose monitoring (CGM) is proposed. Block chain is implemented to save the data encrypted that can be accessed remotely.
Bertsimas et.al.,2016	Prescriptive data analytics for diabetic management using electronic medical records(EMR).	Using k-nearest neighbor algorithm, future diagnostic management for diabetes is achieved.
Ara .,2017	Predictive data analytics, while integrating IoT and Machine learning,streamline data analytics for diabetic management is proposed.	A much faster, smart and economical E-Followup system was achieved with Azure streaming analytics.
Huzooree et.al.,2017	Predictive data analytics is proposed for the diabetic management system.	The Autoregressive(ARX) model is implemented to predict glucose for diabetic patients.
Han et.al.,2008	Predictive data analytics is proposed for diabetic management systems.	A prediction model is built by implementing Rapid-I's and Rapid Miner, data analytics.
Prabhu& Selvabharathi .,2019.	Predictive data analytics is proposed for diabetic management systems using a deep belief neural network.	After applying the normalization technique, a prediction model using deep belief neural network is implemented.

patient's glucose data by securing future data. Similarly, in (Huzooree et.al.,2017), the autoregressive model is proposed for predicting glucose in diabetic patients. The dataset consists of CGM information, Blood pressure(BP),total cholesterol, low -density lipoprotein cholesterol(LDL), high-density lipoprotein cholesterol(HDL).The time series ARX model of prediction is proven to provide the best prediction with exogenous inputs.

Rapid-I's and RapidMiner are implemented in(Han et.al.,2008) for performing data analytics. Dataset extracted from Pima Indian database. With a similar source of the dataset, a predictive model is performed. The deep learning model is implemented for maximum recall of 1, the precision of 0.67 and the F1 measure of 0.808 when compared to other machine learning algorithms (Prabhu & Selvabharathi, 2019).

Real-Time Data Analytics on Diabetic Management System

The data analytics on diabetic management systems can be much explored in this session by considering the real-time dataset.

Table 3 provides the result reported on diabetic management using machine learning. On the real-time PIMA Indian dataset, different AI algorithms have been applied. SVM considered has less computation complexity, but the accuracy is less i.e,75% when compared with other research. Neural Network, Standard deviation k-nearest neighbor and Deep Learning have been considered. Deep Learning depicts the greatest accuracy of 98.07% when compared with Neural Network and k-nearest neighbor.

Table 3. Data analytics results in the diabetic management system

Ref	Method Applied	Measure
Rajeswari& Vijayakumar.,2021	SVM	75%
Khanam& Foo.,2021	Neural Network	88.6%
Patra & khuntia.,2021	k-nearest neighbor	83.2%
Naz&Ahuj .,2020	Deep Learning	98.07%

CHALLENGES FACED WHILE INTEGRATING AI AND IOT IN CLOUD

The challenges that can hinder the performance of integrating AI and IoT in the cloud are discussed below. If these challenges are taken into consideration, a better-performing IoT cloud will be advantageous.

1. Privacy and security with the advent of the blockchain, data can be securely transferred to the cloud and can be accessed at any location by authenticated users. The physical location of the data, SLA and lack of trust in the service provider form trust issues in the IoT cloud that has to be addressed. Apart from that, due to multi-tenancy, due to the addition of more layers, leakage of sensitive information is possible(Pundir et.al.,2016, Atlam et.al.,2017).
2. Interoperability-When aligning with different IoT devices, it is evident that due to the different technologies, there is diversity.The manufacturers should follow the same standards so that as the cloud depends on interoperability and the same standards from all technologies, this requirement is still a challenge(Pundir et.al.,2016, Atlam et.al.,2017).
3. Integration issues-When integrating IoT and AI with the cloud, there is a strong potential for the development of new scenarios and applications. There should be an implementation of a communication method between different devices.A proper communication strategy must be developed that would help to solve integration issues(Pundir et.al.,2016, Atlam et.al.,2017) .
4. Competing standards-To protect the proprietary systems; many companies try to protect their open system proponents. Depending upon the various requirements, power requirements uses, capabilities and device class, standards that is interoperable must be developed. International standards must be applied by the legacy systems (Pundir et.al.,2016, Atlam et.al.,2017).
5. Adequate bandwidth requirement- The data, when transferred from IoT devices to the cloud, requires high bandwidth.Increasing the bandwidth needs enough storage space and computation evolution(Pundir et.al.,2016).
6. Monitoring data from cloud-Monitoring the stored data from the cloud requires a specific velocity and volume, which are a challenge for observing the performance, managing resources, capacity planning, security, SLA's and troubleshooting (Pundir et.al.,2016).

FUTURE OF AI AND IOT DATA ANALYTICS IN CLOUD

With the advent of new technologies every day, the challenges discussed in the above section have research potential for the future of AI and IoT data analytics in cloud integration. This section will throw light on open issues and future research directions. Standard protocols and API's for reliable and heterogeneous devices is the future for a smart IoT-Cloud paradigm. Fog computing acts as a bridge between the edge of the network of IoT devices and the cloud. Implementing fog computing in future applications will reduce the delay and latency issues. Even with encrypted data with blockchain,there is still a possibility of insider attacks. Providing security has the potential in the development of properly secured IoT systems. Issues in SLA violations can be solved by multiple clouds. Multiple clouds increase the costs, question the heterogeneity of multiple platform integration and QoS management support. This remains an open issue to be addressed. There are many machine learning applications (Ponnusamyetal .,2017,Ponnusamyet.al.,2020)that model can be applied for diabetic management. Energy efficiency is still an open issue when integrating IoT and cloud that has a strong research potential in the future to be explored(Atlam et.al.,2017).

CONCLUSION

IoT integrated with the cloud makes any technology empowered by allowing the users to perform computing with the internet and provide real-time analysis and results. This chapter has provided deeper insight into the data analytics when blending IoT and AI.AI with advantages of implementation with cloud and IoT id discussed.Smart applications with Tri union pf AI, IoT and cloud, are discussed further. Data analytics which is the center of processing the acquired data, is discussed in detail with types of data analytics. AI and IoT with data analytics scenarios are also explored by considering different smart applications. Data analytics is much explored with diabetic health care management systems. Data analytics approaches for different healthcare scenarios are discussed. Challenges along with the future potential of research is also elaborated in this chapter. With the amalgamation of IoT and AI with cloud data analytics, improved communication with effective transfer of data efficiently is obtained.

REFERENCES

A performance-aware dynamic scheduling algorithm for cloud-based IoT applications. (2020). *Computer Communications, 160*, 512–520. doi:10.1016/j.comcom.2020.06.016

Abdel-Basset, M., Manogaran, G., Gamal, A., & Chang, V. (2019). A Novel Intelligent Medical Decision Support Model Based on Soft Computing and IoT. *IEEE Internet of Things Journal*, 1–1. doi:10.1109/JIOT.2019.2931647

Abdul Minaam, D. S., & Abd-ELfattah, M. (2018). Smart drugs:Improving healthcare using Smart Pill Box for Medicine Reminder and Monitoring System. *Future Computing and Informatics Journal*, *3*(2), 443–456. doi:10.1016/j.fcij.2018.11.008

Al Bassam, N., Shaik Asif, H., Al Qaraghuli, A., Khan, J., Sumesh, E. P., & Lavanya, V. (2021). IoT Based Wearable Device to Monitor the Signs of Quarantined remote patients of COVID-19. *Informatics in Medicine Unlocked, 100588*, 100588. Advance online publication. doi:10.1016/j.imu.2021.100588 PMID:33997262

Aloi, G., Fortino, G., Gravina, R., Pace, P., & Savaglio, C. (2021). Simulation-Driven Platform for Edge-Based AAL Systems. *IEEE Journal on Selected Areas in Communications*, *39*(2), 446–462. doi:10.1109/JSAC.2020.3021544

Ara, A., & Ara, A. (2017). Case study: Integrating IoT, streaming analytics and machine learning to improve intelligent diabetes management system. *2017 International Conference on Energy, Communication, Data Analytics and Soft Computing (ICECDS)*. 10.1109/ICECDS.2017.8390043

Atitallah, S. B., Driss, M., Boulila, W., & Ghézala, H. B. (2020). Leveraging Deep Learning and IoT big data analytics to support the smart cities development: Review and future directions. *Computer Science Review*, *38*, 100303. doi:10.1016/j.cosrev.2020.100303

Atitallah, S. B., Driss, M., Boulila, W., & Ghézala, H. B. (2020). Leveraging Deep Learning and IoT big data analytics to support the smart cities development: Review and future directions. *Computer Science Review*, *38*, 100303. doi:10.1016/j.cosrev.2020.100303

Atlam, H. F., Alenezi, A., Alharthi, A., Walters, R. J., & Wills, G. B. (2017). Integration of Cloud Computing with Internet of Things: Challenges and Open Issues. *2017 IEEE International Conference on Internet of Things (iThings) and IEEE Green Computing and Communications (GreenCom) and IEEE Cyber, Physical and Social Computing (CPSCom) and IEEE Smart Data (SmartData)*. 10.1109/iThings-GreenCom-CPSCom-SmartData.2017.105

Ayaz, M., Ammad-uddin, M., Sharif, Z., Mansour, A., & Aggoune, E.-H. M. (2019). Internet-of-Things (IoT) based Smart Agriculture: Towards Making the Fields Talk. *IEEE Access: Practical Innovations, Open Solutions*, *7*, 1–1. doi:10.1109/ACCESS.2019.2932609

Bakar, Ab Hamid, Yunus, Zawani, Halim, & Zainuddin. (2020). Descriptive Analysis of Type 2 Diabetes Mellitus Patients Using Data From Hospital. *Information Systems*, *16*, 94.

Barcelo, M., Correa, A., Llorca, J., Tulino, A. M., Vicario, J. L., & Morell, A. (2016). IoT-Cloud Service Optimization in Next Generation Smart Environments. *IEEE Journal on Selected Areas in Communications*, *34*(12), 4077–4090. doi:10.1109/JSAC.2016.2621398

Barcelo, M., Correa, A., Llorca, J., Tulino, A. M., Vicario, J. L., & Morell, A. (2016). IoT-Cloud Service Optimization in Next Generation Smart Environments. *IEEE Journal on Selected Areas in Communications*, *34*(12), 4077–4090. doi:10.1109/JSAC.2016.2621398

Bassoli, M., Bianchi, V., De Munari, I., & Ciampolini, P. (2017). An IoT Approach for an AAL Wi-Fi-Based Monitoring System. *IEEE Transactions on Instrumentation and Measurement*, *66*(12), 3200–3209. doi:10.1109/TIM.2017.2753458

Bertsimas, D., Kallus, N., Weinstein, A. M., & Zhuo, Y. D. (2016). Personalized Diabetes Management Using Electronic Medical Records. *Diabetes Care*, *40*(2), 210–217. doi:10.2337/dc16-0826 PMID:27920019

Bianchi, V., Bassoli, M., Lombardo, G., Fornacciari, P., Mordonini, M., & De Munari, I. (2019). IoT Wearable Sensor and Deep Learning: An Integrated Approach for Personalized Human Activity Recognition in a Smart Home Environment. *IEEE Internet of Things Journal*, *6*(5), 8553–8562. doi:10.1109/JIOT.2019.2920283

Bianchi, V., Bassoli, M., Lombardo, G., Fornacciari, P., Mordonini, M., & De Munari, I. (2019). IoT Wearable Sensor and Deep Learning: An Integrated Approach for Personalized Human Activity Recognition in a Smart Home Environment. *IEEE Internet of Things Journal*, *6*(5), 8553–8562. doi:10.1109/JIOT.2019.2920283

Chen, G., Ding, C., Li, Y., Hu, X., Li, X., Ren, L., Ding, X., Tian, P., & Xue, W. (2020). Prediction of Chronic Kidney Disease Using Adaptive Hybridized Deep Convolutional Neural Network on the Internet of Medical Things Platform. *IEEE Access: Practical Innovations, Open Solutions*, *8*, 100497–100508. doi:10.1109/ACCESS.2020.2995310

Deebak, B. D., Al-Turjman, F., Aloqaily, M., & Alfandi, O. (2020). IoT-BSFCAN: A smart context-aware system in IoT-Cloud using mobile-fogging. *Future Generation Computer Systems*, *109*, 368–381. doi:10.1016/j.future.2020.03.050

Diabetes statistics: Read the facts. (2020, September 29). Retrieved from The Checkup website: https://www.singlecare.com/blog/news/diabetes-statistics/

Dobrescu, R., Merezeanu, D., & Mocanu, S. (2019). Context-Aware Control and Monitoring System with IoT and Cloud Support. *Computers and Electronics in Agriculture*, *160*(May), 91–99. doi:10.1016/j.compag.2019.03.005

Education, K. is passionate to write about A. driving technological change. (2020, June 11). *The Rise of Data: Data Science, Big Data and Data Analytics for Seamless Business Operations*. Retrieved from https://www.analyticsinsight.net/the-rise-of-data-data-science-big-data-and-data-analytics-for-seamless-business-operations/

Fernández-Caramés, T., & Fraga-Lamas, P. (2018). Design of a Fog Computing, Blockchain and IoT-Based Continuous Glucose Monitoring System for Crowdsourcing mHealth. *Proceedings.*, *4*(1), 5757. doi:10.3390/ecsa-5-05757

Forooghifar, F., Aminifar, A., & Atienza, D. (2019). Resource-Aware Distributed Epilepsy Monitoring Using Self-Awareness From Edge to Cloud. *IEEE Transactions on Biomedical Circuits and Systems*, *13*(6), 1338–1350. doi:10.1109/TBCAS.2019.2951222 PMID:31689205

García-Magariño, I., Lacuesta, R., & Lloret, J. (2018). Agent-Based Simulation of Smart Beds With Internet-of-Things for Exploring Big Data Analytics. *IEEE Access: Practical Innovations, Open Solutions*, *6*, 366–379. doi:10.1109/ACCESS.2017.2764467

Gill, S. S., Tuli, S., Xu, M., Singh, I., Singh, K. V., Lindsay, D., Tuli, S., Smirnova, D., Singh, M., Jain, U., Pervaiz, H., Sehgal, B., Kaila, S. S., Misra, S., Aslanpour, M. S., Mehta, H., Stankovski, V., & Garraghan, P. (2019). Transformative effects of IoT, Blockchain and Artificial Intelligence on cloud computing: Evolution, vision, trends and open challenges. *Internet of Things*, *8*, 100118. doi:10.1016/j.iot.2019.100118

Goel, P., Jain, P., Pasman, H. J., Pistikopoulos, E. N., & Datta, A. (2020). Integration of data analytics with cloud services for safer process systems, application examples and implementation challenges. *Journal of Loss Prevention in the Process Industries*, *68*, 104316. doi:10.1016/j.jlp.2020.104316

Goel, P., Jain, P., Pasman, H. J., Pistikopoulos, E. N., & Datta, A. (2020). Integration of data analytics with cloud services for safer process systems, application examples and implementation challenges. *Journal of Loss Prevention in the Process Industries*, *68*, 104316. doi:10.1016/j.jlp.2020.104316

Han, J., Rodriguez, J. C., & Beheshti, M. (2008, December 1). *Diabetes Data Analysis and Prediction Model Discovery Using RapidMiner*. doi:10.1109/FGCN.2008.226

Han, Y., Han, Z., Wu, J., Yu, Y., Gao, S., Hua, D., & Yang, A. (2020). Artificial Intelligence Recommendation System of Cancer Rehabilitation Scheme Based on IoT Technology. *IEEE Access: Practical Innovations, Open Solutions*, *8*, 44924–44935. doi:10.1109/ACCESS.2020.2978078

Huzooree, G., Khedo, K. K., & Joonas, N. (2017, July 1). *Glucose prediction data analytics for diabetic patients monitoring*. doi:10.1109/NEXTCOMP.2017.8016197

Kamruzzaman, M. M. (2020). *Architecture of Smart Health Care System Using Artificial Intelligence*. doi:10.1109/ICMEW46912.2020.9106026

Khanam, J. J., & Foo, S. Y. (2021). *A comparison of machine learning algorithms for diabetes prediction*. ICT Express. doi:10.1016/j.icte.2021.02.004

Kulkarni, P., Mahabaleshwarkar, A., Kulkarni, M., Sirsikar, N., & Gadgil, K. (2019). Conversational AI: An Overview of Methodologies, Applications & Future Scope. *2019 5th International Conference on Computing, Communication, Control and Automation (ICCUBEA)*. 10.1109/ICCUBEA47591.2019.9129347

Kumar, N. M. S., Eswari, T., Sampath, P., & Lavanya, S. (2015). Predictive Methodology for Diabetic Data Analysis in Big Data. *Procedia Computer Science, 50*, 203–208. doi:10.1016/j.procs.2015.04.069

Latif, G., Shankar, A., Alghazo, J., Kalyanasundaram, V., Boopathi, C. S., & Arfan Jaffar, M. (2020). I-CARES: Advancing health diagnosis and medication through IoT. *Wireless Networks*, *26*(4), 2375–2389. Advance online publication. doi:10.100711276-019-02165-6

Linthicum, D. S. (2017). Making Sense of AI in Public Clouds. *IEEE Cloud Computing*, *4*(6), 70–72. doi:10.1109/MCC.2018.1081067

Mahdavinejad, M. S., Rezvan, M., Barekatain, M., Adibi, P., Barnaghi, P., & Sheth, A. P. (2018). Machine learning for internet of things data analysis: A survey. *Digital Communications and Networks*, *4*(3), 161–175. doi:10.1016/j.dcan.2017.10.002

Mahmud, S., Iqbal, R., & Doctor, F. (2016). Cloud enabled data analytics and visualization framework for health-shocks prediction. *Future Generation Computer Systems*, *65*, 169–181. doi:10.1016/j.future.2015.10.014

Mahmud, S., Iqbal, R., & Doctor, F. (2016). Cloud enabled data analytics and visualization framework for health-shocks prediction. *Future Generation Computer Systems*, *65*, 169–181. doi:10.1016/j.future.2015.10.014

Meloni, A., Pegoraro, P. A., Atzori, L., Benigni, A., & Sulis, S. (2018). Cloud-based IoT solution for state estimation in smart grids: Exploiting virtualization and edge-intelligence technologies. *Computer Networks*, *130*, 156–165. doi:10.1016/j.comnet.2017.10.008

Moghadas, E., Rezazadeh, J., & Farahbakhsh, R. (2020). An IoT patient monitoring based on fog computing and data mining: Cardiac arrhythmia usecase. *Internet of Things*, *11*, 100251. doi:10.1016/j.iot.2020.100251

Mujawar, S., & Joshi, A. (2015). Data Analytics Types, Tools and their Comparison. *International Journal of Advanced Research in Computer and Communication Engineering*, *4*(2). Advance online publication. doi:10.17148/IJARCCE.2015.42110

Munoz, R., Vilalta, R., Yoshikane, N., Casellas, R., Martinez, R., Tsuritani, T., & Morita, I. (2018). Integration of IoT, Transport SDN, and Edge/Cloud Computing for Dynamic Distribution of IoT Analytics and Efficient Use of Network Resources. *Journal of Lightwave Technology*, *36*(7), 1420–1428. doi:10.1109/JLT.2018.2800660

Musacchio, N., Giancaterini, A., Guaita, G., Ozzello, A., Pellegrini, M. A., Ponzani, P., Russo, G. T., Zilich, R., & de Micheli, A. (2020). Artificial Intelligence and Big Data in Diabetes Care: A Position Statement of the Italian Association of Medical Diabetologists. *Journal of Medical Internet Research*, *22*(6), e16922. doi:10.2196/16922 PMID:32568088

Naz, H., & Ahuja, S. (2020). Deep learning approach for diabetes prediction using PIMA Indian dataset. *Journal of Diabetes and Metabolic Disorders*, *19*(1), 391–403. doi:10.100740200-020-00520-5 PMID:32550190

Paganelli, A. I., Velmovitsky, P. E., Miranda, P., Branco, A., Alencar, P., Cowan, D., Endler, M., & Morita, P. P. (2021). A conceptual IoT-based early-warning architecture for remote monitoring of COVID-19 patients in wards and at home. *Internet of Things*, *100399*, 100399. Advance online publication. doi:10.1016/j.iot.2021.100399

Patra, R., & khuntia, B. (2021). Analysis and Prediction Of Pima Indian Diabetes Dataset Using SDKNN Classifier Technique. *IOP Conference Series. Materials Science and Engineering*, *1070*(1), 012059. doi:10.1088/1757-899X/1070/1/012059

Peng, W., Gao, W., & Liu, J. (2019). AI-enabled Massive Devices Multiple Access for Smart City. *IEEE Internet of Things Journal*, *6*(5), 1–1. doi:10.1109/JIOT.2019.2902448

Ponnusamy, V., Coumaran, A., Shunmugam, A. S., Rajaram, K., & Senthilvelavan, S. (2020, July). Smart Glass: Real-Time Leaf Disease Detection using YOLO Transfer Learning. In *2020 International Conference on Communication and Signal Processing (ICCSP)* (pp. 1150-1154). IEEE. 10.1109/ICCSP48568.2020.9182146

Ponnusamy, V., & Malarvihi, S. (2017). Hardware impairment detection and prewhitening on MIMO precoder for spectrum sharing. *Wireless Personal Communications*, *96*(1), 1557–1576. doi:10.100711277-017-4256-6

Prabhu, P., & Selvabharathi, S. (2019, July 1). *Deep Belief Neural Network Model for Prediction of Diabetes Mellitus*. doi:10.1109/ICISPC.2019.8935838

Pundir, M., Sharma, M., & Singh, Y. (2016). IJARCCE Internet of Things (IoT): Challenges and Future Directions. *International Journal of Advanced Research in Computer and Communication Engineering*, *5*. Advance online publication. doi:10.17148/IJARCCE.2016.53226

Raja Singh, R., Yash, S. M., Shubham, S. C., Indragandhi, V., Vijayakumar, V., Saravanan, P., & Subhramaniya, S. (2020). IoT embedded cloud-based intelligent power quality monitoring system for industrial drive application. *Future Generation Computer Systems*, *112*, 884–898. doi:10.1016/j.future.2020.06.032

Rajeswari, S. V. K. R., & Vijayakumar, P. (2021). Prediction of Diabetes Mellitus Using Machine Learning Algorithm. *Annals of the Romanian Society for Cell Biology*, 5655–5662. https://www.annalsofrscb.ro/index.php/journal/article/view/6653

Ramesh, S., & Perros, H. G. (2000). A multilayer client-server queueing network model with synchronous and asynchronous messages. *IEEE Transactions on Software Engineering*, *26*(11), 1086–1100. doi:10.1109/32.881719

Reports, V. (n.d.). *Streaming Analytics Market is Projected to Reach USD 52,190.0 Million by 2027 at CAGR 26.8% | Valuates Reports*. Retrieved October 14, 2021, from www.prnewswire.com website: https://www.prnewswire.com/news-releases/streaming-analytics-market-is-projected-to-reach-usd-52-190-0-million-by-2027-at-cagr-26-8--valuates-reports-301287553.html

Sadoughi, F., Behmanesh, A., & Sayfouri, N. (2020). Internet of things in medicine: A systematic mapping study. *Journal of Biomedical Informatics*, *103*, 103383. doi:10.1016/j.jbi.2020.103383 PMID:32044417

Sciarrone, A., Bisio, I., Garibotto, C., Lavagetto, F., Staude, G. H., & Knopp, A. (2021). Leveraging IoT Wearable Technology Towards Early Diagnosis of Neurological Diseases. *IEEE Journal on Selected Areas in Communications*, *39*(2), 582–592. doi:10.1109/JSAC.2020.3021573

Szablewski, L., & Sulima, A. (2017). The structural and functional changes of blood cells and molecular components in diabetes mellitus. *Biological Chemistry*, *398*(4), 411–423. doi:10.1515/hsz-2016-0196 PMID:27768581

Tawalbeh, L. A., Mehmood, R., Benkhlifa, E., & Song, H. (2016). Mobile Cloud Computing Model and Big Data Analysis for Healthcare Applications. *IEEE Access: Practical Innovations, Open Solutions*, *4*, 6171–6180. doi:10.1109/ACCESS.2016.2613278

Wei, J., & Xu, C.-Z. (2006). eQoS: Provisioning of Client-Perceived End-to-End QoS Guarantees in Web Servers. *IEEE Transactions on Computers*, *55*(12), 1543–1556. doi:10.1109/TC.2006.197

Wu, T., Wu, F., Qiu, C., Redoute, J.-M., & Yuce, M. R. (2020). A Rigid-Flex Wearable Health Monitoring Sensor Patch for IoT-Connected Healthcare Applications. *IEEE Internet of Things Journal*, *7*(8), 1–1. doi:10.1109/JIOT.2020.2977164

Chapter 10
Edge Computing for Secured IoT Analytics on the Cloud

S. Meenakshi Sundaram
GSSS Institute of Engineering and Technology for Women, India

Tejaswini R. Murgod
GSSS Institute of Engineering and Technology for Women, India

ABSTRACT

This chapter provides an insight into building healthcare applications that are deployed in the cloud storage using edge computing and IoT data analytics approaches. Data is collected from environments both within or external to the hospital. The devices that are connected enable the healthcare providers to monitor patients at large distances, manage chronic disease, and manage medication dosages. The data from these devices can be added to clinical research to gain an insight into the participant's experiences. Artificial intelligence techniques like machine learning or deep learning can be employed at the edge of the networks for IoT analytics of multiple data streams in online mode. The industrial edge computing is growing rapidly from 7% in 2019 to being expected to reach approximately 16% by 2025. The total market for intelligent industrial edge computing that includes hardware, software, services has reached \$11.6B in 2019 and is expected to increase to \$30.8B by 2025.

INTRODUCTION

Employing Cloud computing approach we process the data in a centralized cloud environment or data centers. In edge computing we use a distributed approach for data processing and analytics in an IoT network that includes smart objects or edge devices. The smart sensors or actuators present in the smart objects enables data storage and analysis employing artificial intelligence techniques. Employing edge computing it is possible to build health care applications using Internet of Things (IoT) technology. Edge computing streamlines the movement of traffic from IoT devices and implements real-time local data analysis.

DOI: 10.4018/978-1-7998-9132-1.ch010

Copyright © 2022, IGI Global. Copying or distributing in print or electronic forms without written permission of IGI Global is prohibited.

The data processing in IoT devices is carried out in the places where it is created instead of moving the data to remote data centres or the cloud. Geographically distributed medical care centres are benefited with the use of edge computing. Computation efficiency is improved in edge computing with reduced response time in milliseconds and also conserves the network resources. Edge computing employing AI techniques provide higher safety and security levels. With enhanced security features and edge AI-powered devices the risk is minimized. The Internet of Things, as it relates to healthcare, allows for real-time data monitoring and analysis using medical devices and wearables connected to a network. The internet-enabled medical monitoring devices found in hospital rooms to wearable devices such as fitness trackers provide vast information streams, with a vast exponential data growth. Edge gateways reduce transfer and storage costs of large data sets by locally processing, buffering, filtering, and securing data. There are seven key characteristics that make modern edge computing more intelligent are open architectures, data pre-processing and filtering, edge analytics, distributed applications, consolidated workloads, scalable deployment / management and secure connectivity.

The primary reason why the edge has become so popular in recent years is because the "edge" as we know it is becoming increasingly intelligent. This "intelligent edge" opens up a whole new set of opportunities for software applications and disrupts some of today's edge to cloud architectures on all the layers of the edge. This according to IoT Analytics' latest research on Industrial IoT edge computing. According to the report, intelligent edge computing resources have replaced "dumb" legacy edge computing resources at an increasing pace. The former makes up a small portion of the market today but is expected to grow much faster than the overall market and thus gain share on the latter. The hype about edge computing is warranted because the replacement of "dumb" edge computing with intelligent edge computing has major implications for various industrial applications including health care.

The benefits of switching from "dumb" to "intelligent" edge computing architectures include an increase in system flexibility, functionality, scalability and in many cases a dramatic reduction in costs. It was analyzed that employing edge computing, there is almost 92% reduction in industrial automation costs by switching to intelligent edge hardware. Cisco was an early thought leader in conceptualizing the term "fog computing" and developing IoT solutions designed to run there. For instance, a telecommunications provider may view the edge as the micro datacenter located at the base of a 5G cell tower (often referred to as "Mobile Edge Computing" or MEC), while a manufacturing end user may view the edge as the vision sensor at the end of the assembly line.

The definitions are different because the goal / purpose of hosting workloads at the edge are different: the telecommunications provider tries to optimize data consumption i.e. performance issues associated with consumers of the data), while the manufacturing end user is trying to optimize data generation (i.e. performance issues associated with transmitting and analyzing the data). IoT Analytics defines edge computing as a term used to describe intelligent computational resources located close to the source of data consumption or generation.

BACKGROUND

There are three types of edges namely thick edge, thin edge and micro edge. The thick edge describes compute resources (typically located within a data center) which are equipped with components designed to handle compute intensive tasks / workloads (e.g., high-end CPUs, GPUs, FGPAs, etc.) such as data storage and analysis. There are two types of computational resources located at the "thick" edge, which is typically located 100m to approximately 40 km from the data source. A Cell tower data centre has rack-based computing resources that are located at the base of cell towers. On major data centers, the rack-based computing resources are located at the same physical location as the sensors generate the data.

Thin edge describes the intelligent controllers, networking equipment and computers that aggregate data from the sensors / devices generating data. "Thin edge" compute resources are typically equipped with middle-tier processors and sometimes include AI components such as GPUs or ASICs. There are 3 types of computing resources located at the "thin" edge, which is typically located at 1m to 1km from the data source namely Computers, which are generic compute resources located outside of the data center, networking equipment, which are intelligent routers, switches, gateways and other communications hardware primarily used for connecting other types of compute resources and Controllers, which are intelligent for controlling the processes.

The Micro edge describes the intelligent sensors / devices that generate data. "Micro edge" devices are typically equipped with low-end processors (e.g., Arm Cortex M3) due to constraints related to costs and power consumption. Since computing resources located at the "micro edge" are the data generating devices themselves, the distance from the compute resource is essentially zero. One type of compute resource is found at the micro edge are sensors / devices, which are physical pieces of hardware that generate data and / or actuate physical objects. They are located at the very farthest edge in any architecture. Modern intelligent edge computing architectures are the driving force behind the move to more edge computing and the value-creating use cases associated with the edge.

Characteristics of Intelligent Edge Computing

The figure 1 given below describes the seven characteristics of intelligent edge computing that include open architectures, data pre-processing and filtering, edge analytics, distributed applications, consolidated workloads, scalable deployment/management and secure connectivity.

1. Open Architectures:

The proprietary protocols and closed architectures have been a common place in edge environments for decades. However, these have often proven to lead to high integration and switching costs as vendors lock-in their customers. Modern, intelligent edge computing resources deploy open architectures that leverage standardized protocols and semantic data structures that reduce integration costs and increase vendor interoperability.

2. Data Pre-Processing and Filtering

Transmitting and storing data generated by legacy edge computing resources in the cloud can be very expensive and inefficient. Legacy architectures often rely on poll / response setups in which a remote server requests a value from the "dumb" edge computing resource on a time-interval, regardless of whether or not the value has changed. Intelligent edge computing resources can pre-process data at the edge and only send relevant information to the cloud, which reduces data transmission and storage costs. An example of data pre-processing and filtering is an intelligent edge computing device running an edge agent that pre-processes data at the edge before sending it to the cloud, thus reducing bandwidth costs.

Figure 1. Seven characteristics of intelligent edge computing

1 Open architectures
2 Data pre-processing and filtering
3 Edge analytics
4 Distributed applications
5 Consolidated workloads
6 Scalable deployment / management
7 Secure connectivity

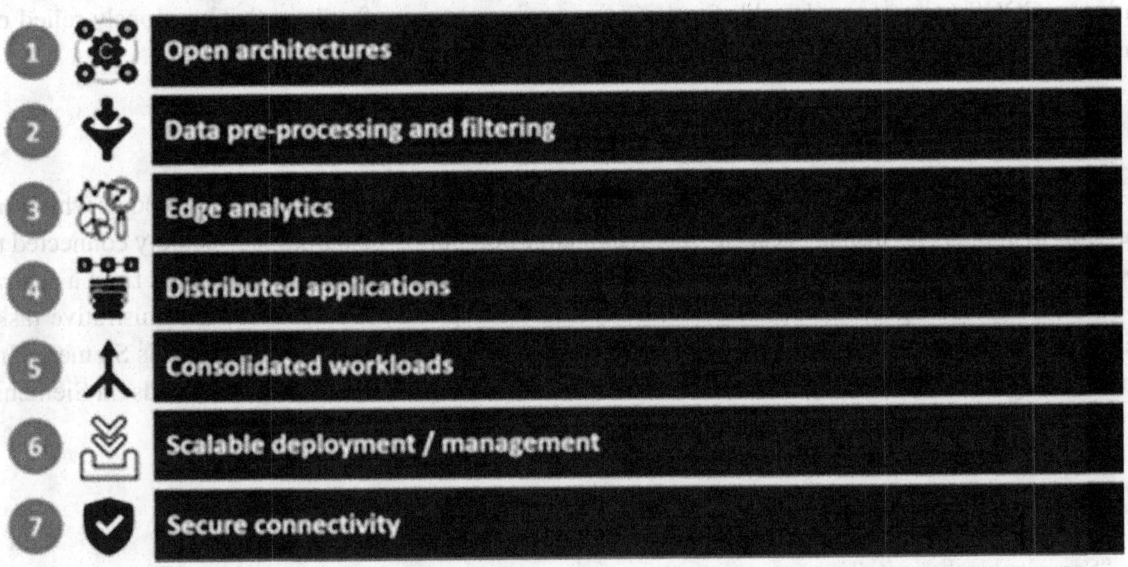

3. Edge Analytics

Most legacy edge computing resources have limited processing power and can only perform one specific task / function (e.g., sensors ingest data, controllers control processes, etc.). Intelligent edge computing resources typically have more powerful processing capabilities designed to analyze data at the edge. These edge analytics applications enable new use cases that rely on low-latency and high data throughput. The networks facilitate the sharing of knowledge between intelligent edge sensors and allow end users to build predictive maintenance solutions based on advanced anomaly detection algorithms.

4. Distributed Applications

The applications that run on legacy edge computing devices are often tightly coupled to the hardware on which they run. Intelligent edge computing resources de-couple applications from the underlying hardware and enable flexible architectures in which applications can move from one intelligent compute resource to another. This de-coupling enables applications to move both vertically (e.g., from the intelligent edge computing resource to the cloud) and horizontally (e.g., from one intelligent edge computing resource to another) as needed.

5. Consolidated Workload

Most "dumb" edge computing resources run proprietary applications on top of proprietary RTOSs (real-time operating system) which are installed directly on the compute resource itself. Intelligent edge computing resources are often equipped with hypervisors which abstract the operating system and application from the underlying hardware. This enables an intelligent edge computing resource to run multiple operating systems and applications on a single edge device. This leads to workload consolidation, which reduces the physical footprint of the computing resources required at the edge and can result in lower COGS (cost of goods sold) for device or equipment manufacturers that previously relied on multiple physical compute resources.

6. Scalable Deployment / Management

Legacy computing resources often use serial (often proprietary) communication protocols which are difficult to update and manage at scale. Intelligent edge computing resources are securely connected to local or wide area networks (LAN, WAN) and can thus be easily deployed and managed from a central location. Edge management platforms are increasingly being used to handle the administrative tasks associated with large scale deployments. An example of an edge management platform is Siemens' Industrial Edge Management System, which is used for deploying and managing workloads on Siemens' intelligent edge computing resources.

7. Secure Connectivity

"Security by obscurity" is a common practice for securing legacy computing devices. These legacy devices often have proprietary communication protocols and serial networking interfaces, which do add a layer of "security by obscurity"; however, this type of security comes at a cost of much higher management and integration costs. Advancements in cyber security technology are making it easier and safer than ever to securely connect intelligent devices. Different levels of security can be provided throughout the product lifecycle depending on the specific needs of the application.

ROLE OF EDGE AND CLOUD COMPUTING IN HEALTHCARE

Edge allows us to manage your connectivity and disperse processing closer to where data is, the advantage is a natural evolution when we optimize some part of our stack in the network with giving more localized services for your application. Moving the analysis of clinical information to edge computing is crucial for healthcare organizations that want to benefit from going digital and the key to digital healthcare Analytics. For example, in the hospital, we collect data from IoT devices, which is monitoring patients and transfer it to the trust's Electronic Health Record (EHR) from the bedside, with the authentication of staff to the IoT devices through proximity cards.

Edge computing entails processing and analyzing data closer to the source of where that data is collected. Instead of a device or sensor sending all of its data over the internet to the cloud or an on-premise data center, it can process this data itself, essentially becoming its own mini data center and deliver this data to a nearby computing device, such as a gateway networking device, a computer, or micro data center for analysis. This is sometimes called fog computing, though edge and fog computing are often used interchangeably. With this new kind of architecture, a vast amount of processing power becomes decentralized from cloud service providers, which can help increase the speed of data analysis and decrease the load placed on internet networks to transmit huge amounts of data.

Edge-computing architectures for IoT are classified according to different factors such as data placement, orchestration services, security and big data (Salam, H. & Moussa, A., 2020). Edge computing solves a few problems related to the transfer of data for IoT technologies, like latency, reduced load on networks, privacy and security, reduced data management costs, and disaster recovery. Latency refers to the time taken to process and analyze the captured data. The latency issue is also extremely important in other time-sensitive situations such as emergency response and patient care. In these scenarios, the ability to process data faster can be the difference between life and death. According to the Cisco Global Cloud Index, the amount of traffic running through cloud computing networks has increased to 14.1 ZB (a trillion gigabytes) per year in 2020. Some of the data-transfer load can be removed from the cloud by processing some of this data closer to where it's collected. Additionally, moving the processing of data away from the cloud can help minimize the network load in places where internet connectivity is not that strong.

Storing large amounts of data in the cloud can be cost prohibitive and downloading this data from the cloud can have high costs as well. Additionally, the more data that we transfer to the cloud, the higher bandwidth costs we will have to pay. As the volume of data collected continues to increase, it makes less sense to copy huge amounts of data from one system to another to process and analyze it, if you don't have to. Storing and analyzing some of this data at the edge might help to cut down on these costs. Only the data that needs to be analyzed in aggregate can be transferred to the cloud. Other devices and IT assets will remain operational if one fails.

The decentralization of computing power that edge networks provide will assure you that if one edge device fails, other nodes and associated IT assets will remain operational. This is similar to the cloud disaster recovery strategy of using multiple Availability Zones and Regions to ensure that your data and applications aren't lost in the event of a catastrophe.

Additionally, edge computing can actually be a form of disaster recovery in the case of an internet outage due to a natural disaster.

While security used to be a primary concern in moving to cloud computing, that fear has largely subsided. The concern isn't so much with the storage of data in the cloud, but more about the transfer of data over a network to the cloud. Especially in situations where devices collect sensitive personal data such as health metrics or location data, the transmission of this data can have privacy, legal, and security ramifications. The various regulations in different countries and regions makes this more complicated. Thus, storing some of this data in or closer to the devices may improve privacy and security. The other side of the security argument is that the edge devices themselves may be more susceptible to a breach. This may be true, so it's important that you take steps to ensure the security of your edge devices, such as encrypting your data, tightly controlling access, and securing the networks.

Even as more data processing and analysis is moved to the edge, cloud computing will still play a big role in making IoT devices smarter and better. There can be a lot of value in aggregating the data collected locally and analyzing it to come up with overarching insights that can be sent back to and shared across all sensors. The cloud is better suited to perform heavier analyses like looking at historical events and very large datasets. Many times the centralized nature and raw computing power of the cloud outperforms decentralized edge networks in terms of speed, scalability, and costs.

So while edge devices may carry the burden of real-time functional analysis, the cloud will shoulder the load of strategic, high-level insight creation to improve the operation of these devices. While edge computing certainly provides many benefits to IoT-based networks, it does add some complexity to architecture and operations. To take full advantage of setting up a combination of edge and cloud computing networks we need to understand the data analysis needs in order to create network architecture. If some of the data is going to be processed and analyzed by the devices that collect it (pure edge computing), and the rest will be sent to the cloud for analysis, then it's a relatively easy architecture. Else to apply fog computing, where there may be intermediate nodes between the edge devices and the cloud, then the architecture may be a bit more complicated.

A cloud computing architecture needs to handle the aggregation and processing of the large amount of data that your IoT network will generate. Setting up the right databases, server types, load balancers, and other cloud components will be important in ensuring an efficient data aggregation and analysis process are the major challenges. After the network architecture has been designed (and eventually implemented), well-defined data policies must be created. These policies include:

- What kind of data will be processed and analyzed at the edge, and what will be sent to the cloud
- Who is authorized to access what types of data
- Data backup schedules for business continuity and disaster recovery

To take advantage of all of the data collected the analytics team, tools, and processes need to be in place.

This includes answers to queries like:

- Who is responsible for moving the data between which repositories?
- What analytics team members will be responsible for what kind of analyses on which types of data?
- What tools will your analytics team use to perform these analyses?
- What are the business goals you'll achieve with your analytics program?

The data is only as good as the insights that can be gleaned from it. So it's important to have top-notch data analysts, tools, and processes in place to garner this knowledge.

As IoT becomes more pervasive, edge computing will do the same. IoT security includes comprehensive security architecture, firewalls, intrusion detection systems, authentication and authorization mechanisms, as well as privacy-preserving designs (Kewei, Sha. & Andrew, Yang, 2020). The ability to analyze data closer to the source will minimize latency, reduce the load on the internet, improve privacy and security, and lower data management costs. The cloud will continue to play a critical role in aggregating important data and performing analyses on this massive set of information to glean insights that can be distributed back to the edge devices. The combination of edge and cloud computing will help to better manage and analyze data and significantly increase the value of your IoT efforts.

The healthcare industry is developing and changing at an incredible rate, with technology becoming the driving force. Yet, the workloads and emerging technology above only touch the surface of what Health IT and medical professionals are experiencing. Technology enables to leap forward in the way healthcare professionals deliver patient care. From quickly pulling up patient health records to sequencing genomes, to digitizing pathology slides, technology is driving progress forward. Data managed in the healthcare industry has grown by 878% from 2016 to 2018 (Source: 2019 Dell EMC Global Data Protection Index Survey)

The average number of connected devices per hospital bed in the U.S. is 10 to 15.1. The intelligent industrial edge computing market is estimated to reach $30.8B by 2025, up from $11.6B in 2020. The Information Technology and Operational Technology architectures have evolving quickly. Organizations that manage physical assets can reap tremendous cost savings and unlock new opportunities by switching to modern, intelligent edge computing architectures. IoT in healthcare has led to a massive amount of data production. In 2020, McKinsey estimated that medical data has doubled every 73 days. To secure IoT services, reliable backup security solutions should be designed in case of failures of Machine Learning based schemes (Zhanyang, Xu. & Wentao, Liu, 2020). Artificial Intelligence (AI) and Machine Learning (ML) make a substantial impact on the speed in which the data is collected and analyzed. Deep Learning thrives off processing more and more data and continues to learn, making algorithms even smarter. The intelligent industrial edge computing will make up an increasingly large share of the overall industrial automation market, growing from ~7% of the overall market in 2019 to ~16% by 2025.

The total market for intelligent industrial edge computing (hardware, software, services) that has reached $11.6B in 2019 is expected to increase to $30.8B by 2025. Also, with real-time information, the increasing unstructured data of which sensor and IoT data are part, traditional approaches does not meet the requirements which are needed. There are various scenarios where speed and high-speed data are the main components for management, power issues, analytics, and real-time need, etc. helps to process data with edge computing in IoT.

EDGE IOT SMART HEALTHCARE ARCHITECTURE

Edge-based IoT healthcare frameworks generally involve remote monitoring systems that exploit different types of smart sensors for the implementation of healthcare systems that are diagnostic, sensitive, and preventive (Akmandor A.O. & Jha .N.K. 2017, Hossain M. & Muhammad. G 2014, Muhammad. G, et al., Masud . M et al., 2012). In most recent studies, fog computing nodes work as local servers: they gather, analyze, and process health IoT sensor data and give rapid-response services (Tang. W & Shen X.S., 2019). For many years, healthcare researchers have been exploring solutions for the remote monitoring of patients and for the transmission of health reports to provide clinicians with patient data in real time. Recent advances in IoT technology have opened a door for intelligent solutions that take advantage of software platforms and system architectures. These solutions, such as for monitoring chronic illness, epidemic surveillance and control, elderly and pediatric care, and management of health and fitness (Alhussein. M & Muhammad. G 2018 , El-Latif. A, et al. 2018, Ali ,Z & Alhamid. M.F 2017 , Muhammad .M, et al. 2011, Hossain. M.S & Muhammad. G 2020, Ghoneim. A, et al.2018), are intended to resolve healthcare issues at various levels. A general edge/fog computing-based approach uses architecture with multiple levels (Al-Fuqaha. A & Ayyash .M , 2015) :

1. Level-1 for edge nodes, where data are collected from IoT body sensors. Low-level processing takes place in hand-held or portable devices like smart watches, smart phones, tablets, or embedded devices or local gateway devices.
2. Level-2 for fog nodes, where data are collected from IoT field sensors or edge devices. Storage and local processing are performed here using servers or PCs.
3. Level-3 for cloud processing, where all the data are gathered and stored. High-level processing takes place here, including the application of sophisticated algorithms and data analysis.

It is not necessary that all three levels of edge architecture are contained simultaneously in the same architecture. In non-dynamic solutions, fog nodes can be used to collect data directly from sensors, and they may be assisted by cloud service providers. Similarly, edge devices explicitly interact with cloud providers in certain complex dyn1mic situations where a fog level cannot be enforced.

EDGE INTELLIGENCE IN IOT HEALTHCARE FRAMEWORKS

While edge computing strives to combine various types of edge devices and servers that can collaborate for the efficient processing of locally generated data, edge intelligence strives to embed AI and cognitive intelligence related to human behavior into edge architectures. Using intelligent AI-based edge in IoT architectures does not necessarily mean that the AI techniques are totally trained and analyzed at the edge layer; they may also involve a collaboration of cloud, fog, and edge computing. The innovation and advancement in IoT devices have made it possible to achieve the Internet of Everything (IoE) (Miraz M.H. & Picking, R. 2015). Huge cloud data centers are distributed worldwide, hence edge intelligence is all the more necessary for processing so much information. AI techniques can be implemented with edge computing using many new platforms and scenarios, such as Industry 4.0, tactile internet, Healthcare 2.0, advanced DL, and territorial control, which could be embedded in IoT healthcare platforms to connect them with humans, which makes information more relevant and intelligible (Mallardi, G & Bellifemine, F. 2017). Similarly, for smart city healthcare applications like AAL (Lin. K , et al., 2019) edge intelligence is proposed to offer healthcare systems based on intelligent agents. These agents can manage the environment according to the situation, provide contextual support to users, adapt to user's preferences, and monitor and control the environment automatically. Intelligent edge platforms are also used in proposals for smart telemedicine systems (Mallardi, G & Bellifemine, F. 2017), and for providing treatment, disease prevention and detection, and medical support to patients using advanced wearable sensors for real time patient monitoring. Fog-based data analytics (Rahmani, A.M & Liljeberg, P., 2018) was also proposed in a recent study for a smart healthcare framework. One study even proposed a cloud-to-fog architecture (Nandyala, C.S. & Kim, H.K. , 2016) for healthcare where intelligent edge nodes were placed in smart hospitals and homes, which made remote interaction easy. Another study used edge intelligence to build a real-time health data gathering and analysis system (Kumari, A & Kumar, N., 2018), for which it proposed a three-layer patient-driven healthcare architecture for real-time data collection, processing, and transmission. This system provides insight into the application of fog nodes and servers in a Healthcare 4.0 environment. An ECG based intelligent edge cognitive framework (Modgil, S., 2009) was also proposed for real-time health monitoring. Cognitive intelligence makes the proposed edge computing system smarter, and allows for optimized resource allocation. Hence edge intelligence is now an element of state-of-the-art IoT healthcare architectures that aim to work with more intelligence, reliability, privacy, and efficiency.

MACHINE LEARNING (ML) AND IOT IN HEALTHCARE FRAMEWORKS

Machine Learning has been applied for multiple applications and domains by a number of researchers all over the world. The use of Machine Learning in the healthcare IoT domain has seen huge interests from researchers recently. Machine Learning helps in remote and real-time monitoring, and treatment of diseases in the H-IoT framework. It has also been used in Assistive Systems to rehabilitate patients after accidents. Machine Learning has been very popular in diagnosis and prediction of cardiac arrest in heart patients, using IoT based smart sensors (Ram S.S. & Shiratori, 2019) In heart patients the ECG signal is monitored continuously and after noise filtering it is sent to Machine Learning algorithms for feature extraction (Ram S.S. & Shiratori, 2019). In the field of Ambient Assisted Living (AAL), there are many applications of machine learning for IoT based healthcare scenarios. Machine Learning has been used for fall detection of patients employing edge and cloud computing architecture (Queralta J.P & Westerlund T. (2019). In AAL domain ML has also been used by researchers for patient's sleep pattern monitoring. For analyzing sleep patterns, a multi-modal data is employed consisting of EEG, ECG, or EOG. With the development and advancements in the field of prosthetics, now Machine Learning is being used for aiding and rehabilitation after accidents or trauma. Deep learning has revolutionized the way Brain-Computer Interfacing (BCI) systems are being developed to improve quality of human life and for providing smart cognitive healthcare. Deep learning is being used to interpret brain patterns by analyzing EEG signals and convert the thought processes to speech (Satija U. & Manikandan M.S., 2017). It is also being used for emotion recognition and classification thereby making machines aware of human emotions. It has enabled humans to control robots using their brains without doing any action. Hence Machine Learning based IoT healthcare systems are being used to help patients with severe disabilities to lead a normal life (Mathur N & Glesk I, 2016).

BIG DATA AND BLOCKCHAIN IN IOT-BASED HEALTHCARE FRAMEWORKS

An enormous amount of data is being generated at every moment, especially in an IoT network. Hence, the processing such a large amount of data needs intensive processing capabilities. Many big data analytics techniques have been suggested in the literature for real-time IoT frameworks. (Verma .S & Kato. N 2017, Ahmed E. et al., (2017), but the need for QoS has not been properly addressed. Machine and Deep Learning (DL) techniques combine with IoT architecture to boost big data processing ability, and advanced DL models in particular are extremely powerful for managing such data (Hossain M. S., et al., 2019). Deep Learning has been applied by researchers for various types of medical big data, including data from wearable body sensors and HER data (Amin S. U., et al., 2019), In order to solve the issues related to big data, IoT health systems can implement block chain to maintain data privacy and safeguard patient's interests. Block chain has helped in the deployment of critical services in IoT healthcare architecture, but challenges like scalability, storage, and combined operation are a major concern (Panarello A. & Puliafito A. 2018 , Xie et al. J. 2019, Makdoom I. & No W.,2019, Hossain M. S. & Muhammad G. 2018). The main healthcare application of block chain is providing access and storage control for private medical information (Xie et al. J., 2019). However, the advantages of block chain have not been realized to the full for IoT healthcare systems

CONCLUSION

The advanced health care equipment generate large amounts of data which include health records, medical imaging and analytical data that are being sent from edge, Internet of Things (IoT) devices and also wearable devices. Edge allows us to manage your connectivity and disperse processing closer to where data is, the advantage is a natural evolution when we optimize some part of our stack in the network with giving more localized services for your application. Moving the analysis of clinical information to edge computing is crucial for healthcare organizations that want to benefit from going digital and the key to digital healthcare Analytics, for example, in the hospital, we collect data from IoT devices, which is monitoring patients and transfer it to the trust's Electronic Health Record (EHR) from the bedside, with the authentication of staff to the IoT devices through proximity cards.

There are seven key characteristics that make modern edge computing more intelligent are open architectures, data pre-processing and filtering, edge analytics, distributed applications, consolidated workloads, scalable deployment / management and secure connectivity. Modern, intelligent edge computing resources deploy open architectures that leverage standardized protocols and semantic data structures that reduce integration costs and increase vendor interoperability. Advancements in cyber security technology are making it easier and safer than ever to securely connect intelligent devices. Different levels of security can be provided throughout the product lifecycle depending on the specific needs of the application.

A cloud computing architecture needs to handle the aggregation and processing of the large amount of data that your IoT network will generate. Setting up the right databases, server types, load balancers, and other cloud components will be important in ensuring an efficient data aggregation and analysis process are the major challenges. As IoT becomes more pervasive, edge computing will do the same. The ability to analyze data closer to the source will minimize latency, reduce the load on the internet, improve privacy and security, and lower data management costs. The cloud will continue to play a critical role in aggregating important data and performing analyses on this massive set of information to glean insights that can be distributed back to the edge devices. The combination of edge and cloud computing will help to better manage and analyze data and significantly increase the value of your IoT efforts.

Data managed in the healthcare industry has grown by 878% from 2016 to 2018 (Source: 2019 Dell EMC Global Data Protection Index Survey). The average number of connected devices per hospital bed in the U.S. is 10 to 15.1. The intelligent industrial edge computing market is estimated to reach $30.8B by 2025, up from $11.6B in 2020. The Information Technology and Operational Technology architectures have evolving quickly. Organizations that manage physical assets can reap tremendous cost savings and unlock new opportunities by switching to modern, intelligent edge computing architectures. In 2020, McKinsey estimated that medical data has doubled every 73 days. Artificial Intelligence (AI) and Machine Learning (ML) make a substantial impact on the speed in which the data is collected and analyzed. Deep Learning thrives off processing more and more data and continues to learn, making algorithms even smarter. The intelligent industrial edge computing will make up an increasingly large share of the overall industrial automation market, growing from ~7% of the overall market in 2019 to ~16% by 2025. Also, with real-time information, the increasing unstructured data of which sensor and IoT data are part, traditional approaches does not meet the requirements which are needed. There are various scenarios where speed and high-speed data are the main components for management, power issues, analytics, and real-time need, etc. helps to process data with edge computing in IoT.

REFERENCES

Ahmed, E., Yaqoob, I., Hashem, I. A. T., Khan, I., Ahmed, A. I. A., Imran, M., & Vasilakos, A. V. (2017). The role of big data analytics in Internet of Things. *Computer Networks*, *129*(2), 459–471. doi:10.1016/j.comnet.2017.06.013

Akmandor, A. O., & Jha, N. K. (2017). Smart health care: An edge-side computing perspective. *IEEE Consum. Electron. Mag.*, *7*(1), 29–37. doi:10.1109/MCE.2017.2746096

Al-Fuqaha, A., & Ayyash, M. (2015). Internet of things: A survey on enabling technologies, protocols, and applications. *IEEE Communications Surveys and Tutorials*, *17*(4), 2347–2376. doi:10.1109/COMST.2015.2444095

Alhussein, M., & Muhammad, G. (2018). Voice Pathology Detection Using Deep Learning on Mobile Healthcare Framework. *IEEE Access : Practical Innovations, Open Solutions*, *6*, 41034–44104. doi:10.1109/ACCESS.2018.2856238

Ali, Z., & Alhamid, M. F. (2017). An Automatic Health Monitoring System for Patients Suffering from Voice Complications in Smart Cities. *IEEE Access : Practical Innovations, Open Solutions*, *5*(1), 3900–3908. doi:10.1109/ACCESS.2017.2680467

Amin, S. U., Alsulaiman, M., Muhammad, G., Mekhtiche, M. A., & Shamim Hossain, M. (2019). Deep Learning for EEG motor imagery classification based on multi-layer CNNs feature fusion. *Future Generation Computer Systems*, *101*, 542–554. doi:10.1016/j.future.2019.06.027

El-Latif, A., Abd-El-Atty, B., Hossain, M. S., Elmougy, S., & Ghoneim, A. (2018). Secure Quantum Steganography Protocol for Fog Cloud Internet of Things. *IEEE Access : Practical Innovations, Open Solutions*, *6*, 10332–10340. doi:10.1109/ACCESS.2018.2799879

Ghoneim, A., Muhammad, G., Amin, S. U., & Gupta, B. (2018). Medical image forgery detection for smart healthcare. *IEEE Communications Magazine*, *56*(4), 33–37. doi:10.1109/MCOM.2018.1700817

Hossain, M., & Muhammad, G. (2014). Cloud-Based Collaborative Media Service Framework for HealthCare. International Journal of Distributed Sensor Networks. doi:10.1155/2014/858712

Hossain, M. S. (2019). Applying Deep Learning for Epilepsy Seizure Detection and Brain Mapping Visualization. ACM Trans. Multimedia Comput. Commun. Appl., 15(1S). doi:10.1145/3241056

Hossain, M. S., & Muhammad, G. (2020). Deep Learning Based Pathology Detection for Smart Connected Healthcare. *IEEE Network*, *34*(6), 120–125. doi:10.1109/MNET.011.2000064

Kumari, A., & Kumar, N. (2018). Fog computing for healthcare 4.0 environment: Opportunities and challenges. *Computers & Electrical Engineering*, *72*, 1–13. doi:10.1016/j.compeleceng.2018.08.015

Lin, K., Li, C., Tian, D., Ghoneim, A., Hossain, M. S., & Amin, S. U. (2019). Artificial-Intelligence-Based Data Analytics for Cognitive Communication in Heterogeneous Wireless Networks. *IEEE Wireless Communications*, *26*(3), 83–89. doi:10.1109/MWC.2019.1800351

Mallardi, G., & Bellifemine, F. (2017). Telemedicine solutions and services: a new challenge that supports active participation of patients. *i-CiTies 2017 (3rd CINI Annual Conference on ICT for Smart Cities & Communities)*.

Masud, M., Hossain, M. S., & Alamri, A. (2012). Data Interoperability and Multimedia Content Management in e-Health Systems. *IEEE Transactions on Information Technology in Biomedicine*, *16*(6), 1015–1023. doi:10.1109/TITB.2012.2202244 PMID:22677322

Mathur, N., & Glesk, I. (2016). A practical design and implementation of a low cost platform for remote monitoring of lower limb health of amputees in the developing world. *IEEE Access : Practical Innovations, Open Solutions*, *4*, 7440–7451. doi:10.1109/ACCESS.2016.2622163

Miraz, M. H., & Picking, R. (2015). *A review on internet of things (IoT), internet of everything (IoE) and internet of nano things (IoNT). In 2015 Internet Technologies and Applications*. ITA. doi:10.1109/ITechA.2015.7317398

Modgil, S. (2009). Reasoning about preferences in argumentation frameworks. *Artificial Intelligence, 173*(9), 901–934. doi:10.1016/j.artint.2009.02.001

Muhammad, G., Hossain, M. S., & Kumar, N. (2021, February). EEG-Based Pathology Detection for Home Health Monitoring. *IEEE Journal on Selected Areas in Communications, 39*(2), 603–610. Advance online publication. doi:10.1109/JSAC.2020.3020654

Muhammad, M. (2011). Formant analysis in dysphonic patients and automatic Arabic digit speech recognition. *Biomedical Engineering*. PMID:21624137

Nandyala, C. S., & Kim, H. K. (2016). From cloud to fog and iot-based real-time u-healthcare monitoring for smart homes and hospitals. *International Journal of Smart Home, 10*(2), 187–196. doi:10.14257/ijsh.2016.10.2.18

Panarello, A., & Puliafito, A. (2018). Blockchain and IoT integration: A systematic survey. *Sensors (Basel), 18*(8), 2575. doi:10.339018082575 PMID:30082633

Queralta, J. P., & Westerlund, T. (2019). Edge-AI in lorabased health monitoring: Fall detection system with fog computing and LSTM recurrent neural networks. In *2019 42nd International Conference on Telecommunications and Signal Processing (TSP)*. IEEE.

Rahmani, A. M., & Liljeberg, P. (2018). Exploiting smart e-health gateways at the edge of healthcare internetof-things: A fog computing approach. *Future Generation Computer Systems, 78*, 641–658. doi:10.1016/j.future.2017.02.014

Ram, S. S., & Shiratori. (2019). A machine learning framework for edge computing to improve prediction accuracy in mobile health monitoring. In *International Conference on Computational Science and Its Applications*. Springer. 10.1007/978-3-030-24302-9_30

Salam, H., & Moussa, A. (2020). Edge-Computing Architectures for Internet of Things Applications: A Survey. *Sensors (Basel), 1*(20), 1–52.

Satija, U., & Manikandan, M. S. (2017). Real-time signal qualityaware ECG telemetry system for IoT-based health care monitoring. *IEEE Internet of Things Journal, 4*(3), 815–823. doi:10.1109/JIOT.2017.2670022

Sha, K., Yang, T. A., Wei, W., & Davari, S. (2020). A survey of edge computing-based designs for IoT security. *Digital Communications and Networks, 6*(2), 195–202. doi:10.1016/j.dcan.2019.08.006

Tang, W., & Shen, X. S. (2019). Fogenabled smart health: Toward cooperative and secure healthcare service provision. *IEEE Communications Magazine, 57*(5), 42–48. doi:10.1109/MCOM.2019.1800234

Verma, S., & Kato, N. (2017). A survey on network methodologies for real-time analytics of massive IoT data and open research issues. *IEEE Commun. Surveys Tuts., 19*(3), 1457–1477. doi:10.1109/COMST.2017.2694469

Xie, J. (2019). A survey of blockchain technology applied to smart cities: Research issues and challenges. *IEEE Commun. Surveys Tuts., 21*(3), 2794–2830.

Zhanyang, X. & Wentao, L. (2020). Artificial Intelligence for Securing IoT Services in Edge Computing: A Survey. *Security and Communication Networks*, 1–13.

Chapter 11
Automated Early Prediction of Anomalies Due to Diabetes Using Fundus Images

Sharmila Devi Sivakumar
Loyola ICAM College of Engineering and Technology, India

Vaishnavi Seenuvasan
Loyola ICAM College of Engineering and Technology, India

Gunasri B.
Loyola ICAM College of Engineering and Technology, India

Balaji Srinivasan
Loyola ICAM College of Engineering and Technology, India

ABSTRACT

Diabetes is one of the common diseases in the world that cannot be permanently cured, but with proper medication one can lead a long and healthy life by curbing extreme complications. The skills and equipment required to identify the conditions take a longer time to provide an accurate result and are not an affordable means for all the income groups. In order to overcome this issue, an ML model is created and deployed in an application so it will be used by many in predicting the presence of the disease. The chapter focuses on detecting the presence of two major anomalies, namely diabetic retinopathy (DR) and glaucoma, which were caused due to diabetes. All the dataset used for the project is gathered from Kaggle and Messidor. Around six machine learning algorithms that fall under supervised learning techniques are executed. Among the many models, the random forest model has a high accuracy of 73% for DR prediction. Simultaneously, glaucoma detection is performed using different algorithms showing that Naive Bayes has the highest accuracy of 98%.

DOI: 10.4018/978-1-7998-9132-1.ch011

Copyright © 2022, IGI Global. Copying or distributing in print or electronic forms without written permission of IGI Global is prohibited.

INTRODUCTION

Diabetes Mellitus can be categorized into four types, namely Prediabetes, Type I Diabetes, Type II Diabetes and Gestational Diabetes. Severity of diabetes leads to complications such as cardiac arrest, kidney failure, diabetic retinopathy, glaucoma, cataract, macular edema etc. The skills and equipment required to identify the conditions consumes time to provide an accurate result and are not an affordable means for all the income groups. In order to overcome this issue a ML model is created and deployed in an application to benefit many. Identifying eye disease in the initial stage and providing right medication and consultation may save people from blindness and various other risks that damage the eye and vision permanently.

Diabetic Retinopathy

Diabetic Retinopathy is one of the major complications stemming from the presence of diabetes. Improper care of blood sugar levels is one of the major risk factors resulting in damage to the blood vessels present in the retina of the eye. Manual methods in clinics are normally preferred for detecting DR and other eye anomalies. Both type I and II diabetes patients are affected by DR which causes visual impairments as it is a progressive disease. The main source of identifying this disease is through the retina. Retina is the back layer of our eyes where the images take form and it is very important for one to have a healthy retina for good vision.

Initial signs of the condition are floaters, blurriness, dark areas of vision and difficulty perceiving colours. Mild cases can be treated with proper diabetes management while advanced cases need laser treatment or surgery. Early prediction of this disease can add great advantage in preventing blindness. By applying appropriate machine learning algorithms accurate prediction of the presence of Diabetic Retinopathy can be done.

Around four hundred and twenty million people worldwide are diagnosed with diabetes mellitus. The prevalence of this disease has doubled in the past 30 years and is only expected to increase, particularly in Asia. Of those with diabetes, approximately one-third are expected to be diagnosed with DR. Early detection, which is critical for good prognosis, relies on skilled readers and is both labor and time-intensive. This poses a challenge in areas that traditionally lack access to skilled clinical facilities. Moreover, the manual nature of DR screening methods promotes widespread inconsistency among readers. Finally, given an increase in prevalence of both diabetes and associated retinal complications throughout the world, manual methods of diagnosis may be unable to keep up with demand for screening services.

According to this study, the main cause of DR is the unusual increase of glucose level. The first signals of DR are tiny capillary dilations known as microaneurysms. It states that DR advancement causes neovascularization, macular edema, exudates and also the cotton wool spot at later phase causes retinal segregation. The four stages of DR are classified as:

1. **Mild Nonproliferative Retinopathy:** The earliest stage where microaneurysms occur.
2. **Moderate Nonproliferative Retinopathy:** As the disease advances, few blood vessels that supply the retina are blocked.
3. **Severe Non-proliferative Retinopathy:** More blood vessels are blocked, which reduces blood flow to the areas of the retina. These areas send signals to the body for growth of new blood vessels for nourishment.

4. **Proliferative Retinopathy:** This is the advanced stage, the signals sent by the retina for nourishment trigger the growth of new blood vessels. This condition is called proliferative retinopathy. These new blood vessels are abnormal and fragile. These blood vessels by themselves do not cause symptoms or vision loss. Since they have thin and weak walls., they can leak blood, causing severe vision loss and even blindness can result. The retinal image is a very important diagnostic tool and helps ophthalmologists by analysing using computers to perform diagnosis, treatment, and screening of various epidemic eye diseases including DR.

Glaucoma

Glaucoma is a group of eye conditions that damage the optic nerve located in the back of the eye, the health of which is important for good vision. This damage is often caused by an abnormally high pressure in your eye. This condition in most cases is not detected early on as it produces no symptoms initially but progressively deteriorates side or peripheral vision.

Glaucoma is one of the leading causes for blindness especially in people above the age of 60. The onset can take place during any age but is more common in the aged population. Glaucoma has a tendency to run in families. In some people, scientists have identified genes related to high eye pressure and optic nerve damage.

There are 3 stages of glaucoma:

1. Early Glaucoma:

If the cup to disc ratio is less than 0.29, then the stage of the glaucoma is early.

2. Moderate Glaucoma:

If the cup to disc ratio is above 0.3 and also it should be less than 0.6, then the stage of the glaucoma is moderate.

3. Extreme Glaucoma:

If the cup to disc ratio is more than 0.6, then the stage of the glaucoma is extreme.

RELATED WORKS (Youbi, 2020)

Automated prediction of Diabetic Retinopathy and Glaucoma already exists.

Some of the existing works are:

- Prediction of DR using Machine Learning where an app named "Deep Retina" helps to capture one's own retinal image and get their result immediately by means of a handheld ophthalmoscope.
- The system framework has been designed for DR screening based on AI, Mobile computing, Cloud computing, and Big data analytics which is aimed to benefit people residing at rural areas and also at places where there is lack of medical resources.

- By using a deep learning method the presence of glaucoma is detected, the fundus images of the eye are obtained and the convolution neural network model is created and the accuracy of the model is obtained around 95%.
- The Relevance vector machine method is one of the most used methods to predict glaucoma and it comes under Bayesian and also decision tree models and could obtain the accuracy of about 85% and with support vector machine it provides the accuracy of about 80%.

But there are situations where accurate results are not obtained or missing some important feature values and also times when the prognostic characteristics are not maintained during image augmentation etc.

Hsin-Yi Tsao, Pei-Ying Chan and Emily Chia-Yu Su (Bhatia et al., 2016), applied Machine Learning by creating four different models are the support vector machines, decision trees, artificial neural networks, and logistic regressions developed and in each the accuracy is obtained with which highest accuracy producing model is used for deployment. Support Vector Machine has accuracy which is better than other models. The support vector has high accuracy with 79.5% and 0.839 area under receiver operating characteristic curve. The purpose of creating this model is to give type 2 diabetes mellitus dataset and perform data mining and find high accuracy.

Sejong Oh, Yuli Park, Kyong Jin Cho and Seong Jae Kim (Fong et al., 2004) developed an Machine Learning model in order to predict Glaucoma and its severity, since it is based on classification category, many algorithms to predict the high results like Support Vector Machine (SVM), random forest and XGboost to predict Glaucoma are used. They got a total of 1624 cases which is splitted into 80% training set and 20% test set. On the whole, about 1306 cases were used for creating and developing the prediction models, and the rest of the cases which were about 318 were used for evaluating the model.

Gargeya, R. and Leng, T (Georgescu, 2018), developed a Deep Learning model to predict Diabetic Retinopathy. Around 75137 fundus images were collected from diabetic patients around different hospitals and were split for training and testing the model. The data used were taken from the clinic where the Diabetic Retinopathy was identified. The model achieved a 0.97 AUC with 94% and 98% sensitivity and specificity respectively. MESSIDOR 2 and E-Ophtha databases achieved a 0.94 and 0.95 AUC score duly and this is the best accuracy compared to other models.

Daniele M. S. Barros, Julio C. C. Moura , Cefas R. Freire, Alexandre C. Taleb, Ricardo A. M. Valentim and Philippi S. G. Morais (Gurudath et al., 2014) applied Deep Learning layers to determine every possibility of Glaucoma and the result percentages are found, in specific they implemented Convolutional Neural network layers to get a firm output and prediction. The training data is 80 percent of the dataset and the rest is used for testing to get a good approximation.

De La Torre, J Valls, A. and Puig, D. (Jones & Edwards, 2010) applied the detection of Diabetic Retinopathy by using the Deep Learning interpretable classifier. The model which was created was trained for 300 epochs, reaching out the values of some components QWK value of 0.814 on the validation set. The accuracy of the model they created is 0.857. Deep learning models which have many layers in which the last layer among the input pixels of the analyzed images are obtained. Additional model is created which is 2D-gaussian prior over the RFs.

Martins, J., Cardoso, J.S. and Soares, F (Lam et al., 2018): In this paper the model which is developed using interpretable Computer-Aided Diagnosis (CAD), which will run offline in smart phones we use. Many models are created in Convolutional Neural Networks(CNN) that perform segmentation and classification tasks. These networks are built using pipeline methodology, which achieved 0.91 and 0.75

of Intersection over Union (IoU). and the accuracy of the model developed is of 0.87 with a sensitivity of 0.85 and an AUC of 0.93 were obtained.

Ashish Bora, Siva Balasubramanian, Boris Babenko,Sunny Virmani, Subhashini Venugopalan, Akinori Mitani,Guilherme de Oliveira Marinho,Jorge Cuadros, Paisan Ruamviboonsuk, Greg S Corrado, Lily Peng, Dale R Webster, Avinash V Varadarajan, Naama Hammel, Yun Liu, Pinal Bavishi (Li et al., 2019), applied two different deep learning methods to implement the diabetic retinopathy detection of three-field or one-field colour fundus photographs. 575431 fundus images collected from patients of different race and ethnicity is used as input for the study.

Amitoj Deep Singh, Sourya Sengupta and Vasudevan Lakshminarayanan (Porwal et al., 2018) Explainable AI, applied Deep Learning is one of the most common solutions applied for predicting medical conditions. Though these models give best results the interpretability and black box nature of the algorithm makes it difficult to understand its working. There are studies comparing explainability methods quantitatively which are discussed previously. The quantitative analysis focuses on theoretical correctness and robustness while missing out on actual clinical usefulness. There is a pertinent need to perform end-user based qualitative comparison of explanations for medical imaging applications. This can help to identify the most relevant techniques for explaining decisions to the clinicians. Such studies can be performed using expert agreement where a panel of experts can be asked to rate the explanations.

Filippo Arcadu, Fethallah Benmansour, Andreas Maunz, Jeff Willis, Zdenka Haskova, and Marco Prunotto (Somasundaram & Alli, 2017), applied Machine Learning techniques to find a good working model for Diabetic Retinopathy. The model used here is Deep Convolutional Neural Network(D-CNN) and has the accuracy of nearly 85% and proven to predict the cases accurately. And at the improvising step they used hypertuning to increase the accuracy of the model deployed.

METHODOLOGY

This section highlights the approach proposed in the current work. This section gives us an idea about using supervised learning algorithms in predicting the presence of anomalies i.e, Diabetic Retinopathy and Glaucoma. Machine Learning (ML) in the field of healthcare is a highly researched area. The early diagnosis and time sensitive results are a few advantages that make ML an ideal technology to collaborate with the medical field. So, we have implemented Machine Learning models which are executed involving the following processes: predictive analytics, and image processing for detecting the presence of such vision impairing symptoms earlier to prevent blindness from setting in.

All the datasets and the images used for the project are gathered from Kaggle and Messidor. Among two diabetic retinopathy datasets one contains 70234 images with 51611 images of normal eye, 4882 images of 1st stage DR, 10580 images of 2nd stage DR, 1745 images of 3rd stage DR, 1416 images of 4th stage DR and the other contains 35126 images respectively. The Glaucoma dataset contains 768 images with 293 images of normal eyes and 475 images of Glaucoma affected eyes. The features present in the dataset for Diabetic Retinopathy are Exudates density, Exudates Count, Exudates Area, Optic Disk, Optic Cup, Cup to Disk ratio, Microaneurysm Area, Blood vessel Area, Blood vessel Density Microaneurysm Count, Haemorrhage Count, Haemorrhage Area and DRLevel. The Glaucoma dataset contains the following columns Age, Diabetes Pedigree Function, Glucose, Blood Pressure, Insulin, Body Mass Index, Cup to Disc Ratio and Outcome. With color fundus photography as input, the goal of our project is to detect DR and Glaucoma using Machine Learning algorithms. The Resulting models will maximize the impact i.e., improving DR detection and for Glaucoma.

The project mainly focuses on predicting DR and Glaucoma from retinal fundus images. Since this problem falls under Supervised learning technique, Six models such as Decision Tree, Random Forest, Support Vector Machines, Bagging Ensemble, Logistic Regression and Naive Bayes models under this category are used to predict the results which come under the Primary modelling. The results obtained from these models show very poor performance and the cause behind that problem is identified as class imbalancement. That problem was overcome by performing Secondary Modelling like Feature Selection, Sampling the dataset, Feature importance etc., Feature Selection was done through Principal Component Analysis (PCA). Retinal features are extracted from the fundus using python code. The dataset obtained was found to be 'multiclass'. Both up sampling (SMOTE) and down sampling was performed to make all the majority and minority classes in the dataset balanced. Also, feature importance of the dataset is found, in order to recover from the class imbalancement. Then six ML models are created, which are used to predict the DR level (0-4) with high accuracy. The result obtained from our predictive tool of different algorithms has the highest accuracy of 73.68% using Random Forest and AUC-ROC value of 50%, RMSE value of 2.07, MSE of 4.31 and finally MAE of 1.43. Using the decision tree algorithm, the obtained results are 55% and using logistic regression & Naive Bayes are 73% and using Bagging Ensemble the accuracy obtained is 73.03%. The SVM model gives an accuracy of 73.58%. Hence it is found out that the maximum accuracy is obtained using the Random Forest model. Glaucoma is predicted using the Cup to Disc ratio. The dataset obtained was found to be 'Binary class'. This problem is also based on supervised learning techniques.

Around six Machine Learning algorithms that fall under supervised learning techniques were executed namely, Decision Tree, Random Forest, Support Vector Machines, Bagging Ensemble, Logistic Regression and Naive Bayes models. The result of the Naive Bayes model gives the higher accuracy of 98.7% and other models give a bit lesser accuracy than Naive Bayes which are Decision Tree gives the accuracy of 81.16, Random Forest gives the accuracy of 77.92, Support Vector Machines gives the accuracy of 84.41, Bagging Ensemble gives the accuracy of 70.12. (Sperandei, 2014) Logistic Regression gives the accuracy of 89.61. The model is deployed as a mobile application for the patients to access easily using smartphones. The application is created in such a way that where patients can enter basic details, the application deployed with ML model trains and tests with the data given, makes accurate predictions and finally gives them their result of whether there is any presence or not.

Proposed Solution

Automated detection of Diabetic Retinopathy and Glaucoma is essential to tackle the time-intensive approach present now. We have planned to develop a novel ML model which performs the early-stage detection by identifying all Microaneurysms (MAs), the first signs of DR, Optic Disc, Optic Cup, Blood-vessel count, Bloodvessel Area, Cup to Disc Ratio, along with correctly assigning labels to retinal fundus images which are graded into five categories. The presence of Glaucoma is detected using Cup To Disc Ratio value. Our aim is to provide a cheaper, easily adoptable model that benefits maximum patients.

Random Forest method was applied to reach high accuracy. The 3 steps involved in this process are Image Preprocessing, Supervised learning and Feature Extraction.

Approaches

The following methodologies are used in our project to predict various eye diseases.

Figure 1.

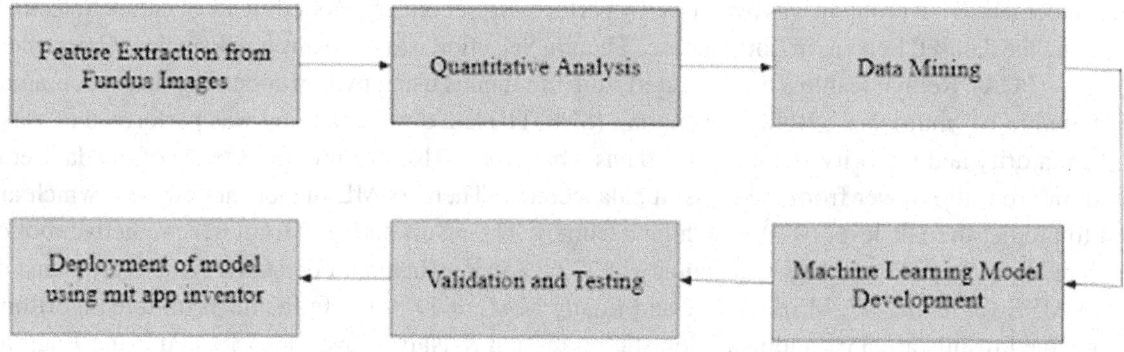

DATASET

Overview of Data Analysis (Kaggle, n.d.)

We have used three fundus image datasets for analysis namely:

- Kaggle - DRDC
- Kaggle - Ocular Disease Detection
- Messidor-2

In our project we have used a dataset from Kaggle DRDC out of the three dataset.

RESULTS AND DISCUSSION

The dataset is passed through various other algorithms and the performance of the algorithms is measured using the performance metrics. Machine Learning classification algorithms such as Naive Bayes (NB), Decision Tree (DT), KNearest Neighbor (KNN), Random Forest, Support Vector Machine (SVM) have been used to predict the occurrence of DR as well as for Glaucoma. However, the results indicate that the Random Forest had the highest accuracy for DR, closely followed by Naive Bayes. Earlier, RF, SVM, DT, NB and KNN were compared for pre-processed data. But here the best performed RF model's metrics for raw dataset and balanced resampled dataset are discussed in detail. For Glaucoma the Naive Bayes model gives a high accuracy of about 98.7%.

Figure 2. Block diagram of this study

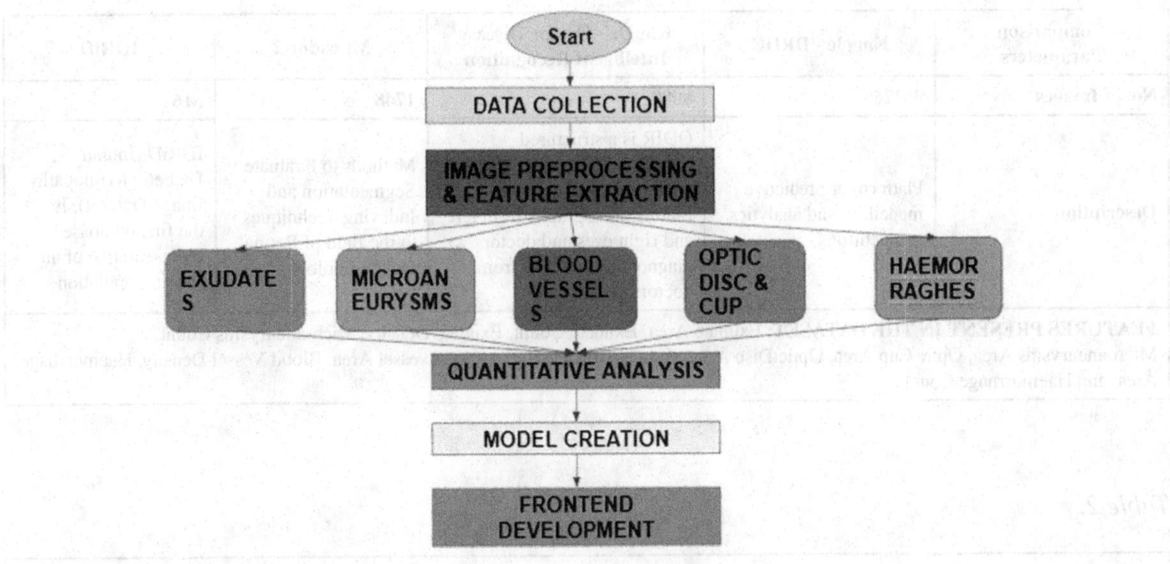

Figure 3. Flow of work

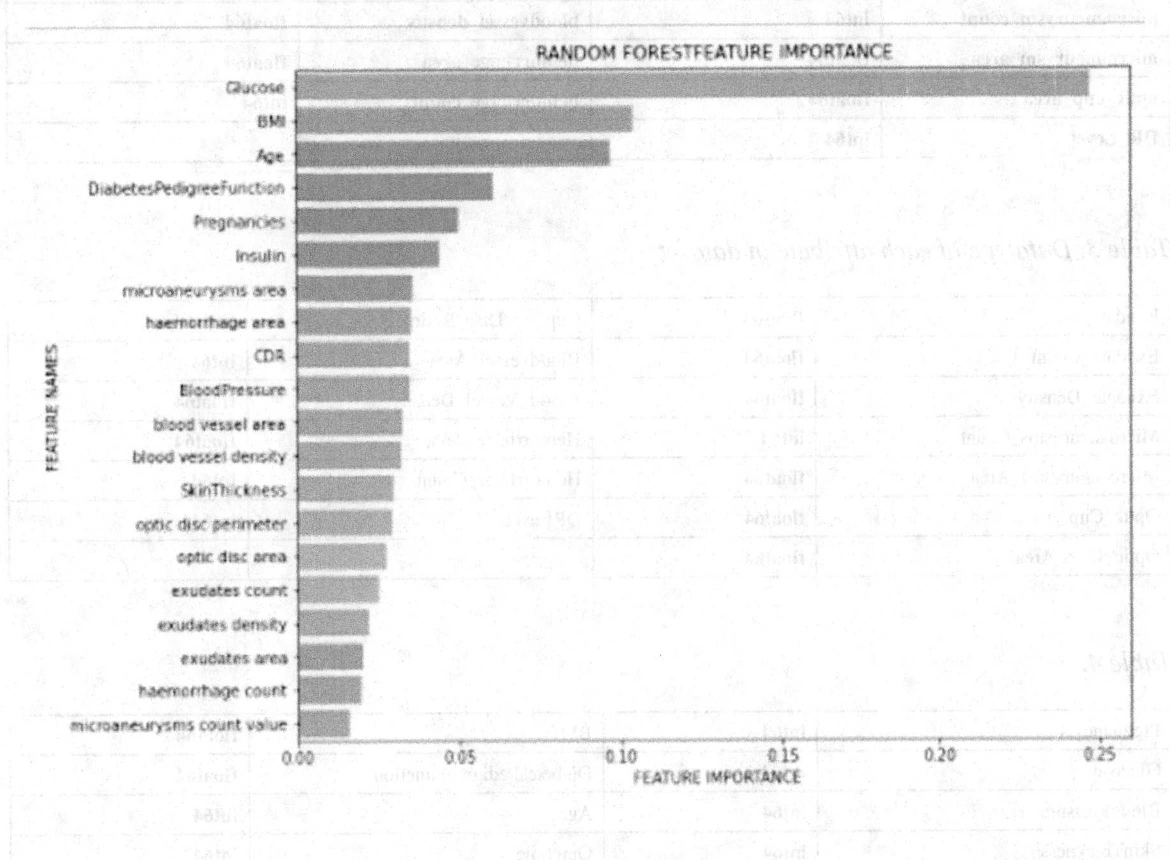

Table 1.

Comparison Parameters	Kaggle - DRDC	Kaggle - Ocular Disease Intelligent Recognition	Messidor-2	IDRiD
No. of Images	35126	8000	1748	516
Description	Platform or predictive modelling and analytics competitions	ODIR is a structured ophthalmic database of 5,000 patients with age, color fundus photographs from left and right eyes and doctors' diagnostic keywords from doctors.	Methods to Evaluate Segmentation and Indexing Techniques in the field of Retinal Ophthalmology	IDRiD (Indian Diabetic Retinopathy Image Dataset), Is the first database representative of an Indian population.
FEATURES PRESENT IN THE DATASET: Exudate Area, Exudate Count, Exudate Density, Microaneurysms Count, Microaneurysms Area, Optic Cup Area, Optic Disc Area, and Cup to Disc Ratio, Blood vessel Area, Blood Vessel Density, Haemorrhage Area, and Haemorrhage Count.				

Table 2.

exudates_area	**float64**	**optic_disc_area**	**float64**
exudates_count	**int64**	**cup_to_disc**	**float64**
exudates_density	**float64**	**bloodvessel_area**	**int64**
microaneurysm_count	**int64**	**bloodvessel_density**	**float64**
microaneurysm_area	**float64**	**hemorrhage_area**	**float64**
optic_cup_area	**float64**	**hemorrhage_count**	**int64**
DR_Level	**int64**		

Table 3. Datatype of each attribute in dataset

Exudate_Area	**float64**	Cup_ to_Disc_Ratio	**float64**
Exudate_Count	**float64**	Bloodvessel_Area	**int64**
Exudate_Density	**float64**	Blood_Vessel_Density	**float64**
Microaneurysms_Count	**int64**	Hemorrhage_Area	**float64**
Microaneurysms_Area	**float64**	Hemorrhage_Count	**int64**
Optic_Cup_Area	**float64**	DRLevel	**int64**
Optic_Disc_Area	**float64**		

Table 4.

Pregnancies	**int64**	BMI	**float64**
Glucose	**int64**	DiabetesPedigreeFunction	**float64**
BloodPressure	**int64**	Age	**int64**
SkinThickness	**int64**	Outcome	**int64**
Insulin	**int64**		

Table 5.

	exudates_ area	exudates_ count	exudates_ density	microaneurysm_ count	microaneurysm_ area	optic_cup_ area	optic_disc_ area	cup_to_disc	bloodvessel_ area	bloodvessel_ density	hemorrhage_ area	hemorrhage_ count	DR_Level
count	70234.000000	70234.000000	70234.000000	70234.000000	70234.000000	70234.000000	70234.000000	70234.000000	70234.000000	70234.000000	70234.000000	70234.000000	70234.000000
mean	190.181664	11.953527	0.008708	3.730287	244.069005	245.419346	3305.942030	4.487491	7052.261782	0.107609	67496.977895	7.092320	0.525970
std	424.872550	15.670882	0.0194540	3.862987	289.207400	291.272711	7127.171856	9.232397	3275.102423	0.049974	2156.637254	3.322378	0.970374
min	0.000000	0.000000	0.000000	0.000000	0.000000	0.000000	0.000000	0.002808	0.000000	0.000000	49357.500000	1.000000	0.000000
25%	0.000000	1.000000	0.000000	1.000000	36.000000	0.000000	0.000000	0.200000	4504.000000	0.068726	65923.000000	5.000000	0.000000
50%	18.000000	6.000000	0.000824	3.000000	139.000000	150.710677	1196.500000	1.118139	7021.000000	0.107132	67140.250000	7.000000	0.000000
75%	52675.75000	168.500000	17.000000	0.007715	6.000000	359.000000	354.651060	4.305049	9399.000000	0.143417	68699.500000	9.000000	1.000000
max	70234.00000	10244.500000	225.000000	0.469071	30.000000	2464.000000	2441.052069	496.204082	18887.000000	0.288193	84690.000000	23.000000	4.000000

Table 6.

	Exudate_Area	Exudate_Count	Exudate_Density	Microaneurysms _Count	Microaneurysms_ Area	Optic_Cup_Area	Optic_Disc_Area	Cup_ to_Disc_Ratio	Bloodvessel_Area	Blood_Vessel_Density	Hemorrhage_Area	Hemorrhage_Count	DRLevel
count	35126.000000	35126.000000	35126.000000	35126.000000	35126.000000	35126.000000	35126.000000	35126.000000	35126.000000	35126.000000	35126.000000	35126.000000	35126.000000
mean	195.273302	13.213432	0.008941	2.835421	188.358780	254.906210	3353.138174	3.508387	5395.561151	0.082330	66965.539714	5.963076	0.265245
std	417.595487	16.572160	0.019121	3.278727	238.233398	277.453531	6537.937449	7.873152	2590.691646	0.039531	1823.594914	2.889101	0.441470
min	0	0	0	0	0	0	0	0.002808	0	0	50480.0	1	0
25%	0	1	0	0	0	0	0	0.200000	3375.00000	0.051498	65649.0	4	0
50%	22.50	8	0.001030	2	100.50000	176.802560	1249.75000	0.749845	5191.00000	0.079208	66658.250	6	0
75%	187.00000	19	0.008562	4	280.50000	375.404109	3798.50000	3.165188	7294.00000	0.111298	67971.0	8	1
max	10244.500000	207	0.469071	26	2042.50000	2175.103804	79846.00000	257.811765	14442.0000	0.220367	76854.0	19	1

Table 7.

	Pregnancies	Glucose	BloodPressure	SkinThickness	Insulin	BMI	DiabetesPedigreeFunction	Age	Outcome
count	768	768	768	768	768	768	768	768	768
mean	3.845052	120.894531	69.10546	20.53645	79.79947	31.992578	0.471876	33.24088	0.34895
std	3.3695	31.972618	19.35580	15.9522	115.2440	7.88416	0.33132	11.76023	0.47695
min	0	0	0	0	0	0	0.07800	0	0
25%	1.000	99.00	62.00	0	0	27.30	0.24375	24.00	0
50%	3.000	117.00	72.00	23.00	30.50	32.00	0.372500	29.00	0
75%	6.000	140.250	80.00	32.00	127.250	36.60	0.62625	41.00	1
max	17.000	199.00	122.00	99.00	846.00	67.10	2.420	81.00	1

Quantitative Analysis

Table 8.

Blood vessels area	● Total no of pixels=width*height of the image ● Black pixel count=total no of pixels-white pixels count ● Total white pixels=np.sum(cv2.bitwise_not(blood vessels))/255
Blood vessels Density	Total white pixel/ (Blood vessel.shape [0]*Blood vessel.shape [1])
Blood vessels perimeter & Blood vessel width	● Applying sobel operator over the extracted blood vessels, edge detected vessels are obtained. ● Blood vessel perimeter = Total white pixels=np.sum(edge detected vessels)/255
Exudate Count & Area	Exudate count and area is calculated by using contours [Cv2.contourArea]
Exudate density	Total white pixel/ (Exudate.shape [0]*Exudate.shape [1])
Hemorrhage Area & count	Hemorrhage area and count is calculated using contours [Cv2.contourArea]
Microaneurysm count & area	Microaneurysms count and area is calculated by using contours [Cv2.contourArea]
Optic Disk & Optic cup area	● Optic Disk Area = Total_white_pixel(optic disk) ● Optic cup Area = Total_white_pixel(optic cup)
Cup to Disk ratio (CDR)	CDR = Optic cup Area/Optic disk Area.

Glaucoma Details

1. Data Review

Table 9.

Pregnancies	Glucose	BloodPressure	SkinThickness	Insulin	BMI	Diabetes PedigreeFunction	Age	Outcome
6	148	72	35	0	33.6	0.627	50	1
1	85	66	29	0	26.6	0.351	31	0
8	183	64	0	0	23.3	0.672	32	1
1	89	66	23	94	28.1	0.167	21	0
0	137	40	35	168	43.1	2.288	33	1

2. Dimension of data : (768, 9)
3. Datatype of each attribute

Table 10.

Pregnancies	**int64**	BMI	**float64**
Glucose	**int64**	DiabetesPedigreeFunction	**float64**
BloodPressure	**int64**	Age	**int64**
SkinThickness	**int64**	Outcome	**int64**
Insulin	**int64**		

4. Descriptive statistics

Table 11.

	Pregnancies	**Glucose**	**BloodPressure**	**SkinThickness**	**Insulin**	**BMI**	**DiabetesPedigreeFunction**	**Age**	**Outcome**
count	768	768	768	768	768	768	768	768	768
mean	3.845052	120.894531	69.10546	20.53645	79.79947	31.992578	0.471876	33.24088	0.34895
std	3.3695	31.972618	19.35580	15.9522	115.2440	7.88416	0.33132	11.76023	0.47695
min	0	0	0	0	0	0	0.07800	0	0
25%	1.000	99.00	62.00	0	0	27.30	0.24375	24.00	0
50%	3.000	117.00	72.00	23.00	30.50	32.00	0.372500	29.00	0
75%	6.000	140.250	80.00	32.00	127.250	36.60	0.62625	41.00	1
max	17.000	199.00	122.00	99.00	846.00	67.10	2.420	81.00	1

5. Class distribution

Table 12.

0	**293**
1	**475**
dtype	**int64**

6. Type of Target : Binary Class

The features are ranked based on the effect they have on the prediction of the disease as shown by Figure 5.1. The ROC-AUC plot in Figure 5.2 shows how correct the prediction performed is.

Figure 4. Feature importance

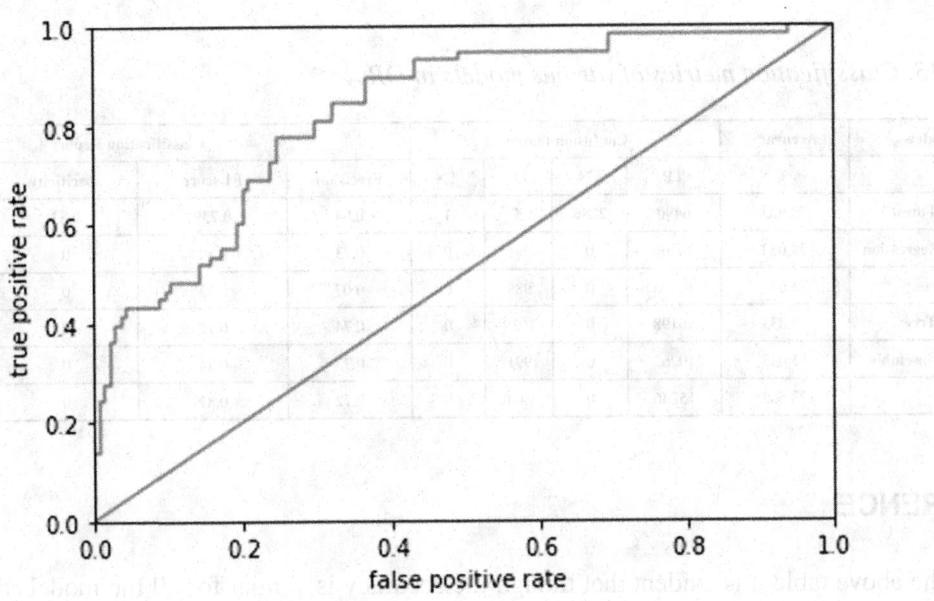

Figure 5. ROC AUC plot

```
Class=0, n=51611 (73.484%)
Class=4, n=1416 (2.016%)
Class=3, n=1745 (2.485%)
Class=2, n=10580 (15.064%)
Class=1, n=4882 (6.951%)
```

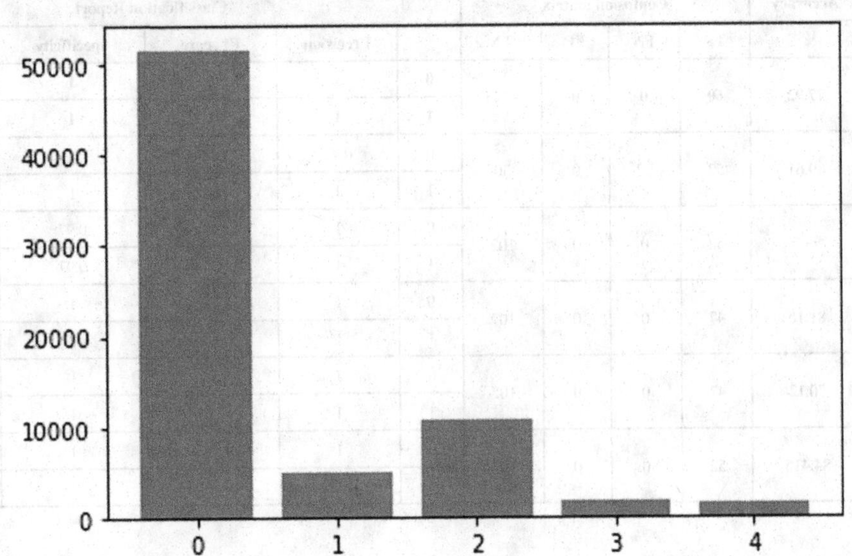

METRICS OF VARIOUS MODELS FOR DR

Table 13. Classification metrics of various models in DR

Models	Accuracy	Confusion matrix				Classification Report			
		TP	FN	FP	TN	Precision	F1 score	specificity	sensitivity
Random Forest	**73.923**	**6490**	**2286**	**5**	**1**	**0.84**	**0.739**	**0.83**	**0.263**
Logistic Regression	73.033	10266	0	991	0	0.73	0.84	0	1.0
Naive Bayes	73.631	10343	0	989	0	0.07	0.13	0	1.0
Decision Tree	55.833	10198	0	1019	0	0.74	0.72	0	1.0
Bagging Ensemble	73.033	10263	0	991	0	0.73	0.84	0	1.0
SVM	72.563	15236	0	1446	0	0.72	0.81	0	1.0

INFERENCE

From the above table it is evident that though the accuracy is similar for all the models the metrics of Random Forest are more efficient.

METRICS OF VARIOUS MODELS FOR GLAUCOMA

Table 14. Classification metrics of various models in Glaucoma

Models	Accuracy	Confusion matrix				Classification Report				
		TP	FN	FP	TN		Precision	F1 score	specificity	sensitivity
Random Forest	**77.92**	**60**	**0**	**0**	**94**	**0**	**1**	**1**	**1**	**1**
						1	**1**	**1**	**1**	**1**
Logistic Regression	89.61	52	72	0	30	0	0.42	0.59	1	1
						1	1	0.45	1	0.29
Naive Bayes	98.7	52	0	0	102	0	1	1	0.97	0.99
						1	1	1	0.97	0.99
Decision Tree	81.16	47	0	0	107	0	1	1	1	1
						1	1	1	1	1
Bagging Ensemble	70.12	47	0	0	107	0	1	1	1	1
						1	1	1	1	1
SVM	84.415	52	0	0	102	0	1	1	1	1
						1	1	1	1	1

INFERENCE

From the above table it is evident that though the accuracy is similar for all the models the metrics of Naive Bayes are more efficient.

Hyper Parameter Tuning

- Changing the hyper-parameters of the Random Forest Algorithm.
- Hyper-parameters are those not included in the dataset but are those present in the algorithm structure.
- Hypertuning is mainly done to improve accuracy of the model.
- In Random Forest parameters like n_estimators,min_samples_split,etc.. are hypertuned and the following results are obtained.

Table 15.

Hyper-parameters	Accuracy	Confusion matrix				Classification Report				
		TP	FN	FP	TN	Precision	Recall	F1 score	specificity	sensitivity
classifier= RandomForestClassifier(n_estimators=500, oob_score=True, min_samples_split=10)	73.753	6470	2280	25	7	0.996	0.739	0.849	0.259	0.739
classifier= RandomForestClassifier(n_estimators=500, oob_score=True, min_samples_split=5)	73.750	6647	2273	48	14	0.996	0.739	1.093	0.260	0.756
classifier= RandomForestClassifier(n_estimators=500, oob_score=True, min_samples_split=15)	73.855	6481	2282	14	5	0.995	0.739	1.093	0.261	0.754
classifier= RandomForestClassifier(n_estimators=500, oob_score=True, min_samples_split=30)	73.912	6490	2286	5	1	0.995	0.739	1.092	0.263	0.756

Table 16.

	Accuracy	Confusion matrix				Classification Report				
		TP	FN	FP	TN	Precision	Recall	F1 score	specificity	sensitivity
classifier= RandomForestClassifier(n_estimators=500, oob_score=True, min_samples_split=30)	73.912	6490	2286	5	1	0.995	0.739	1.092	0.263	0.756
classifier= RandomForestClassifier(n_estimators=100, oob_score=True, min_samples_split=30)	73.923	6490	2285	5	2	0.995	0.739	1.092	0.263	0.756
classifier= RandomForestClassifier(n_estimators=300, oob_score=True, min_samples_split=30)	73.867	6486	2286	9	1	0.995	0.739	1.092	0.263	0.756
classifier= RandomForestClassifier(n_estimators=800, oob_score=True, min_samples_split=30)	73.889	6488	2286	7	1	0.995	0.739	1.092	0.263	0.756

It can be observed that the metrics and accuracy are more or less the same for the model but the most efficient of all can be interpreted with the model having parameters as n_estimators=500 and minimum sample split=30.

After performing all the processes the random forest model seems to give the highest accuracy. So, hyper parameters were chosen and hyper-tuning was done thus giving us the accuracy as 73.923%.

For Diabetic Retinopathy

Table 17.

Metrics	Raw Data	Pre-Processed & Hypertuned data
ACCURACY	73.750%	73.923%
TP	6647	6490
TN	2273	2286
FP	48	5
FN	14	1
PRECISION	0.79	0.84
SPECIFICITY	0.259	0.263
SENSITIVITY	0.756	0.83
F1 SCORE	0.72	0.739
ROC SCORE	0.5	0.56
AUC SCORE	0.5	0.5

For Glaucoma

Table 18.

Metrics	Processed Data
ACCURACY	98.701
TP	52
TN	0
FP	0
FN	102
PRECISION	1.0
SPECIFICITY	0.97
SENSITIVITY	0.99
F1 SCORE	1.0
ROC SCORE	0.9
AUC SCORE	0.98

In our project we predicted the occurrence of DR and Glaucoma using (Narvekar et al., n.d.) data mining techniques. We split the data set into training and testing sets and use the training set to train the model and testing set to test the model. We then evaluate the model performance based on the accuracy metric of the model. This method is not very reliable, as the accuracy obtained for one test set can be very different to the accuracy obtained for a different test set.

Every algorithm has its own limitations and strength specified to the type of application it performs. In the case of our dataset Random forest algorithm worked more efficiently than other algorithms for DR and Naive Bayes algorithm for Glaucoma and obtained the highest accuracy for the above mentioned min_sample_split (500).We selected this algorithm as it is considered as a highly accurate and robust method because of the number of decision trees participating in the process.

Table 19.

Classes	Images	DR Classification
0	51611	Normal
1	4882	Mild
2	10580	Moderate
3	1745	Severe
4	1416	Non Proliferative DR

Our model classifies all the five stages of DR using Kaggle dataset. The accuracy, sensitivity, specificity, precision, and F1-score and other metrics are calculated.

Using the data obtained from the images, the data is divided into two portions that are training and testing. In this we have used an 80-20 ratio during the training and testing of classifiers.

It can be seen that the metrics such as accuracy, cross validation score and specificity are pretty good. But the other important metrics such as precision, sensitivity, AUC and ROC are poor. The main reason is the imbalanced dataset. Hence the dataset is resampled to make it balanced and the metrics were checked. Since class 0 (no DR) is the majority class with approximately 51611 samples and class 4 is the minority class with approximately 1416 samples.

So, we have to either increase the samples of all other classes to match class 0 or reduce the samples of all the classes to match minority class 4. But reducing the samples or under sampling results in loss of vital information from the data. (Pranto et al., 2020) miHence up sampling is the best choice. Thus the dataset is balanced in such a way that 20% samples are present in all the 5 classes.

UPSAMPLED DATA

Hence the models which are trained over raw data (with removed missing and NaN values), k-Fold split pre-processed data and usual split pre-processed data can be considered to predict DR.

Figure 6.

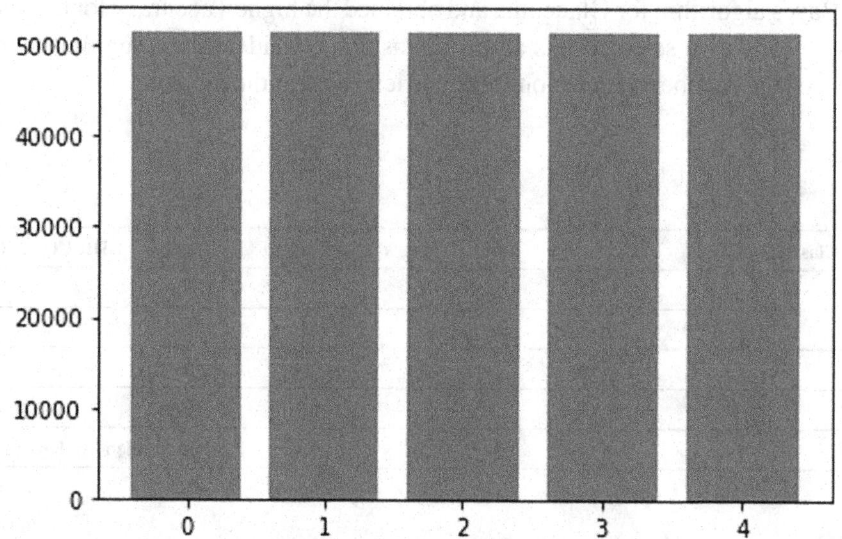

Glaucoma Prediction

As said before Glaucoma is a kind of eye disease which is predicted using Cup-to-Disc ratio.

Depending on the severity the risk of glaucoma can be classified into 3 categories:

1. Early stage. (CDR ratio < 0.29)
2. Moderate stage. (0.3<CDR<0.6)
3. Extreme stage. (CDR > 0.6)

Table 20.

Classes	Images	Glaucoma Classification
0	293	Normal
1	475	Glaucoma

Figure 7.

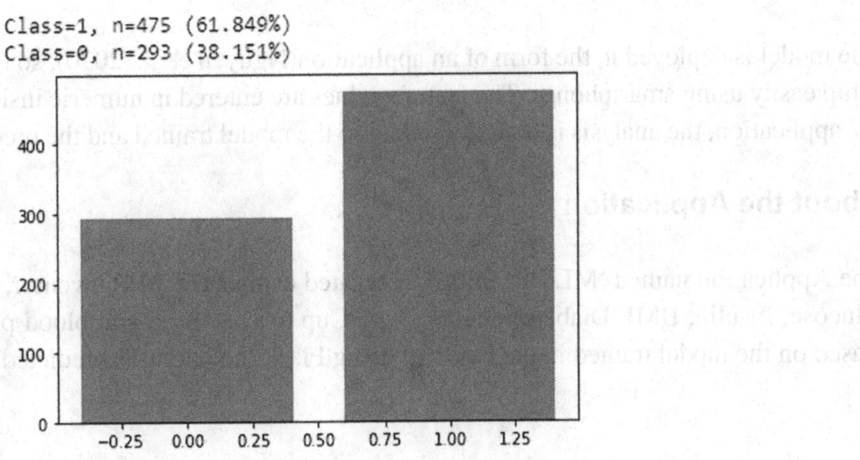

Figure 8.

Model Deployment

The model is deployed in the form of an application(Nguyen et al., 2020), so that people can access the setup easily using smartphones. The feature values are entered in numeric inside the text box present in the application, the analysis is done according to the model trained and the predicted result is displayed.

About the Application

The Application named 'ML PREDICT' is created using MIT APP Inventor, collects information like Glucose, Insulin, BMI, Diabetes degree, Age, Cup to Disc ratio and blood pressure from the patient. Based on the model trained in the backend using Flask the output is predicted.

Figure 9.

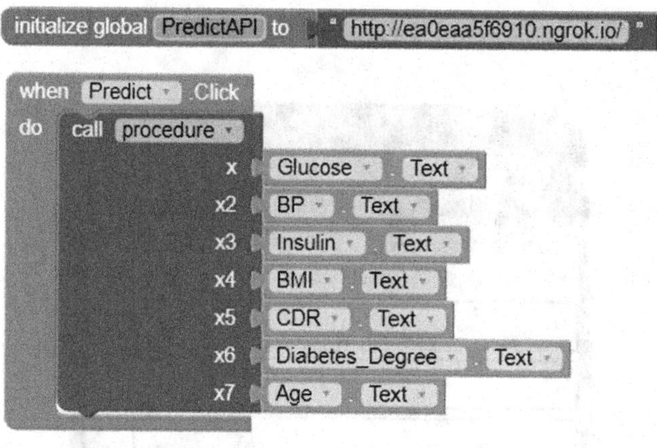

Figure 10.

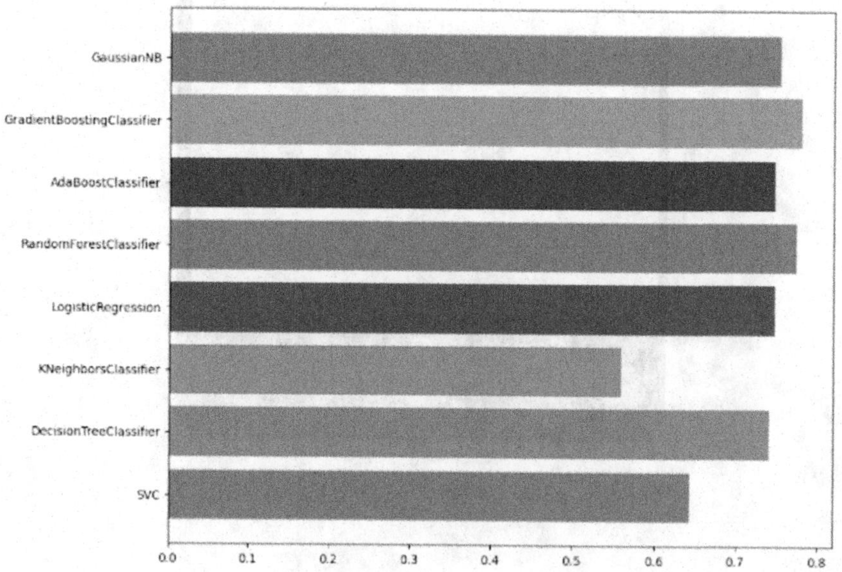

Output Screen

Figure 11.

Output of the Application

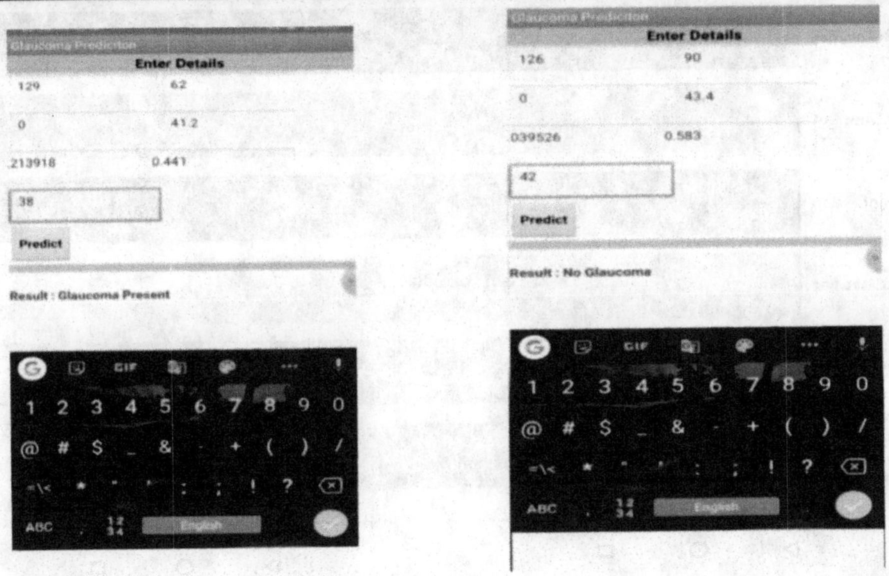

CONCLUSION

An automated solution can be provided for screening the retinal images and predicting the presence of Diabetic Retinopathy and Glaucoma. The datasets used are cleaned, visualised and analysed to get maximum accuracy of prediction.

By performing a Random Forest model we obtained an ROC score of 0.56 and AUC score of 0.5. Performance metrics for this model are as follows, F1-Score is 0.739, Sensitivity is 0.83 and Specificity is 0.263 and Precision is 0.84 ,giving an accuracy of 73% for Diabetic Retinopathy.

Glaucoma prediction is executed using Naive Bayes algorithm, we obtained an ROC score of 0.9 and AUC score of 0.98. Performance metrics for this model are as follows, F1-Score is 1, Sensitivity is 0.99 and Specificity is 0.97 and Precision is 1, giving an accuracy of 98%.

This model is deployed in the form of an application that can be accessed by the public enabling them in detecting the above mentioned conditions.

Figure 12.

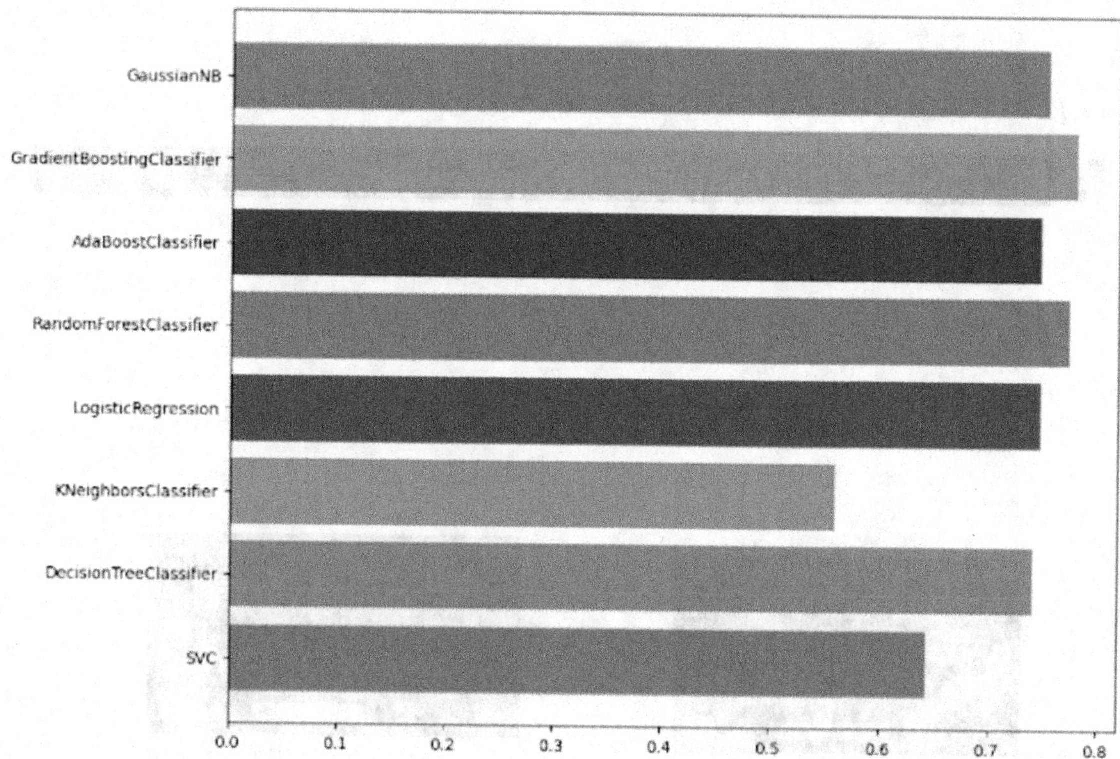
GaussianNB
GradientBoostingClassifier
AdaBoostClassifier
RandomForestClassifier
LogisticRegression
KNeighborsClassifier
DecisionTreeClassifier
SVC
0.0
0.1
0.2
0.3
0.4
0.5
0.6
0.7
0.8

REFERENCES

Bhatia, K., Arora, S., & Tomar, R. (2016, October). Diagnosis of diabetic retinopathy using machine learning classification algorithm. In *2016 2nd International Conference on Next Generation Computing Technologies (NGCT)* (pp. 347-351). IEEE. 10.1109/NGCT.2016.7877439

Fong, D. S., Aiello, L., Gardner, T. W., King, G. L., Blankenship, G., Cavallerano, J. D., Ferris, F. L., & Klein, R. (2004). Retinopathy in diabetes. *Diabetes Care, 27*(suppl1), s84–s87. doi:10.2337/diacare.27.2007.S84 PMID:14693935

Georgescu, L. (2018). *What Artificial Intelligence Is and How It Can Be Used.* Academic Press.

Gurudath, N., Celenk, M., & Riley, H. B. (2014, December). Machine learning identification of diabetic retinopathy from fundus images. In *2014 IEEE Signal Processing in Medicine and Biology Symposium (SPMB)* (pp. 1-7). IEEE. 10.1109/SPMB.2014.7002949

Jones, S., & Edwards, R. T. (2010). Diabetic retinopathy screening: A systematic review of the economic evidence. *Diabetic Medicine, 27*(3), 249–256. doi:10.1111/j.1464-5491.2009.02870.x PMID:20536486

Kaggle. (n.d.). https://www.kaggle.com/c/diabetic-retinopathy-detection

Lam, C., Yi, D., Guo, M., & Lindsey, T. (2018). Automated detection of diabetic retinopathy using deep learning. *AMIA Joint Summits on Translational Science Proceedings AMIA Summit on Translational Science, 2018*, 147. PMID:29888061

Li, Y.H., Yeh, N.N., Chen, S.J., & Chung, Y.C. (2019). Computer-assisted diagnosis for diabetic retinopathy based on fundus images using deep convolutional neural network. *Mobile Information Systems.*

Narvekar, Menezes, Angle, Lotlekar, Naik, & Purohit. (n.d.). *Students Performance Prediction using Data Mining Techniques*. Academic Press.

Nguyen, Q. H., Muthuraman, R., Singh, L., Sen, G., Tran, A. C., Nguyen, B. P., & Chua, M. (2020). Diabetic retinopathy detection using deep learning. *Proceedings of the 4th International Conference on Machine Learning and Soft Computing*, 103-107. 10.1145/3380688.3380709

Porwal, P., Pachade, S., Kamble, R., Kokare, M., Deshmukh, G., Sahasrabuddhe, V., & Meriaudeau, F. (2018). Indian diabetic retinopathy image dataset (IDRiD): A database for diabetic retinopathy screening research. *Data, 3*(3), 25. doi:10.3390/data3030025

Pranto, B., Mehnaz, S. M., Momen, S., & Huq, S. M. (2020). Prediction of diabetes using cost sensitive learning and oversampling techniques on Bangladeshi and Indian female patients. In *2020 5th International Conference on Information Technology Research (ICITR)* (pp. 1-6). IEEE. 10.1109/ICITR51448.2020.9310892

Somasundaram, S. K., & Alli, P. (2017). A machine learning ensemble classifier for early prediction of diabetic retinopathy. *Journal of Medical Systems, 41*(12), 201. doi:10.100710916-017-0853-x PMID:29124453

Sperandei, S. (2014). Understanding logistic regression analysis. *Biochemia Medica, 24*(1), 12–18. doi:10.11613/BM.2014.003 PMID:24627710

Youbi, A. (2020). *Diabetic retinopathy detection through deep learning techniques: A review*. Informatics in Medicine Unlocked.

Chapter 12 Internet of Things-Empowered Next-Generation Healthcare Systems

J. Manga
Sathyabama Institute of Science and Technology, India

V. J. K. Kishor Sonti
Sathyabama Institute of Science and Technology, India

ABSTRACT

Internet of things is seen in many fields like civil engineering, consumer goods, oil and gas fields, smart cities, agriculture, etc. Apart from these, it is applicable to the medical field to detect and treat many kinds of diseases and can find the different health parameters quickly. It became important in the health sector to mitigate the challenges of health problems. Internet of things (IoT) is an amalgamation of pervasive computing, intelligent processing, and real-time response systems. Mechanics, devices, sensors make this machine-to-machine communication a feasible solution to dynamic requirements of tech-aspiring world. This chapter highlights the possibilities of further empowerment of healthcare systems using IoT or in other words IoMT (internet of medical things). Nanotechnology-driven IoT development or internet of nano things (IoNT) has become an added advantage in healthcare applications. So, IoNT with IoMT is another exciting research prospect of the near future. This chapter introduces a technique used in healthcare applications, PUF (physical unclonable function), and it is technique for solving many problems related to privacy and security. Security of data transmission, issues pertinent to reliability, and inter-operability are inherently affecting the progress of IoT-based healthcare systems. This chapter of focuses upon these issues and feasible solutions viewed from the dimension of technology-driven healthcare costs in the modern world and economic implications. The treatment used in this chapter will be more interesting for the casual readers. The analysis of IoMT implications in the near future will be helpful to the ardent learners. The research dimensions of IoT-empowered healthcare systems will add value to the thought process of young researchers.

DOI: 10.4018/978-1-7998-9132-1.ch012

Copyright © 2022, IGI Global. Copying or distributing in print or electronic forms without written permission of IGI Global is prohibited.

OVERVIEW OF INTERNET OF THINGS (IoT):

Internet of things (IoT) changed the way we think, we learn and we live. It will be foretelling that by the year 2025, all devices can be associated with the internet, causes to increase more devices connected to it. From the CISCO point of view, by the year 2030, the no of devices will be connected to the internet can be increased by 500 billion devices. In this regard IoT can be connected to health care devices to mitigate the challenges of health issues. Present health sector became more important with the pandemic situation and humans wants health care virtually rather than consulting a doctor directly. IoT playing a vital role in health sector to connect different health care devices for monitoring of patient's health parameters. In this chapter it is showing that, the IoT is used in healthcare systems for the coming generation. In the IoT system, sensors will be used to connect the devices and can be sensed human body by connecting it to him. There are more technologies has been developed for connecting all devices to the internet like BAN (Body area network), WBAN (Wireless body area network), WSN (Wireless sensor networks), BSN (Body sensor networks), Artificial neural networks etc. by using above methodologies, Ubiquitous computing, resource management, quality of service, real time wireless health monitoring, information security, power savings are possible. The basic IoT architecture is shown in Figure 1.

Figure 1. IoT Architecture

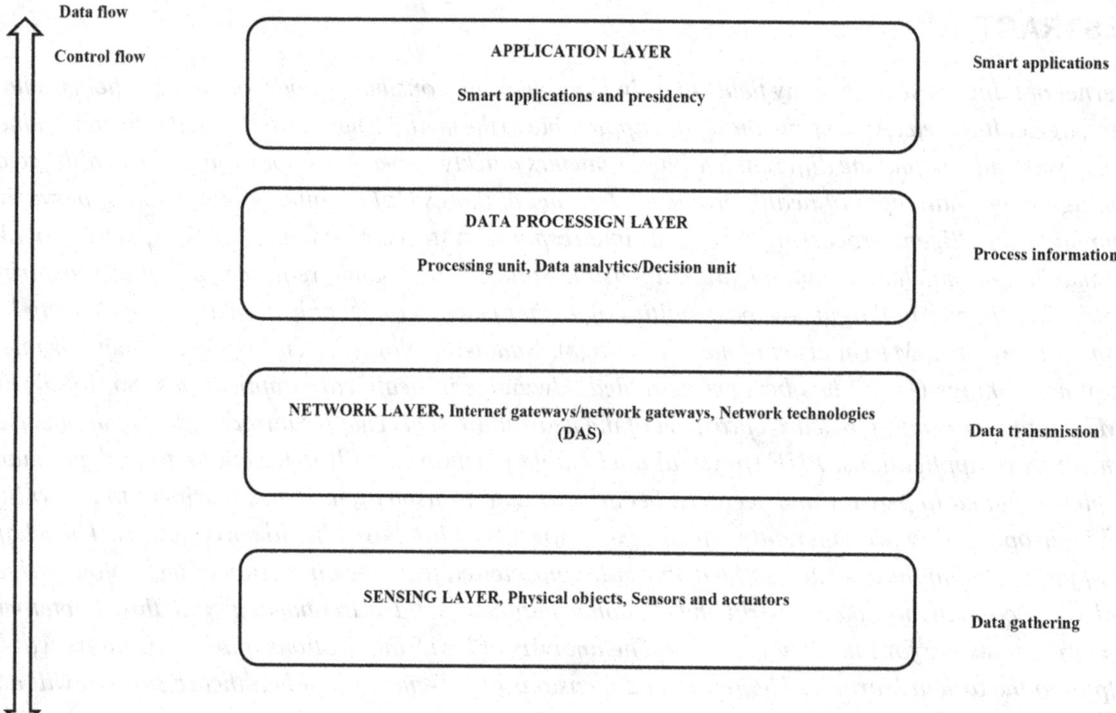

In the IoT architecture, there are four layers viz, sensing layer, network layer, data processing layer and application layer (Pradyumna Gokhale et.al., 2018).

They are explicating as follows:

1. **Sensing layer:** It consists of sensors, actuators, devices and acquires data from corporeal and environs variables, undertaking it and fed to network layer.
2. **Network layer:** this layer consists of internet gateways/network gateways, and data acquisition system. DAS collects the data and converts the data from analog to digital form. Gateways are used to establish the connection between sensors and internet also performs gateways functionalities like malware protection, filtering, decision making and information processing etc.
3. **Data processing layer:** Here data has to be investigated and initialized before sending to application layer where data have been examined by software applications and further it will be monitored and managed.
4. **Application layer:** It is the last layer of IoT model where data centers and cloud management presents can be used at the last stage having applications like healthcare, agriculture, forming, defense and aerospace etc.

ROLE OF IOT IN HEALTHCARE

"Health is Wealth" perhaps the best old lesson learnt in the new normal created by pandemic since 2019. Developed and developing countries are investing huge amount on reinforcement of "Healthcare systems" and obligatory "Health Infrastructure". Few nations are proactive in their health care approach across the globe. The recent ongoing pandemic taught tough lessons to nations about the significance of developing robust healthcare systems.

Day by day healthcare challenges have been increasing with the increase of diseases, aging of population, limited capabilities of hospitals and medical practitioners. Different situations demand different approaches. A situation created by a pandemic is worst to imagine and face. Recently, world has been going through the covid-19 pandemic. The implications and effect on human race are still unmeasured. Covid-19 in other words Coronavirus has affected millions of lives across the globe financially, psychologically and physically.

Hospitals, Psychological counselors, Governments will be overburdened with the work load that is unimaginable and unmanageable. Helplessness and hopelessness rule the society and sometimes rulers. There were studies conducted in Egypt during pandemic on mental health status of general public, administrators and health workers. Stress levels were found increased at work, domestic and financial fronts. Apprehensiveness conquered the mind of the citizens and disturbed the normal life. In recent past, Covid-19 is also causing serious mental and physical illness among the people across the nations.

Unfortunately, there is loss of human life considerably is a major concern. Data scientists, mathematicians and virology experts are engaged in predicting the impact of this pandemic in near future. To overcome these challenges there are many technologies has been developed such as Internet of Things (IoT), Artificial Intelligence (AI), Machine learning (ML) and Data analytics. Among all IoT is has more facilities in healthcare.

According to a report by Aruba Networks, a Hewlett Packard Enterprises subsidiary, the medical sector has the third place in the IoT execution. Healthcare challenges gave better success to healthcare providers to give good quality of service on healthcare (Jaimon T Kelly et.al. 2020). The benefits of IoT in healthcare is continuous monitoring of patients, giving solutions at the collection of patient's details, tracing of the patients and staff etc. IoT can collect any kind of data of the patient. IoT in medical sector have distinctive advantages like, IoT for patients, doctors, health insurers and healthcare providers.

Impact of IoT on Different Infectious Diseases

The IoT has a considerable constructive on human body by detecting different kinds of diseases like corona virus, measles etc. Recognition of disease the first and hard step. In this scenario IoT plays a great role by giving quick caution of the diseases. To accomplish this, it requires interconnection of IoT with artificial intelligence (AI) and ubiquitous computing etc. these are having lot of advantages to recognize the infectious diseases. IoT sensors provide both short term and long-term facilities to healthcare. In the short run, all individuals can be checked and crowded places like airports, borders also be checked. By this can prevent the infections. In the long run, by establishing the global wise detection system which is organized globally so that can prevent infections easily.

TECHNOLOGIES USED FOR IOT HEALTHCARE APPLICATIONS

Sensor Networks

Wireless sensor networks (WSN) are having many applications like industrial automation, healthcare, agriculture, environmental and military applications. Figure 2 shows the sensor node connectivity in a WSN. Wireless sensor networks are the part of ubiquitous healthcare system. Recent years wireless sensor networks (WSN) are used in health care applications due to the advances in medical sensors and low power network system (Mathew. N.O. et.al. 2018).

Figure 2. Components of a sensor node in a wireless sensor network

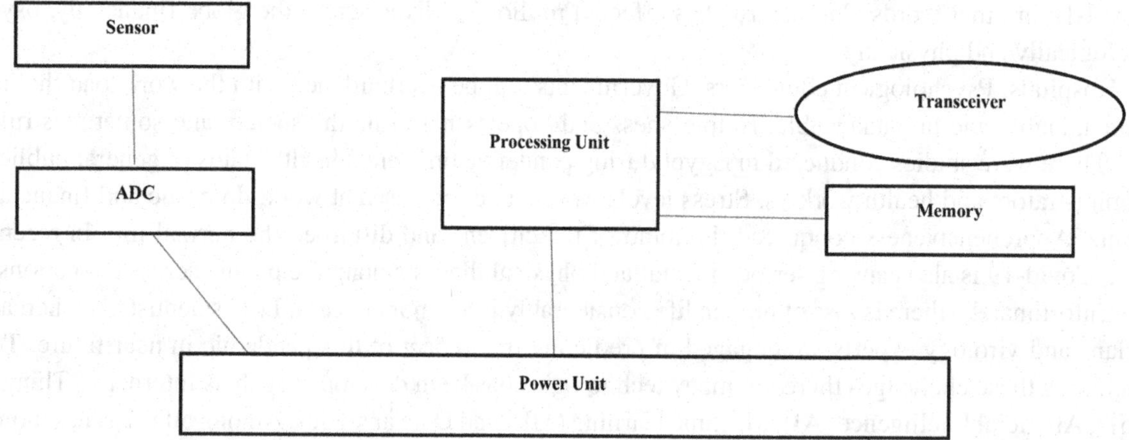

Healthcare industry facing some problems like higher cost, increasing of medical errors, insufficient staffing and aging of population etc. the above problems can be overcome by ubiquitous healthcare system. It helps to reduce the cost and improves the quality of service.

WSN is come to light as a main component for the next generation healthcare systems. WSN's like multi-hop and Zigbee based systems are used for the broadcast or multicast to deliver the information and these are fast and reliable.

The usage of wireless technology has becoming popular because of its simplicity and cost effectiveness. It consists of a large number of sensor nodes connected over a topographic region. Generally, sensors are positioned in high density manner and are large quantities in number. These nodes are light weight, compact, and battery powered devices and can be used virtually. These sensor nodes monitor physical and environmental conditions such as humidity, temperature, noise etc. wireless sensor network can be modified into wireless body area network (WBAN) is used in medical applications for the measurement of different health parameters (Latha.R & Vetrivelan, 2020). These nodes are connected over a human body udder skin or cloth and also very small in size and can reduce the size of the telecommunication equipment.

Physical Unclonable Function Technology

IoT healthcare suffers from privacy and security issues. Patient's health monitoring, timely medical assistance, apt diagnosis and efficient health care systems needs continuous support of technology. This is more significant when it comes to the protection to crucial and sensitive data of a patient.

In this regard, A physical unclonable function (PUF's) is a technique for solving many problems related to privacy and security. PUF is an authentication technique, which is simple but efficient. This acts like a firewall against data attackers. It has IoMT as backbone, cloud that verifies the data origin and authenticated professionals (doctors and medical management team) access. It is robust and having great advantages compared to recent classical cryptographic solutions like it is very compatible with IoT devices and limited computational resources (Armin Babaei & Gregor Schiele, 2019).

Two states are seen in PUF, namely, enrolment and authentication. In the enrolment state all devices are enrolled in the cloud and spread into healthcare system. In the authentication state, authentication process will be done for all devices. A PUF is a module mounted on the cloud generates a response and sent to the PUF module and gives an acknowledgement to the cloud. Then cloud stores all the data that is belongs to devices which are integrated with the PUF module and creates a one- time- password for devices in the authentication process. This technique usage, pros and cons are going to be discussed in this chapter. When patient's health record is needed, and then cloud and all connected devices should be accessed to establish communication for authentication.

In the next step cloud sends a response to the PUF devices, and then the devices also should send a return response to the clod. If both the responses are matched then device authentication cab be completed otherwise it will be denied. Here device authentication is very important to prevent attacks and threats to get security and privacy. Like this healthcare system can get security and privacy using PUF method.

IoT healthcare systems help to get the massive amount of data of the patient's illness, which is not possible always manually. Patient's data is sensitive and should be confidential. Proper encryption systems should be in place while keeping the data safe. There are various algorithms to take this process, but better advancements are needed in the acquisition stage of the data. Therefore, this requirement reminds us the need to develop more sophisticated sensing technology.

Efforts are going in the research arena to design and implement sensors, which can sense data and protect it without getting exploited. This data can be used for statistical study that would support the medical research. Thus, IoT not only saves our time but also mitigates the financial challenges associated with the research. Analysing and predicting medical data helps in developing new drugs, vaccines.

Collection, Analysis, Prediction and Interpretation are the four crucial wings of medical data management. Development of covid 19 vaccination is the best example of recent times. The development of these vaccines is not possible without such medical data analysis in short time. IoMT exactly becomes crucial in these cases, where attention, analysis and inference are almost simultaneously done. IoNT with IoMT is another exciting research prospect of near future.

Security of data transmission, issues pertinent to reliability and inter-operability are inherently affecting the progress of IoT based healthcare systems. This chapter of the book focuses upon these issues and feasible solutions viewing from the dimension of technology driven health care cost in modern world and economic implications. The treatment used in this chapter of the book will be more interesting for the casual readers. The analysis of IoMT implications in near future will be helpful to the ardent learners. The research dimensions of IoT empowered health care systems will add value to the thought process of young researchers.

INTERNET OF MEDICAL THINGS (IOMT)

Virtual learning, remote diagnosis is becoming new normal in academia-medico fields. Remote medicine is not something new, but now it has become almost imperative with the onset of pandemic. Deep Learning plays a vital role in all the fields of Engineering and its applications. In the current trend of information technology, the rate of data grows exponentially. As the size of the data increases it is difficult for the human being to parse the data and build models on top of it. As on date huge volume of unstructured data is available in the health care industry. The IoMT is the combination of intelligent computing, interconnection of medical devices, software applications, healthcare systems wirelessly.

The evolution of IoT technologies, Internet of Medical Things (IoMT) is one in which all prophylactic apparatus is connected to Wi-Fi allows machine-machine interaction. IoMT is also known as healthcare IoT. The growth of IoMT is determined by number of medical devices are increasing and connected the internet for generating the data, information gathering, analyzing and transmitting to the cloud or other sources (Vishnu.S. et.al. 2020).

Eventually, the connectivity of medical devices and sensors improves the medical care productively for human being in inside the walls and remote places. Mainly IoMT is consists of sensors and other circuitry to get the biological information from the patient and process it over a network and stores in a temporary storage device and can be displayed.

Importance of IoMT in Healthcare

The competence of IoMT is exact results of treatment, less inaccuracy and cheaper in cost. IoMT can be connected to smart phone, the technology permits the patient for sending their health records to doctors wirelessly so as to achieve superior observation on patient for different illnesses. This is very much important in current situation to medicate the covid patients wirelessly. IoMT healthcare applications are penetrating into the commercial market with huge potentiality.

The example of IoMT at application oriented is "remote patient monitoring" of people who is suffering from long term illnesses, can track the patient medicines orders and the locality of patients for admit in to the hospitals, wearable mHealth devices used for sending the information to caretakers. In case of Internet of Things (IoT), IoMT has many applications than Near Field Communication (NFC), and Radio Frequency Identification (RFID). In this context for remote patients, it is very much useful for giving medication at their home virtually called

"Telemedicine". It reduces the cost and travelling time to patients to go to hospital and consult a doctor directly. Similarly in health care cost, IoMT is giving services to the human by giving the treatment and medicine virtually instead direct check-ups. So that can decrease the cost. In the study of US healthcare, they are saving $300 billion annually (Mohammed Irfan & Naim Ahmad. S.A., 2018)

With fast increase of covid-19 pandemic, people become more cautious to health and maintains more health tips carefully to protect themselves which results in the growing of eHealth and health devices to monitor health parameters like temperature, cholesterol, sugar levels, heartbeat etc.

By taking above applications IoMT is modelled, which is shown in Figure 3.

Figure 3. Building blocks of IoMT system

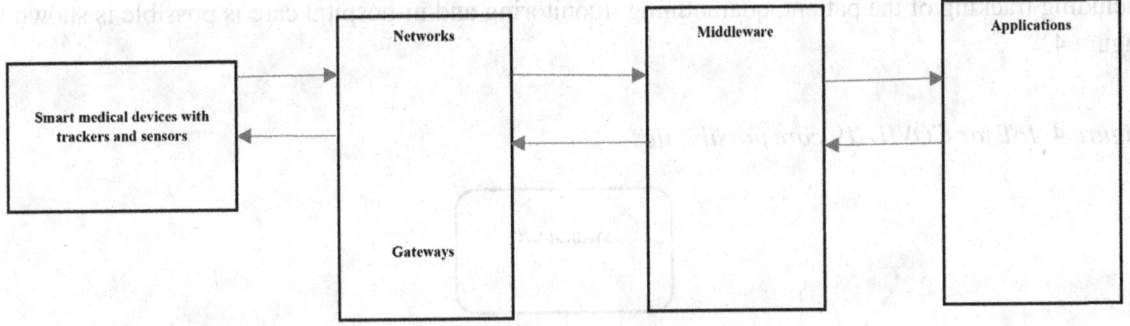

The data extracted from smart medical devices is shared using networks and gateways. Divergent applications are existing using the coordinated system developed in the form of middleware.

The Internet of Medical Things (IoMT) consists of the following layers same as IoT:

- **Perception layer:** This is defined by the smart devices used to collect the all-medical data.
- **Connectivity layer:** Here data transmission can be done between perception layer and cloud and vice-versa through connectivity technologies like networks and gateways.
- **Processing layer:** This layer is represented by the cloud middleware for storing and managing the data.
- **Application layer:** In this layer through software solutions provides the data to the end users.

In fact, Fitbit technology became popular in health applications to get more accurate results for the heart patients by recording simultaneous readings of heart rate and accelerometer data. Fitbit consists of 3-axis accelerometer that can trace the number of steps taken and some other features are also added like distance travelled, calories burned and number of steps climbed. An accelerometer is a kind of sensor used in Fitbit to sense the movement or vibration. For monitoring of heart rate, an optical heart-rate sensor is used in Fitbit by blinking the green LED for number of times to count the human heart beat per minute (BPM) (Azana Hafizah Mohd Aman. Et.al. 2020). Using Fitbit can identify the heart rate zones like peak zone, cardio zone and fat burning zone. This is the one application IoT used in medical field. In this aspect, IoT is offering more applications in healthcare industry by adding its application to nano level. The combination of IoT and nano is called Internet of Nano Things (IoNT). Nano technology offers Scaling of devices, sensors, and systems is much invited without compromising on quality metrics.

The potentiality of IoMT is playing a greater role in the pandemic Covid-19 situation. People died with Covid-19 because of lack of awareness and lack of prompt and timely diagnosis and treatment in hospitals. In this scenario, IoMT is having a greater flexibility to mitigate challenges of Covid-19. IoT is used for different applications to solve the problems of COVID-19 pandemic. IoT can analyze the upcoming occurrences with the advancement of acquired information. Patients can make use of IoT framework for the continuous monitoring of health parameters like pulse rate, glucose level, temperature etc. It serves more clinical opportunities to the individuals to protect themselves.

One of the main problems of IoT innovations in COVID-19 Pandemic is, to fallow the exact treatment for covid patients and particular devices should be used. This makes very complex in serious conditions of the patients. In this regard, by pairing IoT with Artificial intelligence (AI) automatic and scale tracks including tracking of the patient, quarantining, monitoring and in-hospital care is possible is shown in Figure 4.

Figure 4. IoT for COVID-19 care possibilities

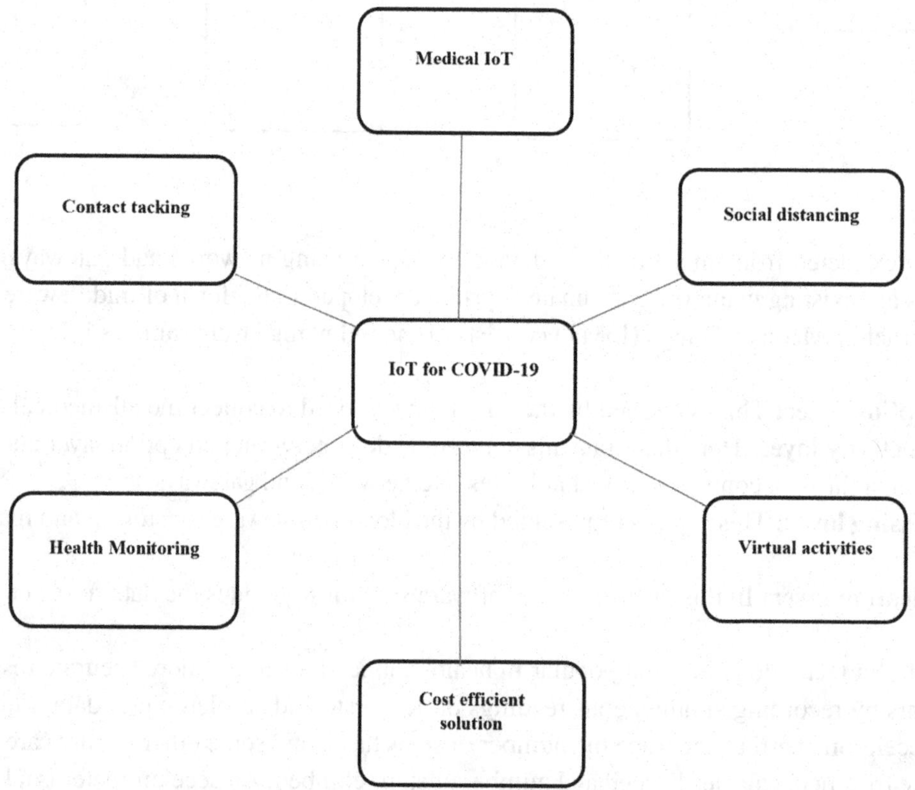

The information about the patient, arrangements of doctors, doctor's notes, and patient past history, X-ray reports and data about different places are produced from different sources, which is acquired using IoT sensors and recorded (The sensor system for medical application has the following stages shown in Figure 5.

Figure 5. Architecture of IoT based sensor system for patient health monitoring system

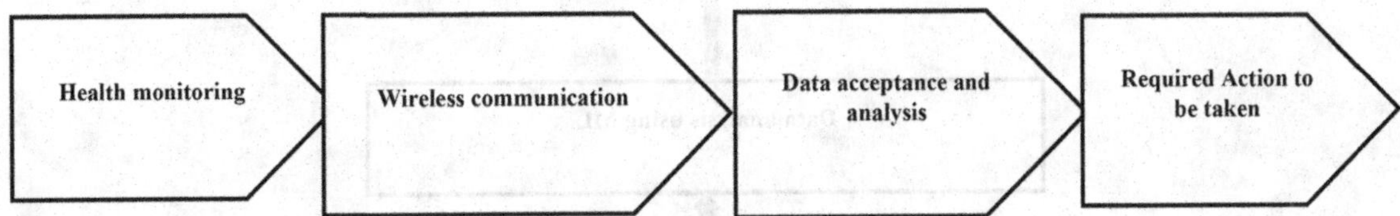

Present day smart phones are implanted with large number of sensors. It is used to sense the daily activities of the patient and can capture the visual information using smartphones. sensors in the smartphones can capture, collect, communicating and stores the large volume of data of the conjecture or COVID-19 patient. Here CT images are scanned by the smartphones and can uploaded to cloud for analysis purposes. It is also possible to examine the multiple CT images for comparison. This can be benefited to diagnose the lungs infection and facilitates to give grade for that. IoT facilitates the sensors to identify the infections from the crowed places like railway stations and clinics (Udgata.S.K. & Suryadevara. N.K. 2021).

Some more applications of IoT are, temperature measurement of employees at their work places. In this non-contact infrared thermometry temperature measures the person's skin temperature. Infrared sensors and thermal cameras are used to measure the skin temperature.

Crowd- based disease tracking (CDT) is one of the applications of IoT where using sensor network people and volunteers can send their sensing data related to disease, symptoms, nearby infection persons, quarantine details etc. through smart phones. using CDT, collected data can be examined for further steps. CDT is less pervasive and needs lot of people intervention and hardware sensors. But it is more reliable and less noisy.

CDT system consists of fallowing components shown in Figure 6.

1. **Data collection:** It consists of a network and users can be connected to it through a smartphone application having stored information and IoT devices (heart rate monitors, thermal scanners, activity trackers). Using this application eligible people can enter their data easily about COVID-19. If the person wants to enter the data, then it facilitates them to enter their location easily and also can share easily.
2. **Data analysis:** This framework can perform some statistical computations on collected data using Artificial Intelligence (AI) and Machine Learning (ML), then analyses infections based on the regions. To maintains the bandwidth and faster computations it can also executes AI algorithms at the end.
3. **Application framework:** At this framework using mobile phone application, it will indicate visually the infected regions. The app can get all the information from the backend of the server and solves the queries of the people (Ex: safe zones of COVID-19, danger zones). Probably, data collection, analysis and application will be done through smartphones.

Figure 6. Overview of the CDT system

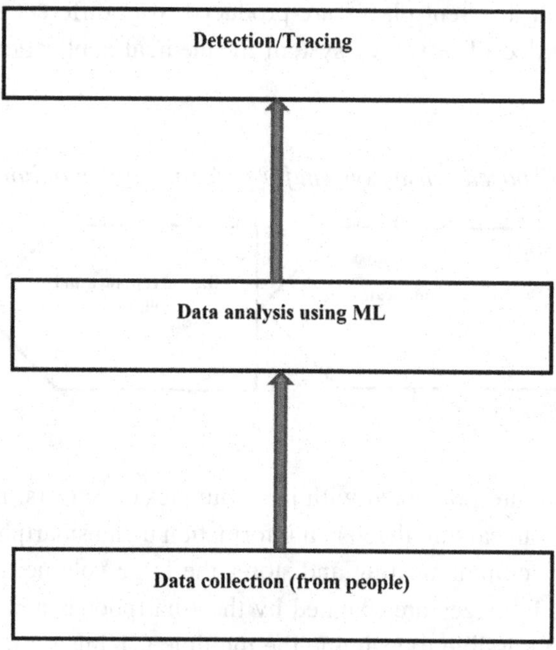

Singapore and south Korea are using this mobile app for security and prevention of COVID-19. And the government of India also launched the app "Arohya Setu" for tracing the COVID-19 from the crowded areas.

IMPACT OF IOMT ON COVID-19 PANDEMIC

IoMT also playing an important role in the present COVID-19 Pandemic situation and also giving opportunities for the next generation healthcare system to live life smartly. The impact of COVID-19 on human is very effective and entire globe suffered from pandemic especially Healthwise. More people died with the lack of medical care in the pandemic. In this regard, IoMT has great advantages to give medical services smartly to the patients. Testing kits has been developed based on detection of COVID-19 using IoMT connected to smart phones. Though there are continuous researches are going on in the entire world, corona second wave has started and again all suffered from this because of lack of awareness about different variants of virus. So, it is necessary to solve all these problems for the next generation. Advantages of IoT and its significance is very much used in the distribution of vaccine supply chain management. Aside from, it is connected for the vehicle tracking, IoT sensors and actuators can be implanted to coolant boxes of vaccine to measure the humidity and temperature. Along with IoT gives security about vaccine details by proving barcodes that send all information to IoT system in the cloud or provides a secret key crypto for sealing the data.

INTERNET OF EVERYTHING (IOE)

IoT composed of only "Things", whereas IoE built with "four pillars", people data, process, things. The term IoE is used by CISCO and QUALCOMM, because it spreads into industrial and business applications to upgrade the lives of people (Mahdi. H. et.al. 2018). The unconnected and nonnetworked devices are connected to the internet such as machine to machine, people to people and people to machine. This is shown in the Figure 7.

Figure 7. Internet of Everything (IoE)

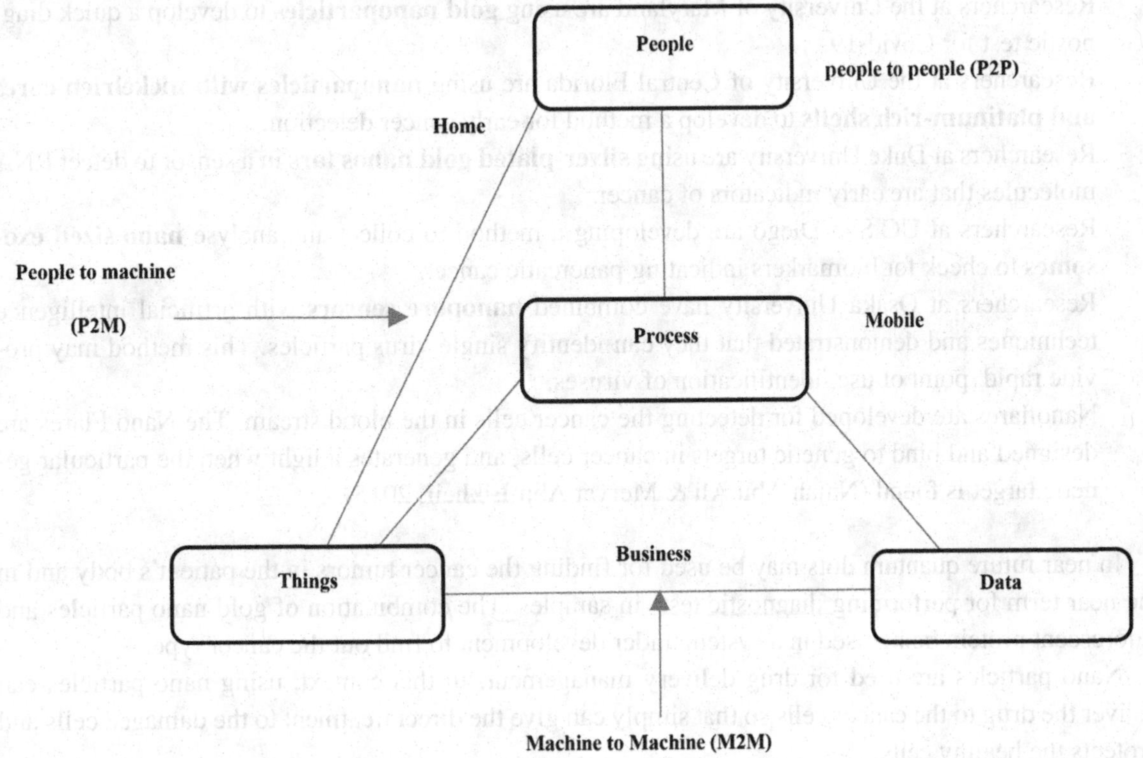

The potentiality of IoE is to extract and analyze the real-time data, senses the data using sensors then apply it to the people-based processor. It also helps in environmental problems, public policy goals and social goals. Next cloud computing facilitates IoE applications to connect everything online. The applications of IoE include, road-embedded sensors, road traffic flow control, agricultural growth monitoring, healthcare and education. It also forms a foundation in the mining industry to dig the fossil fuels and remote monitoring and improves the quality and safety of the system. But IoE failed in implementing the cities to smart communities by adding the features of the smart grid and automation of traffic plan and control. later the IoE has been extended into Nano technology used for the establishment of Internet of Nano Things (IoNT). This can be achieved by using nanosensors in the internet which is connected through a Nano-Network.

NANO IN IOT

Nano technology offers compatible or compact size components. Its applications are diverse in many fields like bio electronics, medical fields, industries etc. along with these, it is applicable in IoT. Nano technology is an extension of existing sciences into nano scale. Nano technology in medicine is playing an important role for the development of nano particles for drug delivery, heat, light and other substances are some specific types of cells such as cancer. Nano particles can heal the diseased cells. This technique can reduce the damage of healthy cells in the human body. Another application of nano is, medical diagnostics is under development.

- Researchers at the University of Maryland are using **gold nanoparticles** to develop a quick diagnostic test for Covid-19.
- Researchers at the University of Central Florida are using **nanoparticles with nickelrich cores and platinum-rich shells** to develop a method for early cancer detection.
- Researchers at Duke University are using **silver-plated gold nanos tars** in a sensor to detect RNA molecules that are early indicators of cancer.
- Researchers at UC San Diego are developing a method to collect and analyse **nano sized exosomes** to check for biomarkers indicating pancreatic cancer.
- Researchers at Osaka University have combined **nanopore sensors** with artificial intelligence techniques and demonstrated that they can identify single virus particles. This method may provide rapid, point of use, identification of viruses.
- Nanoflares are developed for detecting the cancer cells in the blood stream. The Nano Flares are designed and bind to genetic targets in cancer cells, and generates a light when the particular genetic target is found (Najah Abu Ali & Mervat Abu-Elkheir, 2015).

In near future quantum dots may be used for finding the cancer tumors in the patient's body and in the near term for performing diagnostic tests in samples. The combination of gold nano particles and fluorescent protein being used in a system under development to find out the cancer type.

Nano particles are used for drug delivery management. In this context, using nano particles can deliver the drug to the cancer cells.so that simply can give the direct treatment to the damaged cells and protects the healthy cells.

Like this nano technology is used in many health applications such as, chemotherapy, heart diseases, nano medicine, wound treatment etc. In this regard, nano technology merged into IoT and can be using in many applications mainly in medical sector called Internet of Nano Things (IoNT).

Internet of Nano Things (IoNT)

In IoNT, the nano sensors, termed as nano things, connected through a nanoscale network and exchange information using nano communication technology.

Internet of Things not only deployed as the human can see the things but also is involved in nano level as human cannot see. This can be achieved by IoNT and IoBNT. These technologies are not only used in industrial, water purification etc. but also playing an important role in medical applications. The term IoBNT is came from biology and taking the advantages of nanotechnology is a combination of

IoNT with existing IoT health care system and networks. This technology facilitates to reduce the risk of undesired effects on health and/or the environment.

In IoNT nano sensors also called as "nano things" are connected through a nano network and exchange information using nano communication technologies. The basic operation of the nano things is sensing and transmits the sensed data. Nano sensors are embedded into different objects and one object might be incorporated into multiple nano sensors and communicate themselves through nanonetworks. Using wireless sensor networks (WSN) it would be communicates outside the world. Implementation of IoNT is a complemented for other related technologies like IoT, pervasive computing, fog computing, big data analytics, sensor networks, cloud computing etc.

IOT IMPACT DURING COVID-19 PANDEMIC

UAV Based Health Surveillance and Alerting (UHSA)

The impact of IoT, IoMT and IoNT during pandemic can be well understood with the following automatic system.

Unmanned aerial vehicle (UAV) based health monitoring system is a system used to overcome the challenges of COVID-19 urgency. In this system by using sensors (GPS, Thermal cameras, accelerometer, gyroscope) from the Figure 8. it collects the information about the COVID patients remotely. For example, UAVs can detect the infected people in the crowded areas through cameras fixed to it (Joel. J.P.C et.al. 2021).

Figure 8. UAV-based health surveillance and alerting system

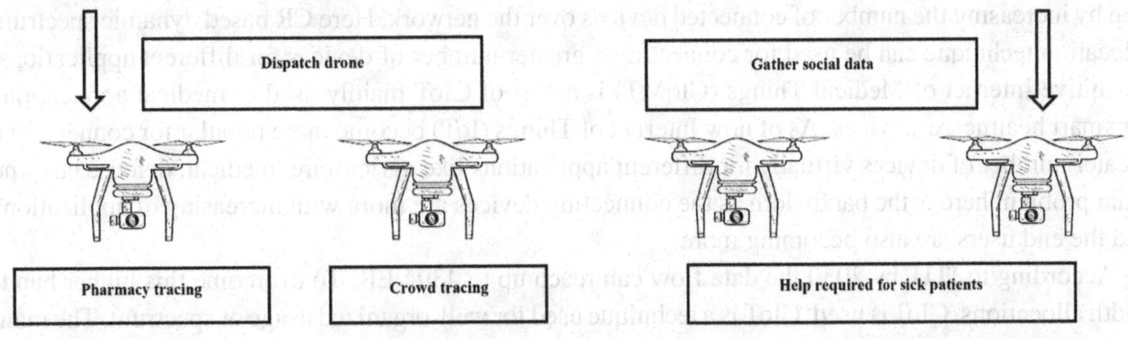

The UAV-based system gives an acknowledgement to Individuals through social signal filtration module or user operated IoT devices about crowded areas. In the next step, the obtained data can be sensed from the backend of the server based on deep learning, machine learning, statistical analysis to get the true data. Then the information can be upgraded over nearby regions by giving alerting messages, alarms that can be installed on UAV system. UAVs are also scan the information based on situation about different regions. Here on-board sensors and image classification algorithms (CNN's) are using in UHSA can detect the people weather they are fallowing the rules or not during the lockdown period.

it also detects the emergency usages like pharmacy tracing and availability of medication. This is the latest application of IoT used in healthcare.

Cognitive Internet of Medical Things

Data flows from every corner of the globe. Scientists, healthcare professionals must be vigilant about the diverse flow of data and the means to process it. Effectiveness and Speed competes each other in these crunch situations. As the domain interest is related to health, ample care must be taken regarding the development of any algorithm, technique or data processing approach.

Most of the times, researchers in the war-room discussions, rely upon the modification of existing algorithms as per the requirement, instead of developing a new method. Computing Science and Engineering has various data-based applications. Newer branches of engineering are emerging with data as a focal point. In this whole process, classification and modelling of data became crucial.

Present technologies like Artificial Intelligence (AI), Cloud Computing, Internet of Things (IoT) are used in health sector in current pandemic COVID-19 situation to solve more health issues (Swayam Siddha. S & Mohanty. C. 2020). Consequently, the technological era is growing with the rapid growth of IoT in 5G technology, combination of AI with machine learning algorithms like decision tree, random forest, reinforcement learning etc., industry 4.0, big data, block chain technology and cloud computing are used for undying solutions to prevent the COVID-19. Also, these technologies can prevent the increase of disease. These technologies use IoT for collection of real time data of the people. The assimilation of this knowledge base is useful in developing another category of IoMT i.e., Cognitive Internet of Medical Things.

Cognitive Internet of Medical Things (CIoMT) is the same type of technology that permits each particular physical object in the world to interface and interchange of information with good quality.

CIoT is a combination of Cognitive Radio (CR) and IoT which holdup machine to machine interaction by increasing the number of connected devices over the network. Here CR based dynamic spectrum allocation technique can be used for connecting a greater number of devices for different applications. Cognitive Internet of Medical Things (CIoMT) is a part of CIoT mainly used in medical applications for smart healthcare services. As of now Internet of Things (IoT) become more popular for connecting a greater number of devices virtually for different applications like agriculture, medical, defense etc., the main problem here is the bandwidth as the connecting devices are more with increasing of applications and the end users are also becoming more.

According to ITU, by 2030 the data flow can reach up to 4394 EB. To overcome this higher bandwidth allocations, CIoT is used. CIoT is a technique used for well-organized usage of spectrum. The main aim of CIoT is to energetically assign radio channels for the information exchange between the related devices connected to it. CIoT is the best suitable approach to present pandemic scenario where more persons are associated and observed over a network. Also because of lock-down and curtailments for the people, more activities become online like e-healthcare, e-learning, e-commerce etc. these activities should be done through wireless communication channel which utilizes more bandwidth. To overcome this problem for getting good bandwidth CIoT is used and having efficient network transmission that transmits short packets by searching the inactive channels and thus improves the bandwidth and make use of spectrum more comfortable.

CIOMT IMPORTANCE IN COVID-19 PANDEMIC AND APPLICATIONS

Present pandemic has transformed a challenge in the entire globe. IoT in particular IoMT become popular to mitigate challenges of COVID-19 Pandemic. The CIoMT is an augmentation of CIoT which is shown in Figure 9.

Figure 9. Development of CIoMT

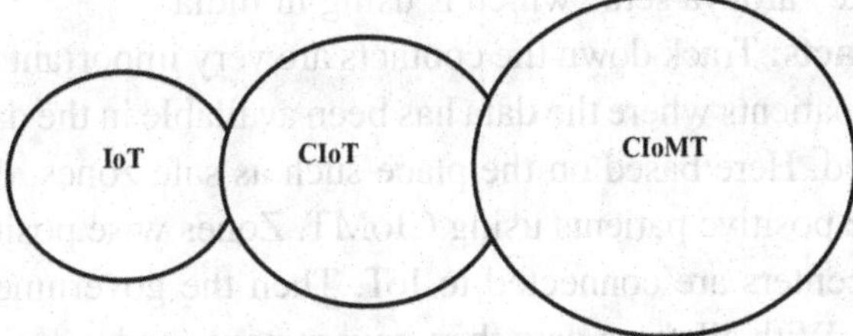

The applications of CIoMT have become popular in COVID-19 Pandemic because of smart allocation of channels and improves the bandwidth facilities for smart healthcare. This technology gives more scope to control the COVID-19 by giving the proper diagnosis and control. Entire world got affected by the COVID-19 and that is not easy to control by individuals until and unless there is a live update about disease (Swayam siddha. S & Mohanty. C, 2020). So, IoMT facilitates to get all the information about diseased people by enabling the sensors, transformation and communicating through the network. In this scenario, IoMT is established in main areas to trace COVID-19 which is shown in Figure 10.

Figure 10. Applications of CIoMT to overcome the problems of COVID-19 Pandemic

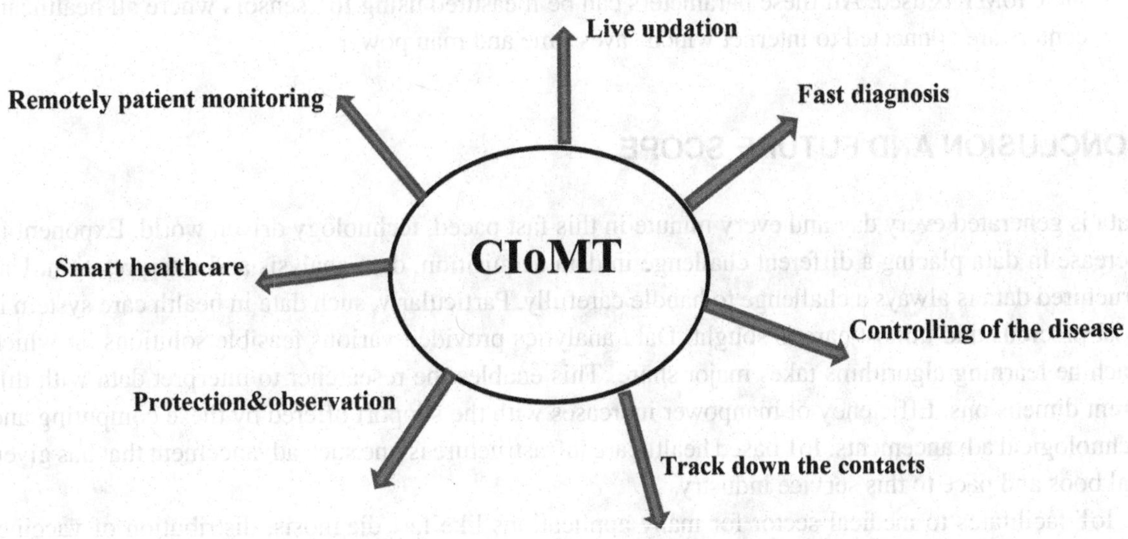

1. **Live updation:** this application belongs to live updates about corona patients like active cases, cured ones, death count can be tracked from various locations using CIoMT technology. Based on the results disease can be analyzed using AI for decision making then further precautions and preparations can be taken and can be updated to persons connected to CIoMT.
2. **Fast diagnosis:** the diseased people and conjecture are isolated even if they are not having symptoms immediate treatment is necessary. In this application CIoMT facilitates the people to get fast clinical treatment by connecting themselves to network for fast and error free results.
3. **Controlling of the disease:** here, the CIoMT is used to give a vigilant to people about diseased ones by using apps like "arohya setu" which is using in India.
4. **Track down the contacts:** Track down the contacts are very important to prevent the virus spread of the corona positive patients where the data has been available in the database in which the health centers can be acquired. Here based on the place such as safe zones, danger zones are upgraded immediately about the positive patients using CIoMT. Zones wise positive cases can be collected when the healthcare centers are connected to IoT. Then the government can analyze these data using AI substructure. With all these data then government can be decided about the lockdown.
5. **Protection and observation:** The inspection of people at hotels, hospitals, crowded areas, airports, railway stations are to be done by facial recognition through CIoMT which is connected to healthcare centers for the observation of corona patients. This can be useful for the prevention of virus spread.
6. **Smart healthcare:** tracing the contacts of COVID-19 patients, giving a treatment and all can be done through CIoMT where limited man power is required and everything can be done remotely, that makes an advantage for the healthy people to protect themselves from virus. Also, patients can get medication remotely from the hospitals.
7. **Remotely patient monitoring:** As the virus is heavily spreading, the CIoMT helps to reduce the intervention of people with doctors directly. Instead, here doctors can take the patients data such as their pulse rate, temperature, computing tomography (CT), X-rays, glucose levels etc. where the CIoMT is used. All these parameters can be measured using IoT sensors where all healthcare centers are connected to internet which saves time and man power.

CONCLUSION AND FUTURE SCOPE

Data is generated every day and every minute in this fast paced, technology driven world. Exponential increase in data placing a different challenge in data acquisition, data analysis and interpretation. Unstructured data is always a challenge to handle carefully. Particularly, such data in health care system is most precious and utmost care is sought. Data analytics provided various feasible solutions, in which machine learning algorithms takes major share. This enables the researcher to interpret data with different dimensions. Efficiency of manpower increases with the support offered by these computing and technological advancements. IoT based healthcare infrastructure is one such advancement that has given real boos and pace to this service industry.

IoT facilitates to medical sector for many applications like fast diagnosis, distribution of vaccine, remotely patient monitoring, smart healthcare etc. Diseased people can be easily identified using IoMT connected with mobile apps. Apart from this, IoT uses cognitive radio technology for the improvement of bandwidth and power savings. Nano technology also can be merged with IoT to provide advanced medical applications for people called Internet of Nano Things (IoNT) for the treatment of diseases like cancer etc. using nano sensors. IoNT provides less space, low power consumption etc. Additionally, the applications of IoT are using in present COVID-19 Pandemic. In this regard, treatment is going on virtually by taking all health parameters using different devices where IoT is connected to it. IoT suffers from security issues. To overcome this problem PUF technology has been developed to provide better security in all aspects. Finally, IoT is used in everywhere as Internet of Everything (IoE).

Cognitive Internet of Medical Things observed to be intelligent and helpful during a typical medical emergency situation such as pandemic. The use of CIoMT in a covid-19 pandemic scenario is explained. In the context of COVID-19, there are some challenges like security; though there are some technologies like PUF technology but still it is facing the problem at security corner in the pandemic situation like many patients' data should be protected. Second one is the network integration. In addition, future scope shall be concentrated on data storage and worthwhile. The importance of prediction models and mathematical models developed, tested and validated across the globe were so significant during Pandemic. The inclusion of more variety and nature inspired algorithms would produce more accurate results and helps to boost our healthcare and administrative systems.

REFERENCES

Ali & Abu-Elkheir. (2015). *Internet of Nano-Things Healthcare Applications: requirements, opportunities, and challenges*. IEEE. doi:10.1109/WiMOB.2015.7347934

Azana, Hassan, Sameen, Bash, Alizadeh, & Latiff. (2020). IoMT amid COVID-19 pandemic: Application, architecture, technology, and security. *Journal of Network and Computer Applications*. Advance online publication. doi:10.1016/j.jnca.2020.102886

Babaei & Schiele. (2019). *Physical Unclonable Functions in the Internet of Things: State of the Art and Open Challenges*. doi:10.3390/s19143208

Bharati, Podder, Mondal, & Paul. (2021). *Applications and Challenges of Cloud Integrated IoMT*. doi:10.1007/978-3-030-55833-8_4

Bin Zikria, Ali, Afzal, & Kim. (2021). *Next Generation Internet of Things (IoT): Opportunities, Challenges, and Solutions Sensors*. . doi:10.3390/s21041174

Dey, Ashour, & Bhatt. (2017). *Internet of Things Driven Connected Healthcare: Internet of Things and Big Data Technologies for Next Generation Healthcare*. Springer International Publishing. doi.. doi:10.1007/978-3-319-49736-5_1

Gokhale, Bhat, & Bhat. (2018). Introduction to IOT. IARJSET, 5(1).

Hatzivasilis, Soultatos, Ioannidis, Verikoukis, Demetriou, & Tsatsoulis. (n.d.). *Review of Security and Privacy for the Internet of Medical Things (IoMT)*. IEEE. doi:. doi:10.1109/DCOSS.2019.00091

Irfan & Naim Ahmad. (2018). *Internet of Medical Things: Architectural Model, Motivational Factors and Impediments*. Dept. of Computer Science, King Khaild University.

Joel, J. P. C. (2021). *Internet of Medical Things in the Context of COVID-19*. Academic Press.

Kelly, Campbell, Gong, & Ham. (2020). The Internet of Things: Impact and Implications for Health Care Delivery. *Journal of Medical Internet Research*. Advance online publication. doi:10.2196/20135

Kumar, Thiwari, & Zymbler. (2019). Internet of Things is a revolutionary approach for future technology enhancement: a review. *Journal of Big Data*. doi:10.1186/s40537-019-0268-2

Latha, R., & Vetrivelan, P. (2020). *Wireless Body Area Network (WBAN)-Based Telemedicine for Emergency Care*. School of Electronics Engineering. *Vellore Institute of Technology, Chennai*. Advance online publication. doi:10.339020072153

Mahdi, Miraz, Ali, & Picking. (2018). *Internet of Nano-Things, Things and Everything: Future Growth Trends*. doi:10.3390/fi10080068

Pradhan, Bhattacharyya, & Pal. (2020). IoT-Based Applications in Healthcare Devices. *Hindawi Journal of Healthcare Engineering, 2021*, 6632599. Advance online publication. doi:10.1155/2021/6632599 PMID:33791084

Sadiku, Kelechi, Sarhan, & Musa Roy. (2018). Wireless Sensor Networks for Healthcare. *Perry College of Engineering, Prairie View A&M University, Journal of Scientific and Engineering Research, 5*(7), 210-213.

Swayam Siddha, S., & Mohanty, C. (2020). Application of cognitive Internet of Medical Things for COVID-19 pandemic. *Diabetes & Metabolic Syndrome, 8*. Advance online publication. doi:10.1016/j.dsx.2020.06.014.8

Udgata, S. K., & Suryadevara, N. K. (2021). *COVID-19, Sensors, and Internet of Medical Things (IoMT), Internet of Things and Sensor Network for COVID-19*. Springer Nature Singapore Pte Ltd. doi:10.1007/978-981-15-7654-6

Vishnu, S., Jino Ramson, S. R., & Jegan, R. (2020). Internet of medical things (IoMT)- Overview. *5th International Conference on Devices, Circuits and Systems (ICDCS).*

Zou, Xu, Wang, Li, Chen, & Hu. (2017). A Survey on Secure Wireless Body Area Networks. *Hindawi Security and Communication Networks*. . doi:10.1155/2017/3721234

Chapter 13
Information Science in the Analytics of Healthcare Data

Sofia Jonathan G.
Lady Doak College, Madurai, India

ABSTRACT

Information science is an interdisciplinary field that deals with the effective collection, storage, retrieval, and use of information for better decision making through related technologies. Today, healthcare organizations are looking for more efficient and sophisticated means of collecting, managing, analyzing data, and delivering medical information to physicians, clinicians, and nurses. The role of information science in the healthcare domain is to improve the quality of patient care, reduce operational cost, and make the entire internal management process well organized for better decision making. Through the application of technology, data analytics and information science practitioners help drive data-informed healthcare decisions. Hence, this chapter covers the techniques that are useful for data analytics and information management in healthcare such as data mining, machine learning, cloud computing, and data visualization.

INTRODUCTION

Information Science is an interdisciplinary field which deals with the effective collection, storage, retrieval and use of information. It also concerns about the analysis, classification, manipulation, movement, distribution and protection of information. It incorporates the recorded information with anticipated knowledge for better decision making through related technologies and services that facilitate their effective management and use.

Historically, Information Science is associated with computer science, Data Science, Psychology, Technology and Intelligence agencies. But now it has been extended to integrate the various aspects of diverse fields which are in need of managing and using information magnificently for their advancement. One such field is healthcare that collects stores and manages huge patient's Electronic Medical Record (EMR) and data pertaining to hospital's administration in order to aid healthcare policy decisions. Today, healthcare organizations are looking for more efficient and sophisticated means of collecting, manag-

DOI: 10.4018/978-1-7998-9132-1.ch013

Copyright © 2022, IGI Global. Copying or distributing in print or electronic forms without written permission of IGI Global is prohibited.

ing, analyzing data and delivering medical information to physicians, clinicians and nurses. The role of Information Science in healthcare domain is to improve the quality of patient care, reduce operational cost and make the entire internal management process well organized for better decision-making. The primary concern is to identify the methodologies to effectively access, process and maintain large volumes of sensitive data catering to the needs.

Today, diagnosis of disease is a vital job in the medical field. It is essential to interpret the correct diagnosis of patient with the help of clinical examination and investigations. Most hospitals have a huge amount of patient data, which is rarely used to support clinical diagnosis (Motilal et. al., 2013). Our healthcare sector daily collects a huge data concerned with patients including clinical examination, vital parameters, investigation reports, treatment follow-ups, drug decisions etc. But very unfortunately it has not been analyzed and mined in an appropriate way. It is just stored as bunches of paper sheet or occupying hard disc space. These valuable data are handled mainly by researches and statisticians at professional level.

Computer information based decision support system that analyze and predict the data can play an important role in accurate diagnosis and cost effective treatment. In future, it will definitely be helpful in various diseases management including effectiveness of surgical procedures, medical tests, medication and the discovery of relationships among clinical and diagnosis data with accuracy.

Health data is collected from a variety of systems and devices, such as online patient portals, electronic medical records, glucometers, health tracking devices, diagnostic systems and genomics. As a result, data exists in different formats, from clinical notes to medical images such as CT scans and at times, the data is unstructured. Through the application of Technology, Data Analytics and Information Science practitioners help in driving data-informed health care decisions. Hence this chapter covers the techniques that provide support for Data Analytics and Information Management in healthcare such as Data Mining, Machine Learning, Cloud Computing and Data Visualization as shown in figure 1. An increased focus on these techniques supports the healthcare system through enhanced decisions for advance care process that can address the public healthcare issues on time. It offers a win-win situation for both the patients and the healthcare providers.

DIGITAL MEDICAL DATA

Health problems impact human lives (Marzyeh Ghassem et. al., 2019). During medical care, health providers collect clinical data about each particular patient and leverage knowledge from it to determine the treatment process of that patient. Clinical data thus play a fundamental role in addressing health problems and improved information is crucial in improving patient care.

In the medical field, huge amount of data is generated, from patient's personal information to medical history, from genetic data to clinical data(Laura Elezabeth et. al., 2018). Medical (clinical) data refers to health-related information that is associated with regular patient care or as part of a clinical trial programme. This clinical data is vital for administrators to determine what areas of their service need to improve and offer more granular information regarding treatment effectiveness, success rates and more. This medical data in the form of digital is a primary source for most health care and medical research. Health care data falls into six major types as shown in Figure 2.

Figure 1. Techniques for data analytics and information management in healthcare

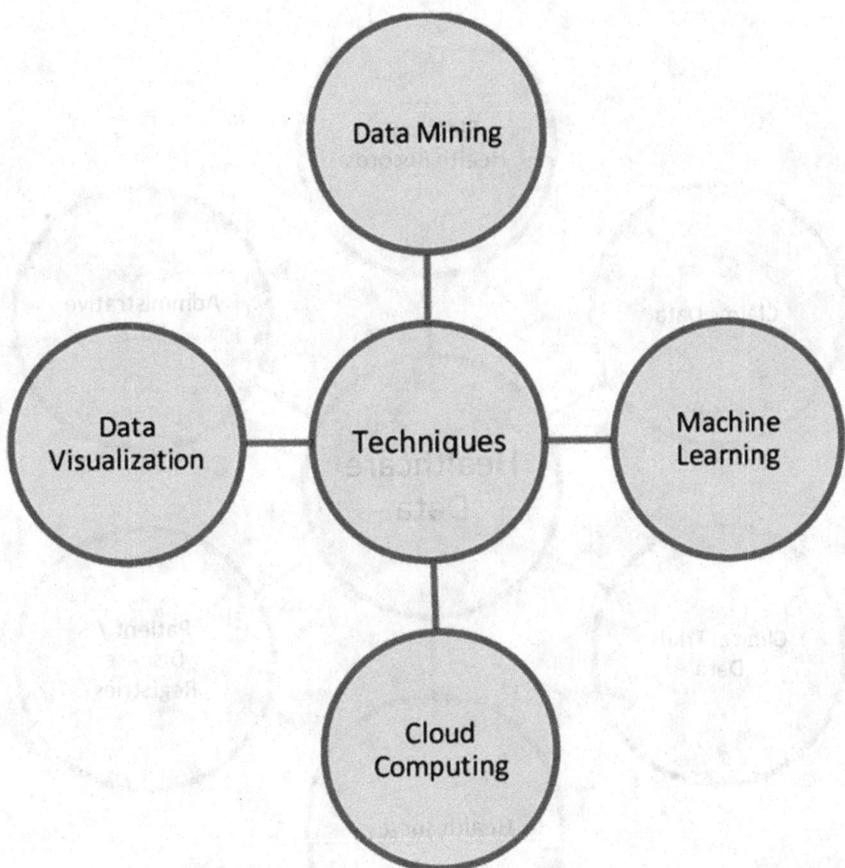

DIGITAL MEDICAL

Electronic Health Record: This is the purest type of electronic clinical data which is obtained at the point of care at a medical facility, hospital, clinic or practice. It is often referred as the electronic medical record (EMR). The data collected includes administrative and demographic information, diagnosis, treatment, prescription drugs, laboratory tests, physiologic monitoring data, hospitalization, patient insurance, etc.

Administrative Data: This non-clinical data focus on record-keeping and other services which is associated with electronic health records. These are primarily hospital discharge information reported to a government / non-government agency.

Claims Data: It describes the information regarding insurance claims. Claims data falls into four general categories: inpatient, outpatient, pharmacy, and enrollment. The sources of claims data can be obtained from the government and/or commercial health firms.

Patient / Disease Registries: Disease registries are clinical information systems that collect and track clinical information of defined patient for certain chronic conditions such as Alzheimer's Disease, cancer, diabetes, heart disease, and asthma. Registries often provide critical information for managing patient conditions.

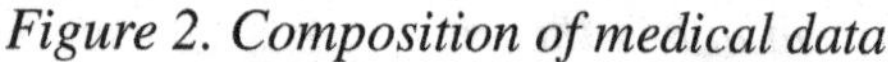

Figure 2. Composition of medical data

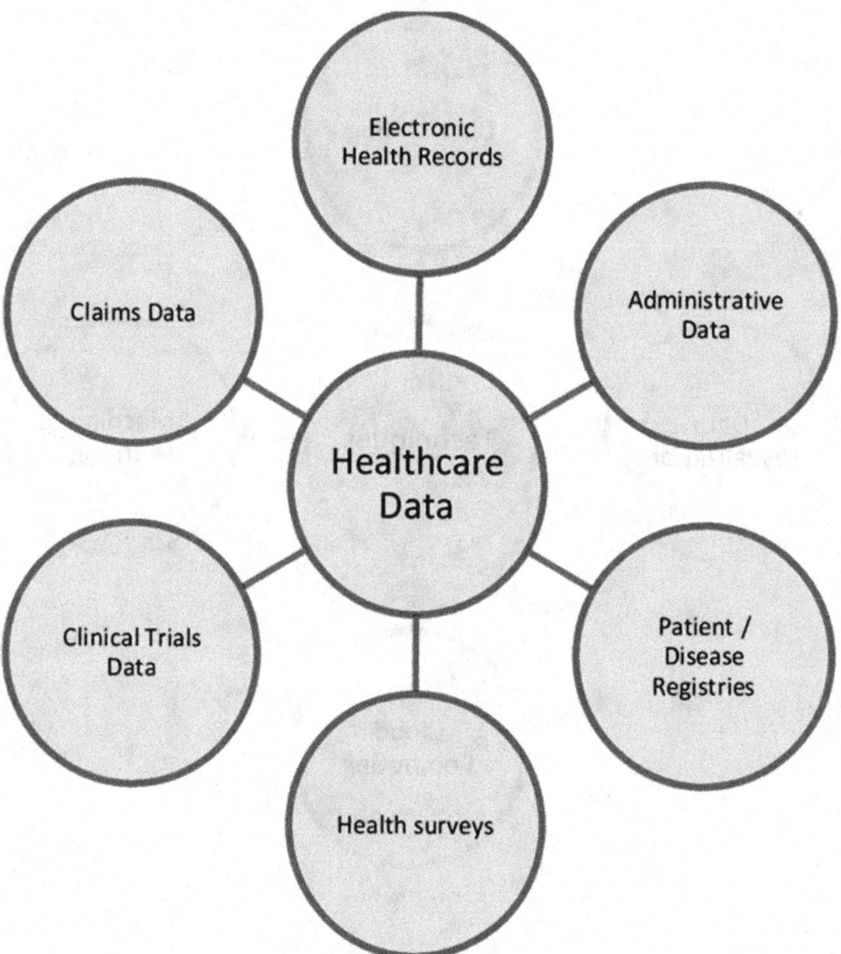

Health Surveys: In order to provide an accurate evaluation of the population health, national surveys of the most common chronic conditions are generally conducted to provide prevalence estimates. National surveys are one of the few types of data collected specifically for research purposes, thus making it more widely accessible. It can help in the analysis of the most common chronic illnesses a nation faces like Covid-19.

Clinical Trials Data: Clinical trial data has been gathered from patients and healthy volunteers who participate in experiment associated with clinical research. Raw data are collected between the time of first participant enrollment and study completion. During the course of the trial, the raw data are abstracted, coded and transcribed.

This medical data generated contains valuable information that can also be utilized for medicinal services and medication regulatory purposes. With this enormous amount of information, significant and dependable inferences can be made which could be helpful for the annihilation of ailments. When this information is analyzed appropriately, it can help to comprehend the causes for sickness and consequently to attain significant leaps in the restorative process. Having computers and technology as an aid, this medical data can be examined quicker in a more accurate way with the help of the technologies. If the medical assumptions deduced from the data are wrong, all the work would be futile.

The digital medical data is not only enormous in amount, but also complex in its structure. Some of the contributing factors to the failure while handling these datasets are given below:

1. The vast variety of structured and unstructured data such as handwritten doctor notes, medical records, medical diagnostic images such as magnetic resonance imaging (MRI), computed tomography (CT)), X-Ray images etc.
2. Existence of noisy, heterogeneous, complex, longitudinal, diverse and large datasets in healthcare informatics.

Hence, there is a need for managing and analyzing such complex, diverse and huge information for enhanced insight and decision-making, within the reasonable time frame and with the available storage capacity. This insight is invaluable which highlights issues like adverse reactions or medical failures quickly, allowing medical personnel to diagnose problems and halt or alter procedures before the problem escalates. It allows medical practitioners to spot the problems precisely and help them to design better processes that improve standards of care and ultimately save lives.

HEALTHCARE ANALYTICS

Healthcare analytics is the process of analyzing current and historical data to predict trends, improve outreach and even better manage the spread of diseases. As healthcare organizations around the world are challenged to reduce costs, improve coordination with care teams, provide more with less, and focus on improving patient care, analytics will be especially important. Hence it focuses on the technologies and processes that measure, manage and analyze healthcare data to provide organizations with actionable insights.

Healthcare analytics is breaking a new vital ground in a sector where the slightest mistake or inaccuracy can have dire consequences. Both practicing physicians and researchers are able to use tools to analyze huge information at speed, drawing out patterns and trends that tell them at glance what's working, what's not and how the patients are responding to the medicines or treatments they've been given.

In health analytics, decision making and problem solving are very vital for proper care of the patients. It enables the practitioners and health workers to make policy, improve working condition with the use of technological base support tools. Building analytics competencies can help healthcare organizations harness big data to create actionable insights that can be used by healthcare providers, hospital and health system leaders to improve outcomes for the people they serve. These insights are developed through analytical disciplines to drive fact-based decision making. In turn, these decisions improve planning, management, measurement and learning. Healthcare organization can also improve their efficiency and effectiveness in the delivery of their duties as it relate to data extraction from patterns in order to make accurate decision by the use of information technology, computer based tools, mathematical computation, statistical tools etc (Ogundele et. al., 2018).

Figure 3 shows the stages of health analytics and the four types of health analytics is given in figure 4.

Clinical data is collected from various sources for analysis. During preprocessing, data will be cleaned to handle missing data and noisy data. Data is transformed to make it better-organized. Transformed

Figure 3. Stages of health analytics

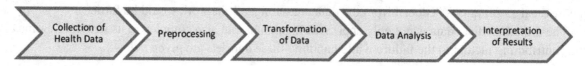

data may be easier for both humans and computers to use. During data transformation, data must be scrubbed, normalized and aggregated into a standard format all can view and manipulate. During data analysis statistical and/or logical techniques will be systematically applied to describe and illustrate, condense and evaluate data. In the last step, interpretation of results is being done by assigning meaning to the collected medical information and determining the conclusions, significance and implications of the findings.

1. **Descriptive analytics** is the most easy and simplest health analytics used by every individual. Descriptive analytics gives overall details of number of patients treated, revenue generated, what are the symptoms of the patients, diseases diagnosed, how are they treated and managed to improve their condition. It gives a summary of the historical data for generate meaningful information. This can be used to diagnose a patient with a particular illness or injury based on the symptoms they're experiencing. Descriptive analytics uses graphical representation for better understanding by the practitioners in healthcare.
2. **Predictive analytics** gives focus on the use of information. Predictive analytics is used to identify future probabilities and trends to predict future occurrences. It defines what could happen in the future. It gathers information from historical background, learn patterns from the dataset and predict the future by extracting useful knowledge. Volumes of complicated data available in healthcare allow predictive analytics of the techniques used in data mining. Health professional could ask, what drugs to be used for the treatment? Who could be affected by this diseases next? It also helps to predict result of a patient and allocate resources appropriately.
3. **Prescriptive analytics** is applied when there are several options in the health problems or choice to deliver the best prescriptive analytics. Prescriptive analytics ask, how do we respond to those potential future events? This has been used in healthcare for treatment and drug prescription. Several drugs might be prescribed by weighing the pros and cons.
4. **Discovery analytics** makes use of the discovered knowledge to come up with new invention and innovation in the field of healthcare. For example, discover new drugs from previously known drugs. This can help to discover new treatment, handle new diseases, and new medication from the known discovery.

DATA MINING FOR HEALTH CARE

Due to its complex features, medical data provide complications for pattern extortion (Saima Anwar Lashari, et. al., 2018). In the last decade, various methods have been used to explore and find patterns and relationships in healthcare data. But from the last few years, Data mining plays a vital role in healthcare industry by exploring more in the sector of health (Ogundele et. al., 2018). It is predominantly used for

Figure 4. Types of health analytics

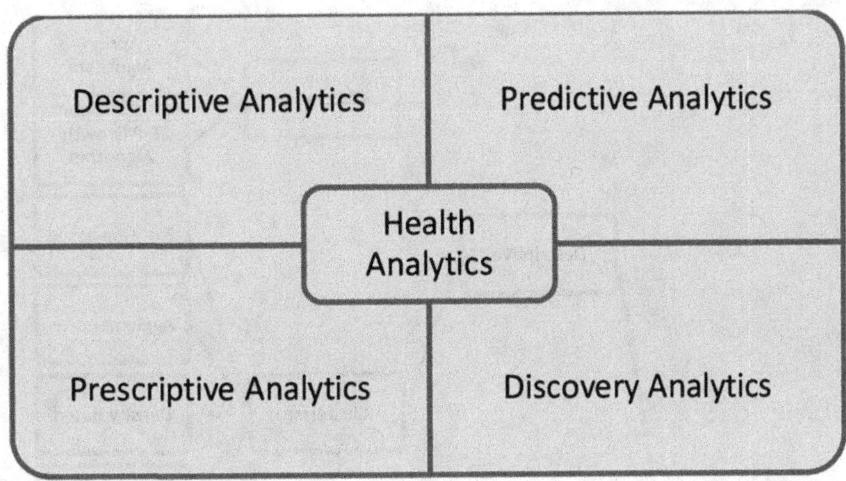

detection and prediction of diseases. Various researchers have also acknowledged the fact that there is a proven need for data mining in healthcare which will help healthcare practitioner to effectively and efficiently provide better services, most especially in prevention, prediction and management of diseases.

In health care industry, data mining helps with the collection and processing of health care data in systemic manner by using computer based programs and subsequent formation of disease prediction. It showed some promise in the use of its predictive analytic techniques and methods to analyze the data related to health issues for improving the services offered in health care industry. The most common data mining algorithms /techniques mentioned in figure 5 are used to predict and analyze various diseases. It can discover and extract hidden knowledge (patterns and relationships) associated with the disease from a historical disease database and assist the healthcare practitioners to make intelligent clinical decisions and provide effective treatments. There are two approaches in data mining: statistical and machine learning algorithms which will be discussed later in this chapter.

Data mining techniques are reliable, practical and effective for the predictive purpose of healthcare data because:

1. It is user friendly and prediction is based on past health records
2. It operates by learning from past health records
3. Data from numerous medical sources is managed and only required data is extracted
4. Models are easily updated by relearning, past medical information and change in trends.

The key phases of data mining such as association, classification and clustering are used by healthcare organization to increase their capability for building appropriate conclusions regarding patient health from raw facts and figures (Sheetal L. Patil, 2015). These techniques are applied in mining medical data, which comprises association rule mining for finding frequent patterns, prediction and classification of diseases and clustering to locate the etiological area. Many researches are doing research on this health care area to analyze the medical data and to develop intelligent decision support systems for more accurate diagnosis and prediction of diseases and also for remote health monitoring.

Figure 5. Data mining techniques for healthcare

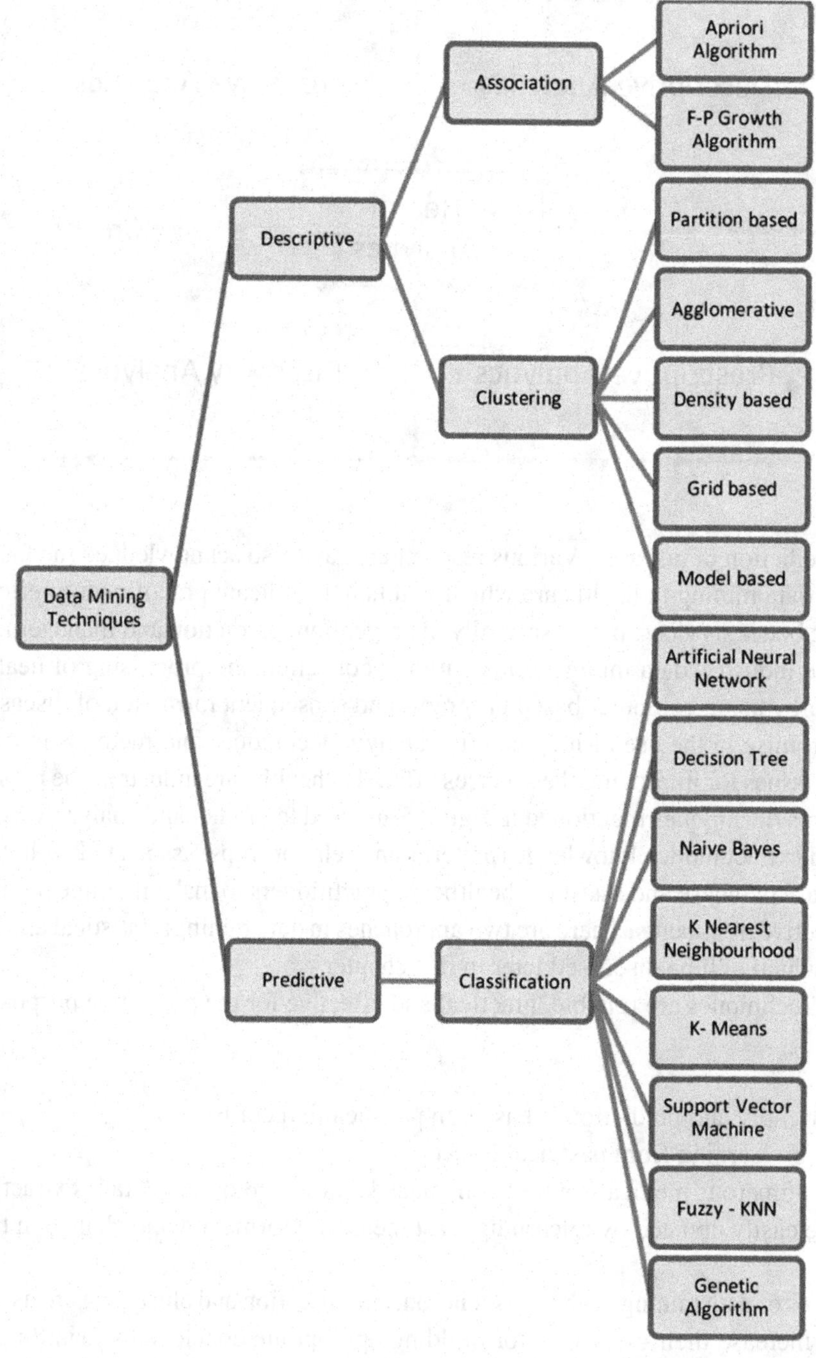

KEY PHASES IN DATA MINING

The detailed description of the key phases in Data Mining shown in figure 6 is given below.

Figure 6. Key phases in data mining for healthcare

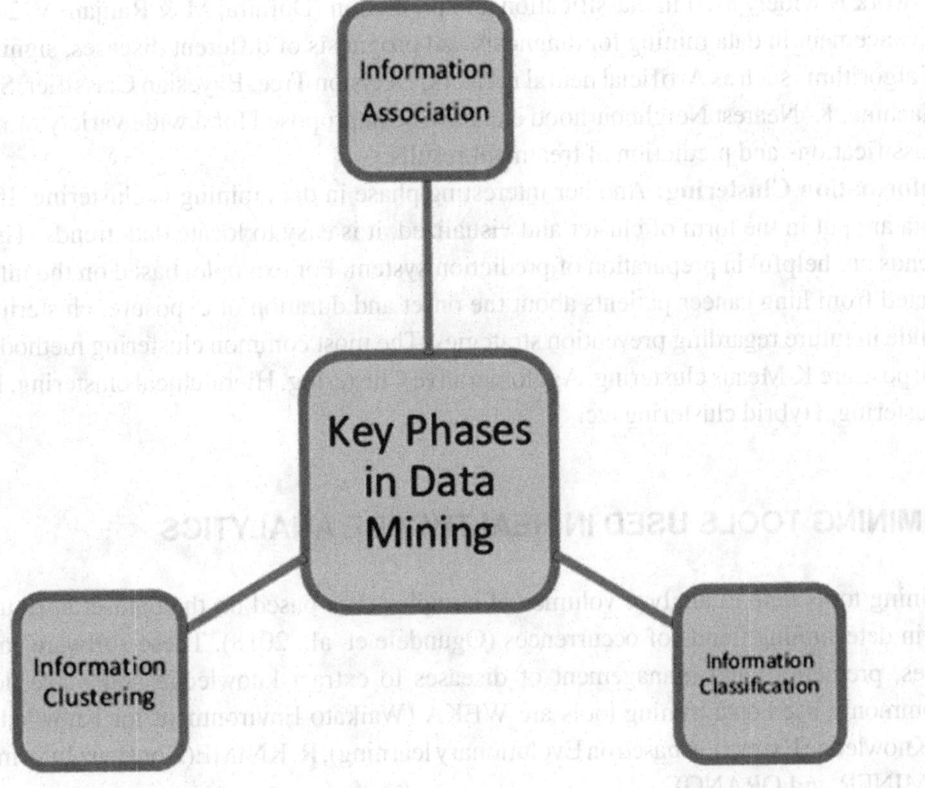

1. **Information Association:** This is the most familiar and straightforward phase. Association finds relationship from datasets in order to predict and give better outcome (Ogundele et. al., 2018). Association also has great impact in the health care industry to discover the relationships between diseases, state of human health and the symptoms of disease (Sheenal Patel & Hardik Patel, 2016). It is used where better accuracy is required. Here association between two or more items or of the same type is identified to formulate specific pattern. For example, it is very well known that there is etiological association between smoking and lung cancer. The data concerned with smoking habit details such as numbers of smoke per day, duration of smoking, type of smoking, specific brands, lifestyle and age of patient etc. are collected and analyzed to find the association between the causes and the disease. Association is useful for identifying the relationship or association among numerous attributes and generates association rules which in turn will help, domain experts for making vital decisions.
2. **Information Classification:** This is second most popular phase. In healthcare industry, the classification provides most widely used methods for detection, prediction and optimization. Here we can classify the collected information according to our objectives like etiological factors, investigation purpose, drug treatment plans and results (Motilal et. al., 2013). Example, the etiological information collected from lung cancer patients can be classified on the basis of the features such as duration of smoking habit, type of exposure, number of exposure, age of patient etc. In classification, features available in the datasets can be classified as low, moderate, high and very high based on the symptoms of the diseases diagnosed (Ogundele et. al., 2018). Patient's survivability

can be analyzed and predicted from the previous knowledge for a period of years. Artificial neural network is widely used in classification and prediction (Durairaj M & Ranjani V, 2013). With the advancement in data mining for diagnosis and prognosis of different diseases, significant number of algorithms such as Artificial neural network, Decision Tree, Bayesian Classifier, Support Vector Machine, K- Nearest Neighbourhood etc. have been proposed for a wide variety of medical image classifications and prediction of treatment results.

3. **Information Clustering:** Another interesting phase in data mining is clustering. If the collected data are put in the form of cluster and visualized, it is easy to locate data trends. These identified trends are helpful in preparation of prediction system. For example, based on the information collected from lung cancer patients about the onset and duration of exposure, clustering pattern can guide in future regarding prevention strategies. The most common clustering methods used for this purpose are K-Means clustering, Agglomerative Clustering, Hierarchical clustering, Density based clustering, Hybrid clustering etc.

DATA MINING TOOLS USED IN HEALTHCARE ANALYTICS

Data mining tools help to analyze volumes of complex data based on the dataset attributes that users specify in determining trends of occurrences (Ogundele et. al., 2018). These software can be used for diagnoses, prediction, and management of diseases to extract knowledge and make decisions. The most commonly used data mining tools are WEKA (Waikato Environment for Knowledge Analysis), KEEL(Knowledge Extraction based on Evolutionary learning), R, KNIME(Konstanz Information Miner), RAPIDMINER and ORANGE.

BENEFITS OF DATA MINING IN HEALTHCARE

The benefits of disease prediction system using data mining techniques is listed below:

1. **Prevention and Diagnosis**(Motilal et. al., 2013)**:** Data mining techniques plays a vital role in strategy preparation for prevention of communicable as well as non-communicable diseases. Lifestyle related diseases like hypertension, diabetes mellitus, cardiovascular diseases, stroke etc can also be easily and accurately diagnosed and it is possible to locate their etiological area using cluster patterns.
2. **Treatment Planning:** Data mining techniques play an important role in working out treatment plan such as surgical procedures, rehabilitation, chronic diseases management plan etc. This would also give assistance to provide long term follow up plan may be easily guided and keen supervision is possible (Motilal et. al., 2013). For example, a patient of hypertension can be managed long term through the patient history and the record of number of patients will direct and guide the practitioner to implement future strategies.
3. **Reduction of cost & Accuracy**: These systems may definitely be helpful in reducing the treatment cost by avoiding unnecessary investigations and patients follow up. It will add accuracy and time management.

4. **Discovery of hidden etiological factors**: Most of our health strategies are planned on the basis of data interpretations from developed countries. Our own systems can be formulated based on the analysis of medical data thereby the geographical errors can be avoided.
5. **Patient Support system:** Computer-based patient support systems benefit patients by providing informational support that increases their participation in health care.

APPLICATIONS OF DATA MINING IN HEALTHCARE

In healthcare sector there is a vast scope for data mining techniques to improve the medical science and also the overall system (Rakhi Ray, 2018). Healthcare industry today generates large amounts of complex data about patients, hospital resources, disease diagnosis, electronic patient records, medical devices etc. There are large data in health industry about patient status on diagnosis, treatment and cost which needs to be analyzed to extract meaningful information and knowledge from it (Ogundele et. al., 2018). The application of data mining in healthcare promises to advance clinical practices such as diagnosis, treatment, prevention, prescription, and optimization thereby ensures fast deliverance. Data mining applications in healthcare are listed below.

1. Treatment effectiveness
2. Healthcare management
3. Customer relationship management
4. Fraud & abuse
5. Hospital Management
6. Pharmaceutical Industry
   a. **Treatment Effectiveness:** The effectiveness of medical treatments can be evaluated by developing data mining applications. By analyzing courses of treatment provided to patients, symptoms of the various disease and contrasting causes data mining can find the effective treatment. Most cost-effective and best treatment can be decided by comparing the outcomes of a group of patients with the same condition or disease already treated using different drug regimens.
   b. **Healthcare Management:** Data mining applications can be developed to better identify and track chronic disease states and high-risk patients, design appropriate interventions and reduce the number of hospital admissions and claims to aid healthcare management. Different medical centers are using data mining techniques to shorten patients' length of stay, minimizing clinical complications, improvement of medical practices, improvement of patients' outcomes and also providing information to the physicians. These eventually improve the quality of healthcare in a cost-effective manner.
   c. **Customer Relationship Management:** Some of the customer interaction in the healthcare system will happen in call centers, reception, billing departments, offices of the physicians, and inpatient settings. Data mining can be used in healthcare to improve the level of satisfaction by determining the usage patterns, future and current needs, and the preference of an individual. This can bring ultimate satisfaction for each individual and also improve hospital profitability.

d. **Fraud & Abuse:** Data mining applications can attempt to detect fraud and abuses by identifying unusual or abnormal patterns of claims by physicians, clinics, or others. They can highlight inappropriate prescriptions or referrals and fraudulent insurance and medical claims.

e. **Hospital Management:** Organizations including modern hospitals are capable of generating and collecting huge amount of data. Data mining applications can be developed to analyze the data stored in a hospital information system which helps to visualize temporal behavior of global hospital activities.

f. **Pharmaceutical Industry:** A deep understanding of the knowledge hidden in the Pharma data is vital to a firm's competitive position and organizational decision-making. Data mining technology is used to help the pharmaceutical firms to manage their inventories and develop new product and services. Data mining can also be used in healthcare to predict the purchase strategies of healthcare customer and hence pharmaceutical companies can also be benefited.

DATA MINING ALGORITHM IN DISEASE PREDICTION

The medical data mining is an extremely important research field due to its importance in the development of various applications in flourishing healthcare domain. The identification of the possibility of heart disease and diagnosis is an important and the most complicated task for medical practitioners as it requires intense medical tests to be conducted. If the risk of a heart attack or the possibility of the heart disease is identified early, it can help the patients to take precautionary measures. Recently, the healthcare industry has been generating huge amounts of data about patients and their disease diagnosis reports that can be taken for the prediction of heart disease worldwide.

Data Mining is a task of extracting the vital decision making information from the collection of past records for prediction. Without data mining, this information may be hidden and cannot be used. Information classification is a data mining technique for making predictions based on the available historical data. Hence the medical data mining integrates the classification techniques that lead to exploring the hidden patterns in the medical data sets which is used for the prediction of the patient's future state.

Consider the heart disease dataset in UCI repository that includes 13 attributes and 270 instances with no missing values. This dataset contains past patient's historical data for various types of heart diseases such as typical angina, atypical angina, non-angina pain and asymptomatic. Figure 7, shows the procedure for the prediction of heart diseases in patients by building a classification model using Naive Bayes Classifier algorithm.

Naive Bayes (NB) is a statistical probabilistic classifier which is based on Bayes rule and it assumes that attributes are independent of each other. The algorithm of Naive Bayes classifier for the prediction is as follows:

- **Step 1**: **Training Phase** - By assuming predictors to be conditionally independent of a class, the parameters of a probability distribution known as the prior probability is estimated from the training data (patient's history).
- **Step 2**: **Testing Phase** - For unknown test data, this method computes the posterior probability of the dataset which belongs to each class. The method finally classifies the test data (new patient's data) based upon the largest posterior probability from the set.

Thus, the type of the heart disease for a new patient can be predicted based on past patient's history and help the health care professionals in the diagnosis of heart disease.

MACHINE LEARNING FOR HEALTHCARE

Health care is one of the most complex, challenging and expensive industry (Jabbar et al., 2018). Machine learning is widely used in health care .Despite of progress made in ICT still there is a need for innovation in health care informatics. Medical data consists of X ray results, DNA sequences, blood samples, vaccination, vital signs etc. Machine learning is able to efficiently obtain, analyze and draw conclusions. Predictive data analysis uses historical data to predict future outcomes, often through machine learning algorithms, which can more efficiently evaluate huge amount of raw data. For example, predictive analytics can consider trends from past viral infection seasons to help predict the severity of an upcoming viral infection season.

The application of Machine Learning(ML) in healthcare is widely anticipated as a key step towards improving care quality and reduction of costs. The digitization in healthcare generates unprecedented amounts of clinical data, which when coupled with modern ML tools provides an opportunity to expand the evidence base of medicine and facilitate decision process. Machine learning can be applied to health care data to develop robust risk models (Jabbar et al., 2018). Healthcare industry is already overburdened with the exploding population and lack of trained doctors. Use of machine learning and artificial intelligence technologies can enhance the productivity and precision of existing ones. Usage of these technologies will help in serving more patients in a less time and also improve healthcare outcomes to reduce the healthcare expense. Interest in machine learning for healthcare has grown immensely, including work in diagnosing diabetic retinopathy, detecting lymph node metastases from breast pathology, autism subtyping by clustering comorbidities, and large-scale phenotyping from observational data etc (Marzyeh Ghassem et. al., 2019).

Statistical techniques have been used to extract implicit information from data, but statistical analysis requires mathematical background. Statistical analysis is time consuming as the analyzer needs to formulate and test each hypothesis, whereas machine learning automates the generation and testing of hypothesis. Machine learning does not promote data reduction but can solve complex problems.

Machine learning in health care is a challenging issue due to large volume and variety of data, challenges related to missing data, task heterogeneity and temporal consistency (Jabbar et al., 2018). Application of Machine learning in Medicine Machine learning yields better results in health care domain. This is due to the faster decision-making, improved efficiency clinical trials, optimized innovation. There are various applications of machine learning in healthcare. Some of them are listed below.

a. Disease Identification/Diagnosis
b. Personalized Treatment/Behavioral Modification
c. Drug Discovery/Manufacturing
d. Clinical Trial Research
e. Radiology and Radiotherapy
f. Smart Electronic Health Records
g. Epidemic Outbreak Prediction

Figure 7. Classification using Naïve Bayes Algorithm

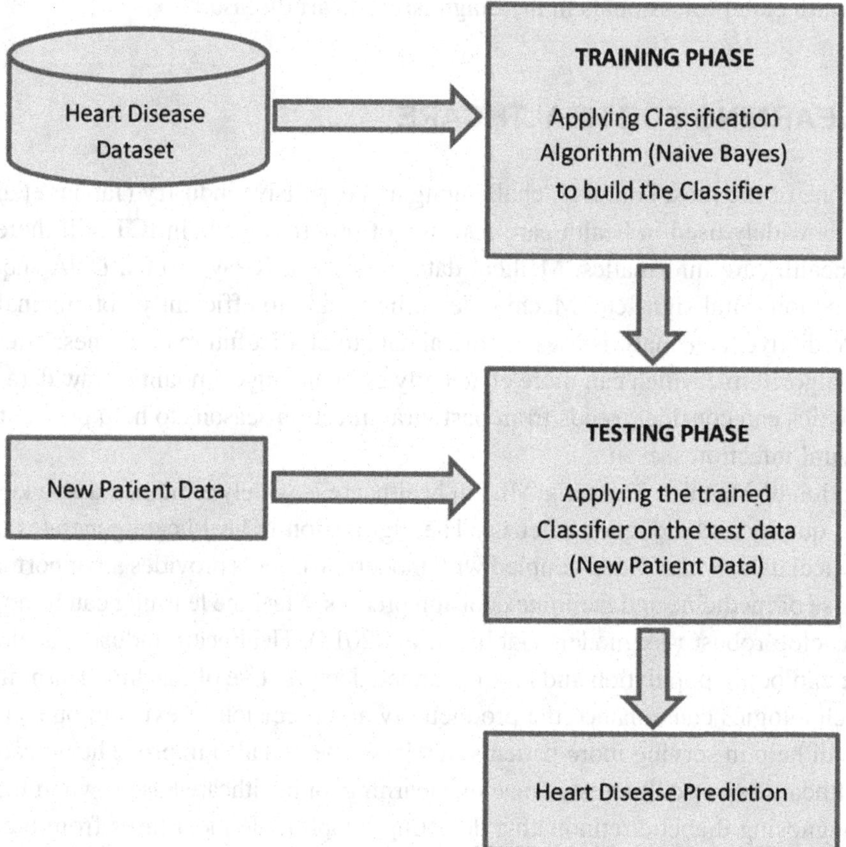

Despite these advances, the direct application of machine learning to healthcare remains fraught with pitfalls. Failure to carefully consider these challenges can hinder the validity and utility of machine learning for healthcare. Many of these challenges stem from the nominal goal in healthcare to make personalized predictions using data generated and managed via the medical system, where data collection's primary purpose is to support care, rather than facilitate subsequent analysis. Existing reviews of machine learning in the medical space have focused on the electronic health record (EHR), which documents the process of healthcare delivery and operational needs such as tracking care and billing and payments. We present a hierarchy of clinical opportunities, organized into the following general categories: automating clinical tasks, providing clinical support, and expanding clinical capacities. We conclude by outlining the opportunities for research in machine learning that have particular relevance in healthcare: accommodating shifts in data sources and mechanisms, ensuring models are interpretable, and identifying good representations.

CLOUD COMPUTING FOR HEALTHCARE

As more medical organizations store data in cloud servers, all medical practitioners and team members can more easily access data from the devices they are connected with. For example, a medical practitioner in the treatment room of the hospital can use his tablet to access a specific patient's health records. A data analyst in another part of the hospital can access those same records and analyze them for visualizing the data.

Cloud computing brings a new business model which enables several advantages that would benefit the general healthcare community. Figure 8, presents cloud driven healthcare service model. This model could be used as a reference to provide various services to the healthcare industry that can improve the traditional healthcare procedures and reduce management overhead.

Figure 8. Cloud driven healthcare services

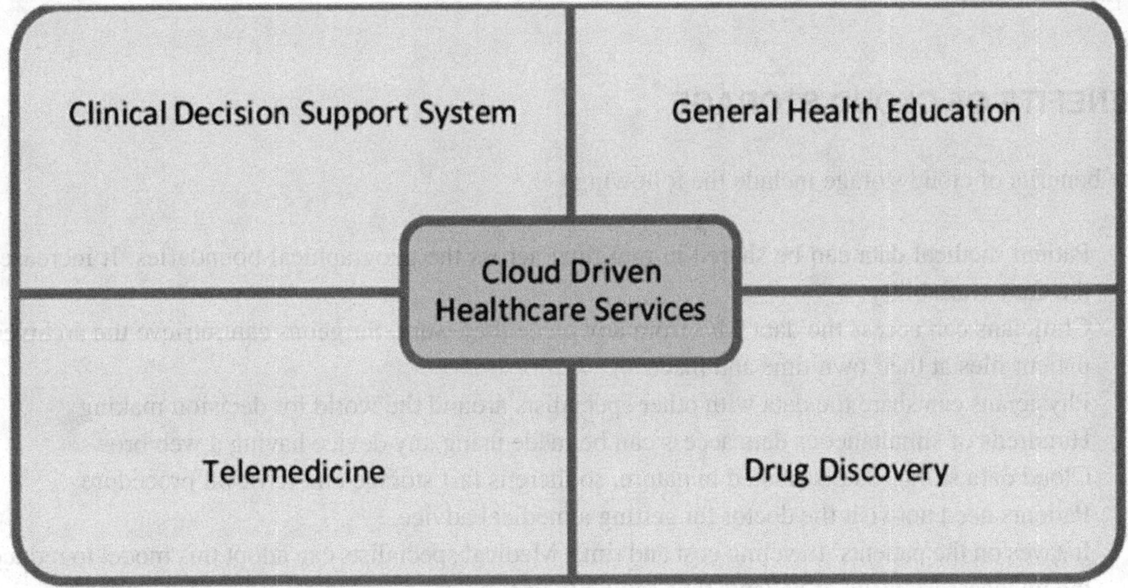

Healthcare industry has been using new technologies to streamline processes, deliver novel patient care applications and ultimately to provid7]\e improved healthcare services (Vaibhav Kamal Nigam & Shubham Bhatia 2016). Using cloud it is quite easy to get healthcare services over the internet using a web browser on a range of devices. By adopting the cloud in medical services both patients and healthcare organizations would obtain a huge benefit in patient's quality of service, collaboration between healthcare organizations as well as reductions in cost. This collaborative approach enables healthcare services to interoperate between them in order to offer a faster and efficient response helping to improve the patient quality of service through sharing information across healthcare organizations. Therefore, hospitals, clinics, imaging centers, pharmacies and insurance companies can efficiently share patient's medical records, prescription information, X rays, test results, physician's references, physicians availability etc. which can be accessed anywhere anytime by authorized entities. All this information would be used for obtaining correct diagnosis, making better decisions and treatments to yield better results. Quality of healthcare services can be improved by scheduling physician's appointments, speeding insurance approval, etc. By adopting the cloud model, also a very important beneficial factor for healthcare organizations is the infrastructure cost. All the infrastructure related processes will be migrated to the remote cloud-computing infrastructure where all the processes will be performed and stored. The new "pay-as-you-go" model allows organizations to pay only for what they use; therefore, there is no reason for acquiring expensive hardware infrastructure, software licenses or to keep/train in-site staff for maintenance, security, replications because the cloud computing providers takes care of them.

Human life is priceless, and medical resources are limited. Therefore, healthcare services adopted by cloud providers match a cost-effective concept where patients and health organizations take advantages of this new technology by improving patients quality of service through a distributed, high-integrated platform, coordinating of medical process, reducing infrastructure investment or maintenance costs which leads to a better healthcare environment. Cloud based software could be developed to make possible the doctor-patient and doctor-doctor interaction as well as to facilitate the transmission and archiving of medical images.

BENEFITS OF CLOUD STORAGE

The benefits of cloud storage include the following.

- Patient medical data can be shared in real time across the geographical boundaries. It increases the data availability
- Clinicians can access the data 24/7 from any place they want. Surgeons can retrieve the archived patient files at their own time and place
- Physicians can share the data with other specialists around the world for decision making
- Hundreds of simultaneous data access can be made using any device having a web browser
- Cloud data storage is distributed in nature, so there is fast storage and retrieval procedure
- Patients need not visit the doctor for getting a medical advice.
- It saves on the patients' traveling cost and time. Medical specialists can adopt this model to reduce the unnecessary visits of patients thus saving their time.

DATA VISUALIZATION FOR HEALTHCARE

Healthcare Data visualization is very important in this data-centric generation and it comes with lot of benefits Clinicians, hospital administrators, and public health officials have long turned to data to drive key decisions. In order to maximize data insights, Healthcare Data visualization helps decision-makers in many ways. Through data visualization, health informatics, and health information management professionals can play a crucial role in offering information and decision support. Visualizing health data allows experts to present key trends and information via graphs, charts, and other visuals that show as well as tell. Visualizing health data is a powerful way to share urgent health information swiftly and effectively and it also opens significant avenues to educate and empower doctors, executives, and the public at large.

For clinical visualizations, much of the needed information may be in unstructured formats rather than structured formats. Organizations attempting to use that information to build visualizations are often perplexed with the process. When healthcare analytics is combined with data visualization tools, it can help managers to operate better by providing real-time information that support decisions and deliver actionable insights. Data visualization strategies help analysts communicate results from analyzed data. Examples in a health care setting can include patient satisfaction ratings in a bar graph, staffing and operations trends in a line graph, and health care effectiveness in a pie chart.

Using tools like Microsoft Excel, Microsoft PowerPoint, SQL, Google Analytics, R, Python and Tableau, hospitals can create data streams and visualizations with the potential to optimize care delivery systems. Data capturing and visualization tools include the following:

- Surveys capture customer feedback and satisfaction ratings that can reveal opportunities for organizational growth.
- Scorecards are used by health care professionals to track the progress of their patients with this strategy.
- Dashboards are customizable and interactive for the healthcare professionals to extract the data required from the analysis and create graphs or charts for presentations.
- Health care professionals use the leverage of data visualizations to illustrate data for different audiences. Visualizations create a clear and succinct story to be demonstrated by the analyst rather than showcasing raw data.

Relevant visualization reports and dashboards will be possible with the potential for previously unattainable results through the new capabilities in cloud services. Increasingly, healthcare is using data visualization to understand the complex networks of data at their disposal. Availability of powerful healthcare data visualization tools transforms the outcome of the analysis into valuable and useful insight. The following steps are to be followed for the successful implementation of data visualization in healthcare.

- Identify the healthcare area of high value and organizational visibility with a high probability of success in which data can be effective.
- Analysts then create a and begin capturing relevant medical data from targeted data sources
- Setting up the transformation of the medical data into system acceptable format
- Using analytical tools, the analyst creates an automated flow for transformed data and perform modeling on it
- Analyst choose a visualization strategy to represent the outcome of the analysis using charts, graphs and other diagrams that simplify rows of data into a graphic and illustrate the data story.
- Data visualizations created from the dashboards can then be exported and used in presentations and reports

Thus the data visualization helps the analyst to communicate their findings in a clear and engaging way to the audience, which could include the health care facility's board of directors or a public health group.

CONCLUSION

Health care industry produces vast amount of data that clutches complex information relating to patients and their medical conditions. There is a huge demand to investigate and analyze them legitimately which can then help in the comprehension of the reason and nature of ailment for the successful diagnosis and prevention of diseases. Though there are many useful applications that have been implemented in the field of healthcare for disease diagnosis, disease detection, infection control, telemedicine and fraud prevention, the usage of technologies such as data mining, machine learning, cloud computing and data visualization plays a vital role in analysis of the healthcare data that can provide solid inferences with regard to wellbeing. This will also enable the medical practitioners to take precautions for high risk diseases by studying the symptoms from the available medical data. The outcomes are dependable and give a good start for the annihilation of illnesses. Though the role of technology for data analytics in the healthcare is indeed complex, its benefit is boundless. Still there are many other directions to be explored, concerning various aspects of healthcare data, such as the quality, privacy, timeliness and so forth. Additionally, the scope and nature of healthcare data can be expanded beyond which may enrich the diagnosis process. Besides, the development in digital diagnostic of diseases, there is a high anticipation on the of impact of these findings which can provide advancement in healthcare and enable all relevant parties to be benefitted. The future of health informatics will also be benefitted from the exponentially increasing digital health data that may benefit the healthcare industry immensely.

REFERENCES

Durairaj, M., & Ranjani, V. (2013). Data Mining Applications In Healthcare Sector: A Study. *International Journal of Scientific & Technology Research*, *2*(10).

Elezabeth, L., Mishra, V. P., & Dsouza, J. (2018). *The Role of Big Data Mining in Healthcare Applications*. IEEE. doi:10.1109/ICRITO.2018.8748434

Ghassemi, Naumann, Schulam, Beam, Chen, & Ranganath. (2019). *A Review of Challenges and Opportunities in Machine Learning for Health*. Academic Press.

Jabbar, Samreen, & Aluvalu. (2018). The Future of Health care: Machine Learning. *International Journal of Engineering & Technology*, *7*(4.6), 23-25.

Lashari, S. A., Ibrahim, R., & Senan, N. N. S. A. M. (2018). Application of Data Mining Techniques for Medical Data Classification: A Review. *MATEC Web of Conferences*.

Motilal, Tayade, & Karandikar. (2013). Role of Data Mining Techniques in Healthcare sector in India. *Scholars Journal of Applied Medical Sciences*.

Nigam & Bhatia. (2016). Impact of Cloud Computing on Health Care. *International Research Journal of Engineering and Technology, 3*(5).

Ogundele, I.O., Popoola, O.L., Oyesola, O.O., & Orija, K.T. (2018). A Review on Data Mining in Healthcare. *International Journal of Advanced Research in Computer Engineering & Technology, 7*(9).

Patel & Patel. (2016). Survey Of Data Mining Techniques Used In Healthcare Domain. *International Journal of Information Sciences and Techniques, 6*.

Patil. (2015). Survey Of Data Mining Techniques In Healthcare. *International Research Journal of Innovative Engineering, 1*(9).

Ray, R. (2018). Advances in Data Mining: Healthcare Applications. *International Research Journal of Engineering and Technology, 5*(3).

KEY TERMS AND DEFINITIONS

Analytics: The systematic computational analysis of data or statistics.

Annihilation of Disease: Completely exterminate the disease.

Association: Relationships among large sets of data items.

Classification: Categorization of data and assigns labels or classes to the items in a collection.

Clinical Data: Information ranging from determinants of health and measures of health and health status to documentation of care delivery.

Cloud Computing: Delivery of different services through the internet.

Clustering: Grouping different data based on the similarity.

Data Mining: Process of analysing large databsets in order to generate new information.

Data Visualization: Graphical representation of information.

Healthcare: Efforts that medical professionals make to restore our physical and mental well-being.

Information Science: Study of processes for storing and retrieving information.

Machine Learning: Concept that a computer program can learn and adapt to new data without human intervention.

Chapter 14
Smart Healthcare IoT Applications Using AI

Hema D.
Lady Doak College, Madurai, India

ABSTRACT

Globally, healthcare professionals strive to diagnose, monitor, and save human lives. An application that advances the medical field to the next level is the need of the hour. Smart healthcare systems using IoT help in the process of monitoring human health by minimizing human intervention. Taking care and monitoring of human health has a significant contribution in declining the mortality rate as well. IoT in healthcare has aided smarter communications and prompt treatment to save lives. Patient data are sensed by sensors/microcontrollers, sent over the internet, stored in the cloud, and received by healthcare professionals during emergencies. Applications of such smart healthcare using IoT are blood glucose meters, medical vehicles, sphygmomanometer, pulse oximeter, Holter monitor, etc. This chapter elucidates several smart healthcare IoT applications using artificial intelligence and cloud computing technology. The chapter also elaborates the importance and functions of various cloud and AI components in designing a smart healthcare application.

INTRODUCTION TO SMART HEALTHCARE

Demand in healthcare system is increasing due to population explosion. Most of the medical services are not feasible and affordable by everyone. Smart healthcare helps people to be health-aware by updating their health status. Smart healthcare came into existence since the inception of telemedicine services. A service system that provides or gathers information promptly, connects people by making use of technology to form a medical ecosystem is considered to be a smart healthcare application. Such applications are developed using Internet of Things (IoT) by incorporating Artificial Intelligence Technology.

The main focus of smart healthcare system is remote monitoring of patients thereby reducing the total treatment cost. In spite of geographical barriers, medical practitioners can extend their services to the patients. End-users of smart healthcare services are Individuals, hospitals, government organizations, clinical research institutes, diagnostics laboratories etc. Smart healthcare aids individual users to self-

DOI: 10.4018/978-1-7998-9132-1.ch014

Copyright © 2022, IGI Global. Copying or distributing in print or electronic forms without written permission of IGI Global is prohibited.

manage their emergency situations. The objective of providing smart health care service is to enhance the quality and efficiency of medical service.

Quality of Service (QoS) in IoT

Functional components in healthcare systems are designed to cater the needs of specific application whereas non-functional components are the aspects through which the quality of a smart healthcare application is determined. The Quality of Service (QoS) for any smart healthcare application should satisfy the following attributes:

1. Reliability- the ability to produce similar results by including fault tolerant methods
2. Low power consumption- ability to work with minimum voltage levels
3. Interoperability- ability to exchange information and data among different information technology systems
4. High speed- ability to communicate data and respond quickly
5. Ambient Intelligent-ability to interact intelligently and unobtrusively with people
6. Sufficient memory-ability to store essential data for computing without any performance
7. Good connectivity- ability to transfer and receive data over a network without latency
8. Small form factor-ability to achieve high functionality using small form factor

IOT HEALTH-CARE SERVICES

IoT is predicted to empower several health-care assistance services where every service renders a combination of health-care solutions. Generally, a service cannot be fairly isolated from a specific solution or application. A variety of IoT health care services in potential areas where an IoT healthcare service or solution requires greater attention is listed by (ahad, Tahir, Aman Sheikh, Istiaque Ahmed, Mughees, & Numani, 2020) and summarized below.

Ambient Assisted Living (AAL)

AAL are concepts, services, and products that enable technologies and the environment to enhance the quality of living. The Motivation of AAL is to provide freedom for elderly people in their ambience safely. AAL administrations provide self-governance and remote assistance at the time of any problem.

Adverse Drug Reaction (ADR)

ADR is the reaction that happens due to the use of a medicine prescribed by the doctor. Typically, ADR is the result of using a medicine in unusual proportion or perhaps the effect of mixing the medicine alongside other medicines. Techniques such as barcode/NFC-authorized gadgets are fixed in patients' body to monitor the ADR. With the help of an intelligent framework to collect pharmaceutical data, smart IoT healthcare services are developed. The data are processed using a processing module for the detection of medicine with the allergy profile along with the electronic history of patient's health.

Community Healthcare (CH)

Community health-care services (CHs) are the foundation local network to provide smart Iot Healthcare application. CHs are system dependent IoT run throughout the metropolitan health-care centers, residential area, sub urban areas or a rural area. Community health-care (CH) is a specific service which includes the aggregate specialized necessities as a suite. Contribution of IoT in rural health-care (Boakye & Olumide, 2020) helps to mitigate the health problems in poor communities, remote monitoring of patients health, increased access to health information and reducing mortality rate. CH networks are acknowledged as helpful network scenarios to uplift rural areas.

Wearable Device Access (WDA)

Non-intrusive sensors have gained popularity in medical health care applications due to the fact that the sensors need not be embedded into the body. Using Wireless Sensor Networks (WSN), medical devices are that are wearable can provide the same services similar to the intrusive devices. Wearable medical services such as smart clothes, smart watches, and smart glasses can be designed with any IoT application. However, the demand for wearable sensors and components is a challenge for the designers and analysts while developing IoT smart medical applications.

Indirect Emergency Healthcare (IEH)

Emergency health-care services deployments are of crucial importance in several situations such as fire accidents, incompatible climate conditions, and in-flight etc. In these situations, IEH arranges for alter notification, data accessibility, record keeping, and post-accident activity. These IEH medical services also help in the mitigation of any future disasters.

Embedded Gateway Configuration (EGC)

As a compositional facility, Embedded Gateway Configuration (EGC) is responsible for the connection of nodes associated with patients in the network, the inter-network to attach the essential servers and customers, and additional systems for medical services. At a service point of view, the gateway has various characteristics, which includes few common integration features.

Embedded Context Prediction (ECP)

To build context-aware (CA) medical health-care applications on IoT network, designers entail bland systems with suitable components known as ECP service. Several challenges in CA health-care system arise when they are overlaid on IoT-based network. Hence, a context predictor must be used for remote health monitoring that based on IoT.

SMART HEALTHCARE IOT APPLICATIONS

Applications of IoT technologies in healthcare help to improve the level of chronic disease management, quality of people life and lifesaving interventions etc. (Yang, et al., 2020). As mentioned in (Yang, et al., 2020), Smart healthcare IoT applications include healthcare monitoring, healthcare information support for patients, service improvement and collection of information resource for big data analytics. Patients' basic health monitoring IoT application (Islam, Rahaman, & Islam, 2020) makes use of five sensors such as heartbeat sensor, room temperature sensor, body temperature sensor, Co Sensor and CO2 Sensor to capture the data from hospital environment which is then communicated through Wi-Fi to medical staff from the server. Along with sensors, there is a need for processor/ microcontroller such as ESP32 to transfer data using SDIO or UART interfaces.

Diabetes is a chronic and prominent disease in recent days with major economic and social impact. An advanced opto-physiological assessment technique (R. S. H., S, N. Y., & A, 2011) is used for designing a mobile IoT (IP based networking) for non-invasive glucose level sensing to manage diabetes in patients. Heart diseases in human can also be diagnosed using ElectroCardioGram (ECG) based on IoT. Electrocardiogram (ECG) signals are collected from patient's body by wearable sensors and the data is stored in a database which can be accessed only by authorized personnel to provide security (Shaown, Hasan, Mim, & Hossain, 2019). Such system is found to be reliable and helps to reduce the mortality rate due to cardiovascular diseases. Human Body temperature is a decisive vital sign in the maintenance of an individual homeostasis. An infrared body temperature sensing module detects the body temperature of a patient through infrared rays. Later, an Open Service Gateway Initiative (OSGi) packages and sends the detected temperature data in an M2M (Machine to Machine) format (Junjian, Zhanli, & Zhuang, 2012).

During the period of Pandemic like Covid-19 etc., Contactless Body temperature monitoring has also become an essential part of healthcare services. In future, designing a contactless IoT based wearable body temperature monitor would be appreciated to reduce the transfer of infection. Human body blood pressure can also be monitored (Guanjing, 2012) using IoT based application. To facilitate data exchanging, a Bluetooth communication module is arranged on the blood pressure instrument. Once the data is collected, it is stored in either mobile phone or a computer. Further the data is analyzed and mined using a processor to diagnose the patient's condition. Pulse oximeter to check the oxygen levels of the human is also the need of the hour during covid-19 like diseases. An integrated carry-on blood pressure/pulse rate/ blood oxygen monitor along with a location module (Jianxin, Min, & Mingjie, 2012) is developed to monitor the patient's condition. This IoT Application uses a Global Positioning System(GPS) and a GPS antenna to locate the position of the human. There is a data communication device that encompasses a Subscriber Identity Module (SIM) and a General Packet Radio Service (GPRS) module to transmit the measure data. A maximum health monitoring system is developed (Imran, Iqbal, Ahmad, & Kim, 2021) for elderly patients' at home, ambulance, and hospital environment. This IoT application detects and notifies deteriorating conditions to the experts based on biomedical sensors for faster and prompt interventions. Biomedical sensors used are wearable ones that can monitor body temperature, blood glucose level, heart rate, and patient body position. Machine learning-based approaches and Thresholding techniques were used to detect anomalies in the sensing health data.

IOT PLATFORMS FOR SMART HEALTHCARE

Knowledge about what a typical IoT architecture comprises of is an essential one before designing any IoT smart healthcare application and to select the ideal platform. Irrespective of the application area, IoT architecture is a multi-layered structure which has several tools for carrying out different activities phase by phase without any delay. IoT provides faster service over other technology especially in health-care services which is why they are smart applications. It is because IoT executes data communication without store and send technique. It directly sends sensed data to the cloud and alerts the medical staffs.

The first stage in any IoT application is data collection and the platform must provide multiple ways of doing this using cloud technology. Patients or environment should be constantly connected to sensors and the network so that critical data is not lost. This will also ease in providing prompt medical help. Once the data is collected from sensors, it should be converted from analog form to digital (A-D Conversion). This conversion will enable the data to be stored, processed, and analyzed for further action and responses. IoT platform must provide a robust engine for real time analysis of incoming data that can take care of all the rules to be applied. The IoT architecture not only should perform data collection but also should take care of back-end management of these devices, such as software updates, remote device management, network management, database management etc. It becomes a crucial function of any IoT platform to store the important data sets in order to perform the analytics because at instances, it affects the action that must be taken as per the data collected. There are several IoT platforms which are usually cloud services like Microsoft Azure IoT Suite, Google Cloud's IoT, Salesforce IoT Cloud, IBM Watson IoT, Cisco IoT Cloud Connect, AWS IoT, Kaa IoT etc. Few of them are free of cost and few require additional cost to be paid. There are several factors that must be considered while selecting the most suitable IoT platform as listed below:

- **Stability –** The IoT platform for any healthcare application for use must be stable under all circumstances most of the time.
- **Security –** All the processes, collected data and information should be secure while selecting a platform to design a smart healthcare IoT application.
- **Suitability –** The IoT platform should be appropriate for the requirement of the smart medical service. It would be ideal if the chosen platform has previously been used for a similar medical application.
- **Scalability –** The major advantages of using IoT for smart healthcare application is the ability to scale up as per the requirement. It must always be considered to select a platform that provides maximum scalability.
- **Data ownership –** Most often, the service provider will take care of owning the data. It is not always the fact that if the smart healthcare application is owned by a person, he owns the data. Hence, while selecting a platform, make sure the data is owned by the application owner and not the service provider.
- **Cost – Several** IoT platforms typically use cloud for storing, processing, and displaying information. The widely used payment type is pay as per the usage. Careful understanding of the pricing model with its caveats and loopholes ensures that there is not too much to pay for a smart health-care application than anticipated.
- **Performance –** It is very essential to enquire about the past performance of the platform that is considered for designing IoT smart healthcare application. The IoT Platform should have always

Figure 1. 3 stage architecture for IoT based smart healthcare application

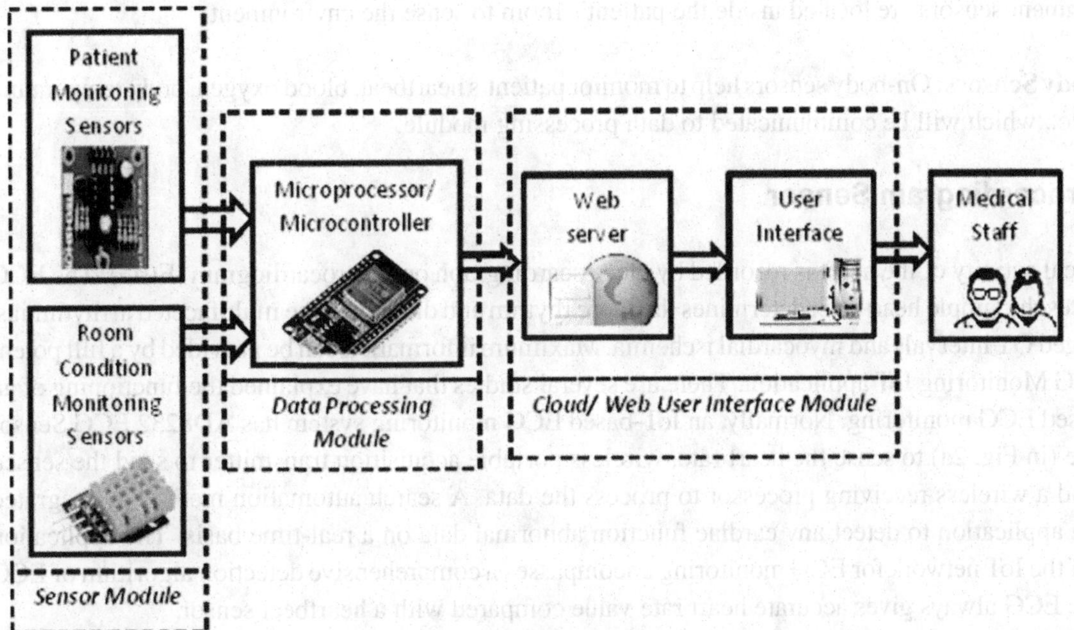

a throughput of 100% without any delay so that the application users do not face any technical glitches at any point of time. The IoT platform must also be fault tolerant so that it can handover the responsibility to alternate service provider in case of failure.

- **Supporting packages and tools –** The platform should provide adequate supporting packages that the developers can use to create their own customized tools, applications, reports, and interfaces for any smart healthcare applications.

DESIGNING A SMART IOT HEALTHCARE APPLICATION

There are several requirements such as the medical equipment, connectivity methods and management type that enable the appropriate design of any IoT supported smart healthcare applications. It is customized by grouping options from the different requirements to serve the need. A 3 stage architectural framework namely Sensor module, Data processing module and Web User Interface constitutes a Smart healthcare IoT Application as depicted in Figure-1.

SENSOR MODULE

The devices that sense or collect data to be sent to the medical practitioners are known as Sensors. A sensing module contains sensors, the primary component using which the rest of the smart healthcare system is designed. A *sensor* is an electronic device which measures physical input from its environment and then converts it into data that can be inferred by a human or a machine. Sensors can be classified into on-body sensors and Environment sensors. On-body sensors are located on patient's body whereas environment sensors are located inside the patient's room to sense the environment.

On-Body Sensors: On-body sensors help to monitor patient's heartbeat, blood oxygen, body temperature etc., which will be communicated to data processing module.

Electrocardiogram Sensor

Electrical activity of the heart is recorded by electrocardiograph or electrocardiogram (ECG). The ECG measures the simple heart rate, determines the basic rhythm and diagnoses the multifaceted arrhythmias, prolonged QT intervals and myocardial ischemia. Maximum information can be provided by a full potential ECG Monitoring IoT application. There are several studies that have explained the functioning of an IoT-based ECG monitoring. Normally, an IoT-based ECG monitoring system has AD8232 ECG Sensor Module (in Fig. 2a) to sense the heart rate, wireless portable acquisition transmitter to send the sensed data and a wireless receiving processor to process the data. A search automation method is integrated to such application to detect any cardiac function abnormal data on a real-time basis. The application layer of the IoT network for ECG monitoring encompasses a comprehensive detection algorithm of ECG signals. ECG always gives accurate heart rate value compared with a heartbeat sensor.

Heart Beat Sensor

The heartbeat sensor is developed based on the theory of plethysmography which measures the changes in volume in different parts of the body. MAX30100 is an integrated pulse oximetry sensor and heart-rate monitor sensor that is widely used in the market. Such Sensors measure pulse waves by discharging red or infrared light from the body surface and subsequently detects the change in blood flow during heart beats as there is a change in the amount of light transmitted through the body. Pulse Timing is more critical in systems where the heart pulse rate should be tracked. The rate of heartbeats reflects the distribution of blood volume, the signal pulses are equal to the pulses of heartbeat when the light is consumed by the blood. The heart beat sensor MAX30100 is depicted in Fig. 2b.

Glucose Level Sensors

Diabetes is a one of the metabolic diseases where there is a high blood glucose (sugar) levels observed over a prolonged period in a human body. Monitoring Blood glucose reveals individual patterns of blood glucose variations and helps in the planning of activities, meals, and medication times. Configuration of Glucose sensors for an IoT application can be both invasive and noninvasive with respective to a patient's body. A noninvasive glucose sensing IoT configuration method on a real-time basis is proposed by (R. S. H., S, N. Y., & A, 2011). In this technique, sensors from patients are connected through IPv6 connectivity to suitable healthcare providers. The utility model designed by (Guanjing, 2012) reveals a transmission device for the communication of collected somatic data on blood glucose levels based on IoT networks. This smart healthcare application includes a blood glucose collector, a computer or a mobile, and a processor. Glucose level sensing IoT application is a great relief to diabetes affected community especially the elderly ones.

Body Temperature Sensor (LM35)

When viruses and bacteria enter human body, they will have a hard time surviving at temperatures greater than the normal body temperature. Hence, when the human body detects a bacterial or viral infection, it reluctantly increases the body temperature and increases blood flow to speed up the body's defense actions which helps to fight the infection. However, increased body temperature also causes harm to the body and so the high body temperatures should be sensed and treated. MAX30205, a body temperature measuring sensor is incorporated into an IoT healthcare service to monitor patients' body temperature as a mobile application (S, P, & M, 2018) to communicate the information to medical staffs. The LM35 is another IoT temperature sensor is an optimized accurate temperature circuits with output voltage. The output voltage is linearly relative to the temperature in centigrade. LM35 is shown in Fig. 2c.

Environment Sensors: IoT smart healthcare application not only involves the patients' body sensors, it also requires several adjoining environment sensors. Environment sensors in IoT smart healthcare application aids in monitoring the real time quantities such as the air temperature, humidity, gases present under the area of investigation.

Room Temperature Sensor (DHT11)

Room temperature Monitoring is important aspect for IoT enabled smart healthcare services. DHT11 is a sensor for measuring temperature and humidity which is commonly used. The room temperature sensor comes with a temperature measurement NTC Thermistor and a microcontroller for the processing of humidity and temperature values. The DHT11 sensor is depicted in Fig. 2d.

Gas Sensor (MQ-9, MQ-135)

Gases present in atmosphere such as Carbon monoxide, Carbon-dioxide, Methane can be detected using Gas sensors. Environment Gases are another important factor to be considered in the smart healthcare services which can interfere in the patients' body condition. MQ-135 sensor can detect the presence of Carbon dioxide, Benzene, smoke, Nicotine and ammonia. MQ-9 Sensor is appropriate for detecting LPG (Liquefied Petroleum Gas), CO (Carbon monoxide) and CH4 (Methane) detection. This sensor has high sensitivity and fast response time through which measurements can be taken promptly. The sensor's sensitivity can be modified using a potentiometer for further processing. The MQ-9 sensor is shown in Fig. 2e and MQ-135 sensor is depicted in Fig. 2f.

CO2 Sensor (MQ-135)

MQ-135 gas sensors are used for NH3, Nicotine, Benzene, Smoke, and CO2 detection to monitor the air quality. The MQ-135 sensor module with its digital pin enables this sensor to work without a microcontroller which is found to be beneficial for detecting specific gases in the environment. The gasses in Parts-Per-Million (PPM) are calculated by analog pins. The TTL powered analog pin works on 5 V, and hence it is easy to incorporate with modern microcontrollers.

Figure 2. Different sensors in IoT healthcare application

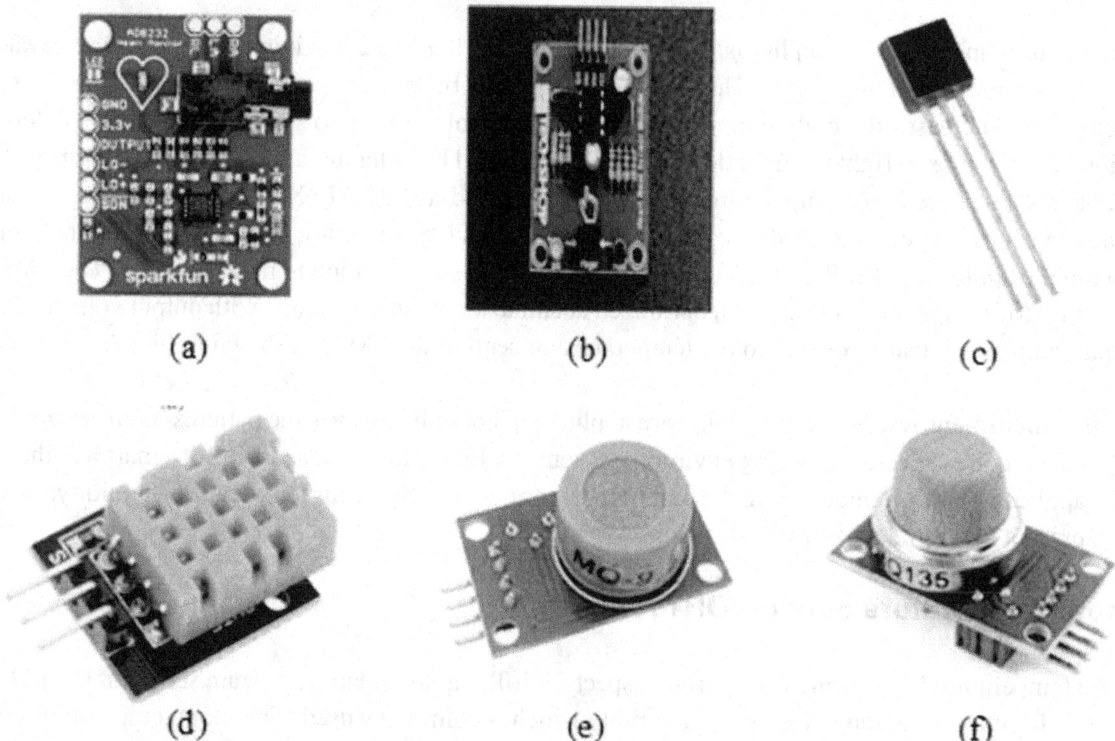

CONNECTIVITY METHODS

Connectivity is the key aspect of the IoT that assists the "things" to communicate and transfer data. The connection methods can either be wired or wireless depending on the needs. However, wired network is found inadequate for most IoT applications because of the wire's reachability and additional hardware support. IoT applications usually require huge range and hence wireless connectivity is preferred for designing such applications.

There are many elements and factors to be considered when selecting a wireless connectivity option such as range (maximum distance that is covered to send data), power consumption (battery life and usage), bandwidth (amount of data that can be sent), cost overhead, reliability, and availability etc., The connectivity method is optimal when it is of high range, low power consumption, high bandwidth and low costs. It is very hard to find such a connectivity technology. For instance, increasing the connectivity range will increase power consumption, and increasing the bandwidth usually increases costs. There are few essential connectivity methods such as 5G Network, BLE/Wi-Fi, Zigbee, LPWAN, Satellites, NFC etc which are enumerated below.

- **5G Network**: People are in the use of 3G and 4G connectivity technologies, however it is not sufficient for building highly dynamic and time-sensitive IoT health care applications. Therefore, the 5G networks technology is designed to fulfill the diverse communication requirements for IoT health-care applications. IoT devices with improved network performance and enriched cellular coverage are merged together to form 5G assisted smart health-care networks. There are several connectivity challenges to be taken into account such as massive number of devices, energy-efficiency, standardization, security etc.

- **BLE/Wi-Fi**: Bluetooth or Wi-Fi connectivity methods come in handy with short-range communication that is utilized in IoT healthcare applications. Bluetooth/Wi-Fi connectivity has lower power consumption and higher bandwidth over other connectivity methods. An enhanced version of Bluetooth, called Bluetooth low-energy (BLE) needs only a fraction of the energy required by a traditional Bluetooth and thereby still reduces power consumption. An interesting IoT smart healthcare application that uses multiple Bluetooth/WiFi access points is tracking Hospital asset using by means of Triangulation.
- **ZigBee**: Zigbee is a low-cost, low-power wireless technology developed to address the special needs of the wireless IoT networks. ZigBee is a wireless mesh network standard for battery-powered IoT devices and applications in wireless control. This connectivity provides low-latency and hence there is a minimal delay in data communication. ZigBee connectivity chips are integrated with radios and microcontrollers as a part of IoT applications.
- **Cellular/Mobile**: Cellular or mobile connectivity is a feasible way of driving communications in IoT appications. It is a method of connecting devices and things like sensors to the internet with the same Network that is used in the smartphone. Instead of creating a new private network for IoT smart healthcare applications, the M2M (Machine to Machine) data can piggyback on the same cellular/mobile network as used in smartphones. This reduces the burden of deploying a additional connectivity option.
- **Satellites:** Satellite connectivity method delivers high bandwidth communication along with high range, but it also consumes very high power. The satellite communication works anywhere on Earth and that is what makes it more preferable by end users. Hence, Satellite communication is perhaps the only option to receive information about shipping and logistics containers while they are travelling on an ocean.
- **LPWAN**: A few countries have new Low-power wide-area networks (LPWAN), such as LoRa and Sigfox available nationwide. It is expected that 75% of the countries will have LPWAN coverage in the next decade. LPWANs possess two important qualities such as low power consumption(due to long lasting small batteries) and long distance communication. LPWAN technology works on the principle of transferring small amounts of data intermittently and that's how the low power consumption possible. An instance of intermittent data communication for low power consumption is trash bin sensors sending signals only when it is to be emptied.
- **NFC (Near-Field Communication)**: NFC is a short-range wireless technology is a very smarter and quick way of connecting and transferring data between devices with a single touch. This connectivity transmits data using electromagnetic radio fields that helps two devices to interlink with each other. For both devices to transfer data, they must contain NFC chips. Further, NFC-enabled devices should be physically touched for the data transfer to occur. NFC connectivity reduces the chance of human error it is because the data is received immediately when it is transmitted. Hence, NFC is very quick way of transferring data in a smart IoT healthcare application that requires instant attention.

DATA PROCESSING

The collected data from sensors is sent to a cloud service using any of the connectivity methods. In the recent decade, the volume and the speed of the data being produced is unbelievable. All the massive amount of data collected by IoT sensors must be processed. The data processing is done to manipulate the collected data to produce meaningful information. This phase is essential to convert the raw data to something very informative. Data is raw, unorganized facts, and it is normally useless till it is processed. After the data being processed, it is called as information. The input of data processing step is data and the output of data processing is information. The information is presented in several forms, such as plain text files, spreadsheets, charts, or images etc.

Data Processing Cycle

The data processing technique follows a 3 stage cycle such as input, processing, and output. While all 3 steps are essential, the key aspect to keep in mind is the clean input to be provided for processing.

- **Input:** This is the first stage of the data processing cycle. In this stage, data collected is converted into a machine-readable form for the computer to process it. As mentioned, this is a crucial stage because the data processing output is entirely dependent on the input data. In simple terms, "garbage in – garbage out". If unclean data is given for processing, the output is definitely irrelevant and non-responsive especially for Smart IoT healthcare applications.
- **Processing:** This data processing stage enables the computer or machines to transform the raw data into information. Various data manipulation techniques are used for such transformation that includes the following:
    - Data Classification: Categorizing data into different groups.
    - Data Sorting: Arranging the data in a certain form of order.
    - Data Calculation: Performing arithmetic and logical operations on data.
- **Output:** The output is received in this last stage after processing. In this stage, the processed data is converted into human-readable form. The useful information after conversion is presented to the end-users. The output data can also be saved in different formats for future uses.

CHARACTERISTICS OF DATA PROCESSING CYCLE

As a Programmer, it always important to consider the following traits for this data processing cycle to be successful and informative.

- **Desired Output:** Before starting with the input stage, it is recommended to think about the desired output of the IoT application under deployment. For instance, what is the information that is relevant for an IoT application such as a Patient Body Temperature Monitoring. One use case would be A Medical staff receiving an alert message when the Temperature exceeds a threshold limit.
- **Data Storage:** Having clarity on the desired output, the next concern is to obtaining and storing the data. The data collected by the sensor devices should be stored in an appropriate form and be

transformed into the required information. Assume, a patient body temperature sensor sends data periodically (e.g. for every 5 minutes). The received data could be used to detect trends among that data, and produce estimations about when is the body temperature likely to go high or low or could sustain int the same level. Due to this potentially massive amount of data the sensors collect, investing in a scalable cloud service will enable to store the data. A data retention policy might also be developed so that holding the IoT data forever in cloud service becomes absurd. The cost of storing huge amount of data for a longer period in the cloud is of high cost. Less data provides no useful information. Hence, prioritizing and balancing between costs and amount of data is a challenging task for IoT based smart healthcare applications.

- **Frequency of Updates:** Before applying data processing, it is significant to decide a good balance between the frequency of data updates and the resources consumption (e.g. calculation power, capacity). There might be scenarios to understand the impact of collected data on the output which is a resource-consuming data processing task. On the other hand, it might be enough to process the collected data like once a day. The "good balance" totally depends on the Smart IoT healthcare use case.

DATA PROCESSING TOOLS AND SERVICES

There are numerous data processing tools and software solutions available for different IoT smart healthcare applications. These software solutions are capable of processing data and presenting the information in an easily understandable form to the end user. There are IoT Platforms that help us to build a data storage and create customized reports. Data can be sent to a cloud service for processing or the data can be processed before sending it to the cloud. The later process is known as edge computing. Edge computing permits the data to be processed close to its origin such as the sensor devices. The data is transmitted from sensor devices to a local edge computing system that processes and stores the data and then sends it to the cloud. Edge computing is preferred in many applications it is because it sends only the important information over the network. Such data is passed on to the data center or cloud-based systems known as IoT Edge Platforms or simply IoT Platforms. Hence, the edge processing is quick, requires less bandwidth from the network and also retains the life of the sensor devices' batteries. There are several IoT Platforms offered by various companies at a price based on the requirement of the IoT application. They include Google cloud, IBM Watson IoT, Amazon AWS IoT Core, Microsoft Azure IoT suite, Oracle IoT, Cisco IoT Cloud Connect etc.

- **Google Cloud**: Google cloud delivers multi-layered architecture applicable for organizing, managing, and sharing data. It has built-in AI/ML capabilities and supports real time IoT applications are very smart.
- **IBM Watson IoT:** This cloud service allows IoT applications to collect, collate, and communicate data from smart and embedded devices, wearable devices etc.,. It provides domain expertise that is used to develop flexible and customized solutions. It is considered to be highly secure platform for the price that is offered.
- **Amazon AWS IoT Core**: Amazon offers AWS, a software suite designed to deliver end to end IoT solutions such as sensors, connectivity, storage, data processing, and user interface. It is also a highly secure platform that helps to track and communicate even when the devices are offline

ie, while not connected to internet. Hence, this connectivity is preferred due to its uninterrupted connectivity.

- **Oracle IoT**: Oracle IoT cloud connects devices to the cloud so that the data is collected, analyzed in real time, and transmit the data to enterprise applications and web services. It is also used to extend existing systems like supply chain management, retail management, ERP, human resource management, and customer handling.
- **Microsoft Azure IoT Suite**: Microsoft Azure suite is used in developing Smart IoT solutions due to its flexibility. This cloud service is used to develop solutions for industries such as health care, retail to transportation, manufacturing, predictive maintenance, and smart connected spaces.
- **Cisco IoT Cloud Connect**: Cisco developed IoT cloud connect, a mobility solution which is stuck with its core competence of networking. It is intended for mobile operators to secure communication channels, optimize their network, and manage data effectively.

USER INTERFACE IN IOT SMART HEALTHCARE APPLICATION

Delivering the information to the end user is done through *user interface* (UI). Examples of user interfaces are applications and softwares on computers and smartphones. The user interface includes features like screens, pages, icons, buttons, forms, etc., by which a user interacts with a computer system. A screen is not mandatory for a user interface. For instance, a TV remote has a user interface which consists of several buttons and gadgets such as Amazon Echo is controlled with voice instructions. There is another term close to the user interface known as the *user experience* (UX). UI refers to the things a user actually sees and interacts with whereas UX is the user's overall experience about a product. UX might be about the application, website, packaging of hardware, installation, etc.

METHODS OF USER INTERFACE

There are various ways by which a user can communicate and interact with an IoT solution. Depending on the use case, one might adopt the sensors and connectivity. Picking the right interaction also depends on the use case. The methods to interact with an IoT solution are receiving auto notifications, proactive monitoring, remote controlled system,

Automatic Notifications

With IoT smart healthcare application, when something unusual happens, doctors and medical staff should receive notifications or alert messages. For instance, if a patient's body temperature exceeds a threshold limit or if the room temperature is too cold or hot, it should be notified. Such information can be sent as SMS, email, phone call, or push notification.

Monitoring Information

In smart healthcare IoT applications, there might be a need to monitor information proactively. An IoT application to track the location of a patient's vehicle or an ambulance might monitor location information even when nothing unusual happens. A mobile or computer application is used for monitoring such information.

Remote Controlled System

The user interface can also allow the user to remotely control the smart healthcare IoT application. For example, the patient's relative could turn on, off or adjust lights, air conditioner in the patient's room via mobile application. This operation can automatically be done by the application itself based on the guidelines.

UI DESIGN CONSIDERATIONS

Building an intuitive UI in IoT solution is challenging taking the complexity to a whole new level. When designing UIs for IoT, there is a list of issues to be considered that are summarized below.

- **Connectivity:** It would be a great idea to design a User Interface (UI) that informs the user clearly of how often is the data processed or sent to the cloud. For example, the UI could send a message to the user such as "Last message received 1 hour ago- next message expected in the this 1 hour"
- **Physical UI**: A user interface that tells the user that the device is on is a physical UI such as a smart Light or small LED light. In some smart IoT healthcare applications, physical UI is essential but it is restricted to extend the battery life.
- **Simplicity:** Delivering the information to the user is much appreciated when it is simple. The information processed from the IoT application must be meet the user's needs. Limiting information for different user groups and showing them only what they need would make the IoT UI very simple to use. Data visualization makes the information much easier to understand.
- **Performance:** Efficient **data processing also involves** massive amount of information to be presented in the user. Performance of the UI should also scale high for larger usage. Graphs are the best way to present a huge amount of data which can be meaningful and also increase the UI's performance. This has to be taken into account when designing the UI, because otherwise the performance of the UI might not scale for larger usage. Graphs are a great way to present large amount of data in a meaningful way, and they also help with the performance of the UI. Pagination technique to display only part of the data at a time in UI will also reflect a stable UI performance.

AI APPLICATIONS IN SMART IOT HEALTHCARE

Artificial Intelligence (AI) is gaining wide attention in many real time applications including self-driving cars, Image tagging, human speech to text conversion, Spam filtering, weather prediction and rainfall estimation, stock prediction etc. It also has enormous applications in healthcare services like a machine monitoring patients' condition and responding accordingly to save the patient in case of an emergency.

Artificial Intelligence (AI) consists of a device or software program that can interpret complex data, including text, images, video, speech etc., and interpret information to achieve a specific goal. AI researchers and vendors have initiated to tackle provide some useful IoT solutions across the health sector.

The health sector continuously faces elevating costs and requires assistance to achieve better outcomes with inadequate resources. Healthcare sector unlike the other sector currently demands disruption. The healthcare sector should evolve solutions to deliver high-quality consistent care and value. There are different types of AI applications such as drug discovery, delivering pre-primary care information to patients, finding patients for clinical trials, recording notes for electronic health records (EHRs), predicting deteriorating heart conditions apnea or asthma in patients, and alerting medical staffs to probable 'code blue' emergencies hours even before they occur. IoT is a boon to such medical applications that are really smart by incorporating Artificial Intelligence (AI) techniques. AI vendors try to implement the necessary infrastructure or devices to deliver actionable analytics using smart IoT solutions. With human lives potentially at stake, AI vendors need to get proper regulatory approval before attempting to implement in hospitals. Once implemented and scaled, data curation is needed through managed services in hospitals that lack data scientists and analysts. AI in IoT solution should improve the efficiency and productivity of the medical staffs to help them deliver higher quality care. In some fortunate instances, AI applications could produce more operative drugs thereby saving doctors' time patient's lives. There are some smart IoT applications using AI techniques in medical sectors that reduce human man power. Machine learning and deep learning techniques have taken the healthcare sector to next level of monitoring patient's condition without the need of medical staffs. The major constraint in applying machine learning and deep learning techniques in medical field is the lack of medical dataset for certain medical conditions. However, these smart IoT healthcare devices are much preferred because they can be worn by patients anywhere anytime and periodical information can be reported to doctors.

- **Blood Pressure Monitoring:** Blood Pressure is another important health condition that reflects the overall well-being of human body. Blood Pressure must be regularly monitored and controlled remotely for which IoT applications are really helpful. The combination of a (Keep In Touch) KIT blood pressure (BP) meter and a NFC-enabled KIT mobile phone for Blood Pressure monitoring IoT application is proposed in (A, R, M, D, & G, 2010). BP Monitoring IoT application is composed of a BP apparatus body with data transfer module and internet connectivity. A location-intelligent terminal for carry-on BP monitoring along with other healthcare conditions monitoring (Jianxin, Min, & Mingjie, 2012) is also very popular because people need not be in hospital atmosphere.
- **Oxygen Saturation Monitoring**: During the period of a Pandemic like Covid-19, Pulse oximetry is a noninvasive device for nonstop monitoring of blood oxygen saturation. The IoT application with pulse oximetry is useful for technology-driven smart healthcare services. Wearable pulse oximeter like WristOx$_2$ developed by Nonin is readily available in market recent days. WristOx$_2$ 3150 USB provides accurate, fast oxygen saturation and pulse rate readings in challenging conditions. A drop in normal oxygen level reflects poor functioning of Lungs due to diseases like Asthma, Chronic bronchitis. Lung dysfunction can be monitored using Spirometer which can also be used in Smart healthcare applications. A low-power & low-cost Microphone based Mobile phone application, SpiroSmart (Larson, Goel, Boriello, Heltshe, Rosenfeld, & Patel, 2012) is developed to monitor the lung function that uses machine learning regression technique.
- **Hand Hygiene Monitoring:** Conventionally, there hasn't been a healthcare facility to ensure that the patients and other people inside hospital washed their hands properly and sanitized it. This should be monitored to minimize the risk of spreading contagious diseases. In the recent days, most of the hospitals and other health care sectors use smart IoT devices to remind the patients

and people to sanitize their hands inside the hospital rooms. The IoT devices will also instruct on the best way to sanitize and mitigate a particular risk in the near future. The major constraint in this IoT solution is that it will only remind the people and not sanitize on their behalf. However, research suggests that these smart IoT solutions will help to decline the infection rate by atleast 50 percent in hospitals.

- **Depression/ Mood Monitoring**: Patient's depression and mood information is a complicated data to be monitored and collected continuously for the medical professionals to understand the patient requirements. Most often healthcare providers periodically ask the patients about their feelings and emotions, but they were unable to predict sudden mood swings. It is also because patients don't report their moods and feelings accurately. Hence, "Mood-aware" IoT devices are designed to address these issues. These devices collect and analyze heart rate and blood pressure to infer information about the mood of the patient. There are advanced IoT healthcare devices that perform mood monitoring by tracking the movement of patient's eyes. In (D & S, 2021), machine learning technique that extracts Patch-SIFT facial features and modeled using an ensemble approach recognizes human emotions from facial images with a recognition accuracy of 98%. Such applications can be incorporated within IoT solutions to monitor patient's mood or emotions. The key challenge here is that the IoT devices are not yet found accurate as that of traditional in-person mental assessment.
- **Parkinson's Disease Monitoring**: To treat Parkinson's patients effectively, medical professionals should be able to assess severity of their symptoms and fluctuation throughout the day. Smart IoT sensors make this task much easier by collecting the parkinson's symptoms continuously. The best feature about this IoT solution is that it gives patients the freedom continue with the daily life at their own homes instead of making them to stay in hospital for observation. This smart IoT medical healthcare solution is a wearable solution that connects the patients and medical staffs irrespective of their location.

IOT HEALTHCARE DEVICES

There are other possible IoT healthcare devices that provide treatment along with monitoring data by living in or on the patient. Examples of such IoT healthcare solutions are **Connected Inhalers:** Medical Conditions such as Chronic Obstructive Pulmonary Disease (COPD) or asthma involve unexpected attacks with mild warning. Diagnosing the frequency of the attacks and collecting the data about the environment is also significant in this case. IoT-connected inhalers help healthcare professionals to understand the symptoms and causes of such attack. These connected inhalers will also alert the patients when they leave it at home or when it is used improperly.

- **Connected Contact Lenses:** Connected contact lenses collect healthcare data in a non-intrusive, passive way. These lenses come with micro cameras that allow wearers to take pictures with their eyes effectively. Such connected lenses have been patented by companies like Google. Smart lenses are one of the powerful tool that can be implemented for digital interactions and also to improve health outcomes.
- **Ingestible Sensors:** Data collection within human body is complex, messy and disruptive. For example, a camera or probe struck into a patient' digestive track is much annoying and undesirable.

To address such issues, ingestible sensors collect information from their digestive tract in a less invasive way. They deliver useful insights such as information about digestive and other human systems or even identify the source of bleeding. Such ingestible sensors should be small enough to be swallowed easily and reside in human body for a while. Further, they must be capable of dissolving and passing through the human body cleanly on their own.

- **Surgical Robots:** Deploying small robots inside the human body can help surgeons to perform complex operations that are difficult to manage by human hands. This is a less invasive process because robotic surgeries by small smart IoT devices reduce the size of incisions required for a surgery. It also supports in quicker healing for patients. The limitation is that the IoT device must be small enough and reliable to perform surgeries without any disruption. The IoT devices must also interpret complex conditions inside patient bodies to make the right decisions during a surgery. Recent survey reflects that all these challenges are adequately addressed since its usage is found in the real time hospital surgeries.

CASE STUDY- PREDICTIVE ANALYSIS OF HEALTHCARE SYSTEM USING AI

Treating any disease at an early stage would be more simple and cheap. Artificial Intelligence in Clinics aid in data extraction, management, analysis and predicting various factors involved to make the healthcare system smarter. Healthcare analytics has the ability to reduce treatment costs, predict outbreak of pandemic, avoid preventable diseases and improve life quality. This is the reason for the increase of the average human lifespan globally. Healthcare professionals and entrepreneurs collect massive amount of data and implement best strategies to accomplish healthcare analytics. One such Patient's Dashboard of St. John's Clinic with several Key Performance Indicators (KPI)/metrics for a single month is given in Figure-3 which can be used to predict the upcoming month KPI/metrics.

Figure 3. Monthly healthcare report of St. John's Clinic

PATIENT DASHBOARD | ST. JOHN'S CLINIC | MONTHLY REPORT				
GERIATRICS	GYNAECOLOGY	ORTHOPAEDICS	PEDIATRICS	CARDIOLOGY | SURGERY
Occupancy		**Forecasted patient turnover**		**Satisfaction & service indicators**
Current bed occupancy rate- 76%	Current Patients- 811	Patient turnover rate Present- 3.49% Previous month-5%		Patient Satisfaction-81% Previous month-78%
	Number of beds- 1077	ICU	3.14	**Follow up rate by the departments**
		Other	3.51	
Efficiency & Costs				Geriatrics- 26%
Avg. total cost per patient-$1,424	Staff to patient ratio-0.26	Room turnover- 48 min		Gynaecology-29%
Drug cost per patient by department		**Equipment utilization rate**		Orthopaedics-29%
Surgery- $900	Pediatrics-$850			
	Cardiology -$700 | Orthopaedics- $660	Simple spirometry-40%		Pediatrics-31%
	Gynaecology - $510 \| Geriatrics -$ 445	Ultrasonic Nebulizers-43%		
		Wheelchairs-45%		Cardiology- 32%
		Electrocardiogram-46%		Surgery- 33%

Conventionally, Patients data is collected in bits and bites, archived in hospitals, clinics, surgeries with the impossibility to communicate properly. Digitizing the clinical ambience and communications has created several treatment models. Gathering huge amount of data for medical use has been costly and time-consuming. With improved IoT and AI technologies, it is not only easy to collect data but also to create comprehensive healthcare reports to derive critical insights for better care. Doctors can easily understand about a patient's condition over a period and can pick up warning signs of serious illness. KPI's are collected using IoT devices, transferred to cloud over a period and then a monthly or a weekly summary can be prepared. Based on the KPI analysis, healthcare professionals can manage to draw a picture of patient's status and let the insurance provide a package for treatment. Though few KPI given in Figure 3 doesn't need IoT solution, it is still significant to get the overall summary to for improved treatments.

Figure 4. Predictive analytics of Key Performance Indicators (KPI's) using IoT

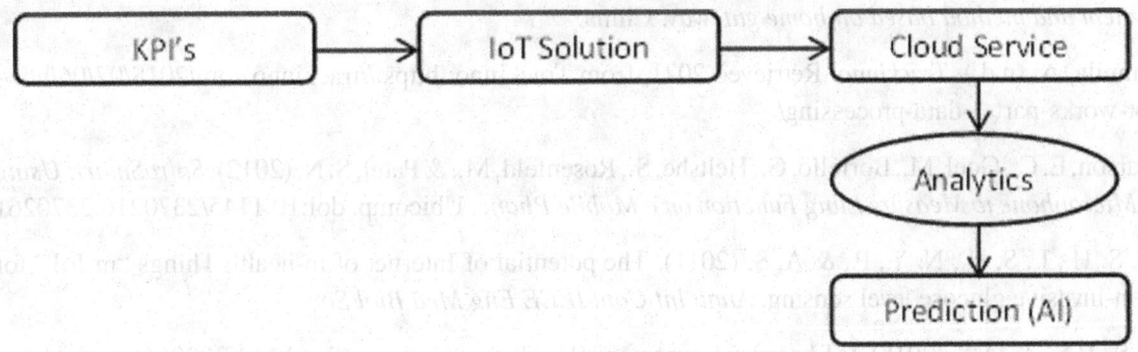

Data driven findings using AI supports to predict and solve a problem, assess methods for quick treatments, track inventory, educate patients with their own health and empower them. AI and IoT based smart healthcare can create healthy living space for human being.

REFERENCES

A, D., R, M.-O., M, D., D, H., & G, S. (2010). The Internet of Things for Ambient Assisted Living. *Seventh International Conference on Information Technology: New Generations,* 804-809.

Ahad, A., Tahir, M., Aman Sheikh, M., Istiaque Ahmed, K., Mughees, A., & Numani, A. (2020). Technologies Trend towards 5G Network for Smart Health-Care Using IoT: A Review. *Sensors*.

Boakye, A., & Olumide, O. B. (2020). The role of internet of things (IoT) to support health services in rural communities. A case study of Ghana and Sierra Leone. *Transnational Corporations Review*.

D, H., & S, K. (2021). Patch-SIFT: Enhanced feature descriptor to learn human facial emotions using an Ensemble approach. *Indian Journal of Science and Technology*, 1740-1747.

Guanjing, Z. (2012a). *Patent No. CN202821362U-Internet-of-things human body data blood pressure collecting and transmitting device.* China.

Guanjing, Z. (2012b). *Patent No. CN202838653U-Somatic data blood glucose collection transmission device for internet of things.* China.

Imran, I., Iqbal, N., Ahmad, S., & Kim, D. H. (2021). Health Monitoring System for Elderly Patients Using Intelligent Task Mapping Mechanism in Closed Loop Healthcare Environment. *Symmetry, 13*(2), 357. doi:10.3390ym13020357

Islam, M., Rahaman, A., & Islam, R. (2020). *Development of Smart Healthcare Monitoring System in IoT Environment*. SN Computer Science. doi:10.100742979-020-00195-y

Jianxin, T., Min, B., & Mingjie, J. (2012). Patent No. CN202875315U-Carry-on blood pressure/pulse rate/blood oxygen monitoring location intelligent terminal based on internet of things. China.

Junjian, Z., Zhanli, K., & Zhuang, M. (2012). *Patent No. CN102811185A-Temperature measurement system and method based on home gateway.* China.

Junnila, A. (n.d.). *Trackinno*. Retrieved 2021, from Trackinno: https://trackinno.com/2018/07/06/how-iot-works-part-3-data-processing/

Larson, E. C., Goel, M., Boriello, G., Heltshe, S., Rosenfeld, M., & Patel, S. N. (2012). *SpiroSmart: Using a Microphone to Measure Lung Function on a Mobile Phone*. Ubicomp. doi:10.1145/2370216.2370261

R. S. H., I., S, H., N. Y., P., & A, S. (2011). The potential of Internet of m-health Things "m-IoT" for non-invasive glucose level sensing. *Annu Int Conf IEEE Eng Med Biol Soc.*

S, S., P, S., & M, S. (2018). IoT based measurement of body temperature using MAX30205. *International Research Journal of Engineering and Technology*, 3913-3915.

Shaown, T., Hasan, I., Mim, M. R., & Hossain, S. (2019). *1st International Conference on Advances in Science, Engineering and Robotics Technology (ICASERT)*. Academic Press.

Yang, X., Wang, X., Li, X., Gu, D., Li, C., & Li, K. (2020). Exploring emerging IoT technologies in smart health research: A knowledge graph analysis. *BMC Medical Informatics and Decision Making, 20*(1), 260. doi:10.118612911-020-01278-9 PMID:33032598

KEY TERMS AND DEFINITIONS

Electrocardiogram: A graph of voltage with time to record the electrical activity of hart using electrodes placed on skin.

Ingestible: Any object that can be consumed into human body.

Invasive: Tends to spread very quick harmfully or undesirably.

Near Field Communication: Radio frequency-based contact-less communication technology.

Non-Intrusive: Medical inspection method to examine human body without opening the organ.

Plethysmograph: An instrument to measure changes in volume within an organ or whole body.

Pulse Oximetry: A medical test to measure the oxygen level saturation of the blood.
Sensor: A device to detect events or changes in environment or human body.
Spirometer: Breathing test to measure the amount of air in lungs.
Zigbee: An IEEE wireless technology used in IoT networks.

Chapter 15
Futuristic Research Perspectives of IoT Platforms

Dhaya R.
King Khalid University, Saudi Arabia

Kanthavel R.
King Khalid University, Saudi Arabia

ABSTRACT

Future IoT innovation patterns will assist offices with getting the greatest proficiency and efficiency out of their hardware and assembling parts. IoT is an essential element of digital transformation enterprises in business and industrial sections. Service suppliers and utilities have also been taking on IoT to get pioneering services to keep competitive. Services with security, power management, asset presentation, healthcare effectiveness, and threat and agreement management must be resolved properly in order to enhance the IoT effectively and efficiently. As new tech turns up, hackers prepare to capture the benefits of its potential flaws, and this is precisely why enhancing the precautions of associated strategy is the top IoT technology development. Objectives of this chapter are to analyze and access the future of IoT in healthcare, security, education, and agriculture. This chapter will focus on edge computing, a hybrid approach to process the data that allows connected devices to distribute, compute, examine, and maintain data locally.

INTRODUCTION

Today, more organizations are exploiting and recognizing the advantages of IoT than any time in recent times. With the touchy development of IoT uses and reception, there are some incredible open doors for organizations that join the IoT upset early. The companies who figure out how to change and enable themselves through the advantages of IoT could make unquestionable upper hands.

The fate of IoT can possibly be boundless. Advances to the modern web will be quickened through expanded organization deftness, incorporated man-made brainpower (AI) and the ability to send, computerize, coordinate and secure assorted use cases at hyper scale. The ascent in innovation and IOT permits

DOI: 10.4018/978-1-7998-9132-1.ch015

Copyright © 2022, IGI Global. Copying or distributing in print or electronic forms without written permission of IGI Global is prohibited.

instructive foundations to embrace savvy classes and the better method of educating. With e-getting the hang of, instructing is simpler. It additionally guarantees the security of their grounds, assets and upgrades admittance to data. The parts of home bots and their effect on our lives will be different and range from some fundamental undertakings like cleaning the windows to more unpredictable obligations like bookkeeping, training or family overseeing.

The stage that will oversee the savvy house will fill in as a reason for the coordination of other brilliant apparatuses, and simultaneously will cooperate with the client by giving a coherent interface. With respect to the advancement side, it will not shock anyone that Apple, Amazon, Google, and Samsung are flow improvement leaders. Yet, not just our homes or work environments can be keen. What about entire urban areas intended to handle gridlock, stopping issues or even make our way of life greener. The expansion of the populace makes the need to rediscover the way we live, and fabricate better conditions that are canny, productive and maintainable. Indeed, the appropriation of IoT advances in shrewd urban areas involves accommodation. And yet, they are prepared to do a lot more. Like structure a savvy economy and administration, improving the foundation, upgrading wellbeing, reducing energy utilization and expense, and decreasing ecological effect (Dhaya & Kanthavel, 2016).

IoT innovation is equipped for deciding the streets, rails, and scaffolds that need to go through reproduction, just as the degree of their debasement, outrageous temperatures that may cause harm. Heavy traffic and clog are perhaps the greatest torment of any huge megalopolis. In any case, it is likewise something IoT is now handling (Kumar et al., 2019). For example, Tel Aviv saves one path on occupied streets for transports and transports. The fretful driver can utilize the path too; just it will cost them a chunk of change. Sensors incorporated into the black-top can get the drivers' tag and consequently charge them. Another normal traffic issue – stopping is being managed in London with the assistance of shrewd advances. The framework permits drivers to find void parking spaces without cruising all over roads looking for void space. A keen city is a protected city. With face acknowledgment and biometric frameworks are only one method of making us protected at home, work or the roads. Yet, there are significantly less difficult brilliant methods of causing us to have a sense of security in the city. For example, a light that turns extra brilliant in the event that it recognizes slamming or hollering. The fate of IoT has a huge chance of unfurling in the car business. The primary motivation behind IoT in the working environment is to make the lives of laborers more advantageous and productive. At this moment, we are investigating the eventual fate of IoT where brilliant gadgets will set the correct AC temperature in shared office spaces, help us book the most advantageous for everybody meeting room, and besides, consider the room inclination by setting the correct temperature, lighting, consequently restock office supplies(Zhou et al., 2017). The advancements of edge computing techniques like concurrent neural network and recurrent neural network have been already ruling their presence firmly in terms of accuracy and reliability for the better decision making lines. This chapter has two strong parts, namely the platforms of IoT and the part of edge computing in IoT along with the integration of both technologies by means of case studies.

NEED OF STUDY OF IOT IN FUTURE

Internet of things in easiest terms is where things are associated with one another through the Internet. Figure 1 says the purpose of the IoT. Every one of these things can meet and share information. This information is then additionally investigated and used to get significant data and improve the other associated gadgets' exhibition (Gaona-Garcia et al., 2017). The ability to turn anything as little as a chip

Figure 1. Purpose of the IoT

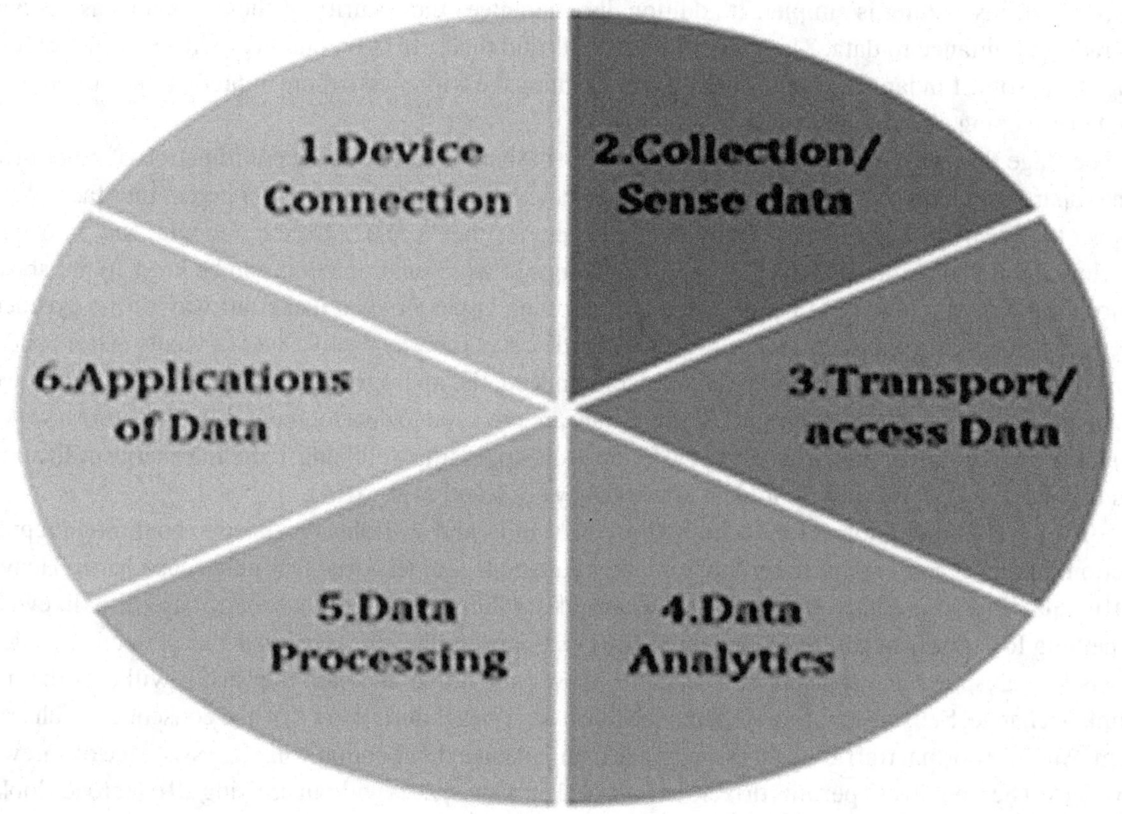

or even a entire city into an operational IoT platform is the future of IoT. According to statista.com, the Internet of Things could potentially interconnect and over 50 billion products by 2030.

Within 2030, Twenty Thousand Million IoT Electronic Gadgets Might be in Use for Every Reason: A diminutive glance demonstrates the usage of IoT devices will be for the upcoming years with aggression.

Cybercriminals to Maintain by Means of IoT Devices to Authorize DDoS Attack: The globe has been recognizable with the essential "Internet of Things" malware by a sprain of harmful indoctrination that can disgrace interconnected devices. This scrupulous sprain of malware is allocated "open source," which gathers the set of laws is obtainable to anybody to modify (Behrendt, 2019).

Further Metropolitan/Brilliant Networks to Convert into Sharp: Buyers will be the distinct ones with IoT devices. Metropolitan stunning organization and relations strength sensibly get grasp of bright enlargements to put the moment and funds (Zanella et al., 2014).

AI Manages the Globe into Something Other Significances: The novel information has the alternative to assist the appliance "acknowledge" what your tendencies are and change itself properly. For instance, when a video site recommends a motion picture anyone likes, it has been most likely in use in inclination dependent on the precedent options (Weber, 2010).

Switches to Maintain Receiving Splendid Safety: Because nearly all purchasers of IoT machines survive in the residence but without safety measures they may be incapable beside attack.

5G Networks to Carry on Satisfying the Expansion of IoT: Considerable far-away carter goes on revolving on relations of fifth-Generation cell in order to make sure instantly recognizable pace and the boundary border (Heer et al., 2011).

Vehicles to Acquire Essentially Additional Clever as Elegance: The fifth generation may modify the means of transportation industry into a advanced matter.

5G's Emergence Lucid the Pathway for Original Assurance Concern: New 5G IoT procedures relates to the fifth connection than throughout a local area wireless control. On an extensive level, the comprehensive dependence on cloud-based boundary renders aggressor awareness to challenge to split.

IoT-Buit up DDoS Assaults to Further Dangerous Structures: IoT gadgets can be made use to support diverse attack and there may be activities to electronic devices (Liu et al., 2012).

Precautions and Safety Issue Will Force Appeal and Directorial Deed: The improvement in IoT mechanism is only a introverted details of safety and confirmation apprehension are increasing.

The Importance of Fog Computing in the Internet of Things: As a device or software produces or gathers high amounts of information, storage of data become progressively complex and costly. Internet speed becomes costly when dealing with much data, necessitating the use of huge data centers to keep and give the data. Fog computing has developed as a viable substitute for traditional data management methods. Fog computing collects and distributes processing, storage, and internet connection programs and services. It saves a huge amount of energy, decreases time and computational complexity, and improves the usefulness and effectiveness of the data.

The Role of Quantum Computing in IoT: Quantum Computing and the Internet of Things (IoT), often known as Quantum IoT, is a theory of increased security architecture that uses quantum physics constraints to control IoT protection. It also assures that storage of data, computation, transmission, and data dynamics are all safe.

FUTURE OF IOT IN HEALTHCARE

Healthcare has the most likely utilization of IoT than some other area. The mix of IoT and Healthcare will have tremendous advantages like ailment checking, self-care, finding new strategies for illness counteraction and control assessments and determination (Kanthavel, 2018).

IoT can make healthcare less expensive and productive later on. It can help in the formation of more redid and patient-situated gear. In addition, IoT will likewise empower patients to improve admittance to information, customized care.. Figure 2 shows the IoT In healthcare market size by 2004-2025. The development of 5G networks, which give 100 times higher connectivity speeds, is key to the future of IoT in healthcare. Connectivity is required for IoT devices to communicate and transfer data between the patient and the care provider. Faster cellular data transfer gives IoT devices more flexibility in terms of the amount of data they can send and receive, as well as at a faster rate. Gadgets that help people with adherence to treatment at home, sleep monitoring devices that can check heart rate, oxygen levels, and movements for high-risk patients, and remote temperature monitoring tools are among the new healthcare IoT uses that have emerged as a result of these advancements.

Figure 2. IoT in the healthcare market (source: www.grandviewsearch.com)

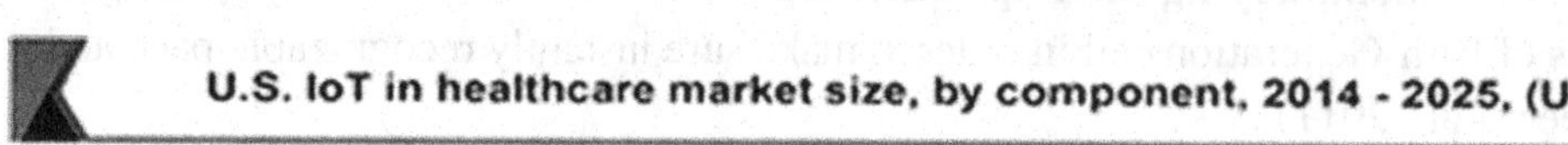

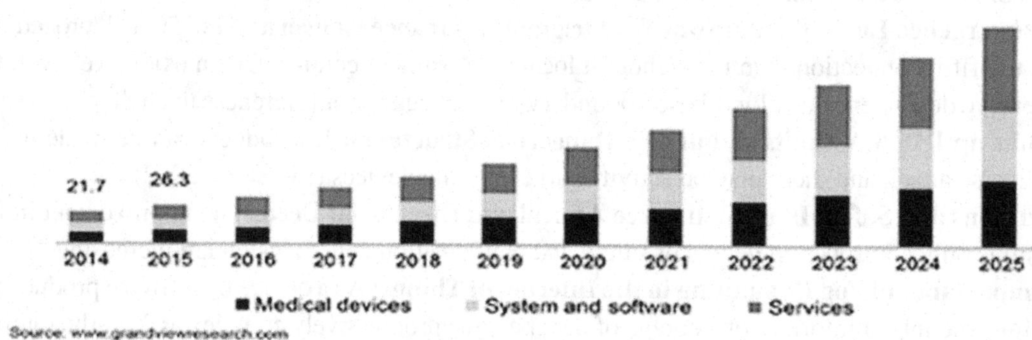

Future Uses of IoT in Healthcare

Remote Observation: Tweak software and gadgets will peruse information from clinical cards of patients progressively and help specialists in directing a superior investigation of the patient's wellbeing (Ammar et al., 2018).

Wearable's: Various contraptions that can consistently screen every day exercises of the patients and store the information are accessible on the lookout. These gadgets educate patients about their proactive tasks. They can likewise help in forestalling crisis, as the patient's data would be shipped off the specialist right away

Quality Checking: IoT can help in giving capacities and regulators to different fundamental hardware in the clinic. Imperfections in the gadgets can likewise be sorted out progressively; in this way, decreasing the odds of inappropriate treatment (Dhaya & Kanthavel, 2020a). Figure 3 shows the potential capacity of IoT in the Healthcare

Future Benefits of IoT in Healthcare

Enhanced Control and Exposure: Continuous oversight through IoT gadgets can save lives in health related crises, for example, asthma assaults, cardiovascular breakdowns and so forth the associated gadget can gather basic information on the patient's wellbeing and move it to the doctor continuously. An investigation directed by the Center for Connected Health strategy recommends that there was a half decrease in re-affirmation pace of patients because of distant oversight.

End-to-End Relationship: IoT can robotize the work process of patient consideration with the assistance of healthcare versatility arrangements. It enables interoperability, M-M Connections, data improvement and data swap over while assembling medical care transport extra beneficial. Diverse network conventions in the gadgets permit medical clinic; work force to mark early on the indications of sickness in the patients (Anirudh et al., 2017).

Figure 3. The potential capacity of IoT in healthcare

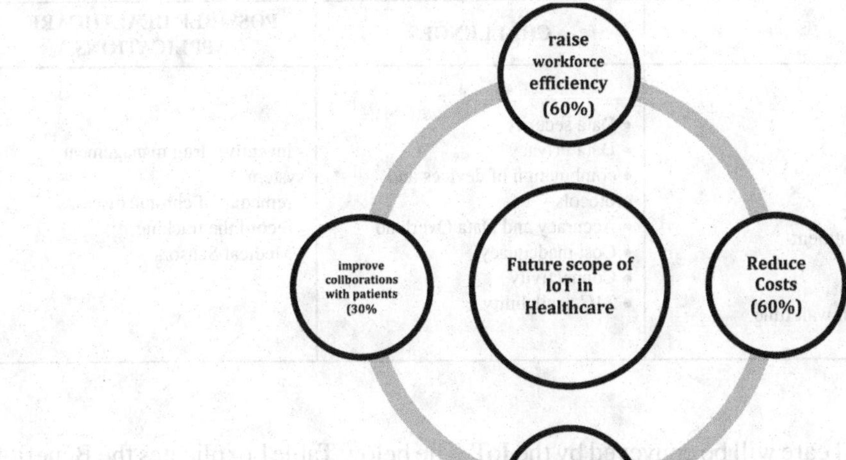

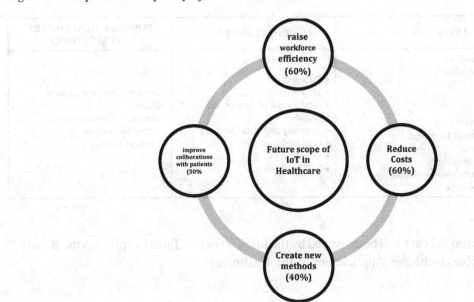

Data Investigation: IoT gadgets collect description and break down the broad information gathered in brief timeframe, require of its stockpiling. This will permit medical suppliers in zeroing in on important information needed to treat the patient. The information driven experiences will accelerate the dynamic cycle of specialists.

Mindful and Follow: Convenient alerts can be imperative in case of risky conditions. IoT licenses clinical contraptions to collect basic data and move it to experts consistently. The reports give an ideal assessment related to the patient's situation.

Lesser Costs: The associated gadgets and wearables will permit patients to interface with specialists from their residences. The customary call for various checks and exams will be limited. This will keep expenditure and season of patients consistently (Arias et al., 2015).

Drug Management: With the assistance of shrewd remote pill bottles, the following prescription timetable will turn out to be simple. This will help individuals who neglect to take as much time as necessary. The IoT empowered prescription administration cycles will likewise furnish specialists with examination for contributing improved consideration to the patients.

Outlook Confronts of IoT in Medical Field

With the expansion on the lookout for healthcare IoT, the difficulties will undoubtedly increment. Putting away heaps of information gathered by numerous gadgets will represent a test to the healthcare organizations. As this information will likewise be traded among different gadgets, the security concerns will likewise increase. Unapproved admittance to linked procedure can make damage the patient's safety. Consequently, legitimate verification and authorization will be significant to create the development with IoT(Bodeau et al., 2010). Applications that IoT has to bring to the table are not completely grown at this point. The far and wide of associated gadgets in the medical configuration is additionally inadequate. IoT and medical jointly will drastically modify the administration contributions in the emergency clinics.

Table 1. Benefits, challenges and possible healthcare applications of IoT healthcare

BENEFITS	CHALLENGES	POSSIBLE HEALTHCARE APPLICATIONS
• Real time Health Monitoring • Connectivity & Affordability • Quick Analysis • Data collection • Alert & Tracking • Professional Remote Assistance • Reduced Cost & Improved Treatment • Quick diseases diagnosis • Drug & Equipment management • Reduced emergency rooms with wait time • Next level patient experience	• Data security • Data Privacy • combination of devices and protocols • Accuracy and Data Overload • Cost inadequacy • Connectivity • 24/7 availability	- inventive drug management system - remedial of chronic diseases - record the tracking - Medical Sensors -

The digitalization in medical care will be conveyed by the IoT. The below Table1 explicates the Benefits, Challenges and Possible Healthcare Applications of IoT Healthcare

FUTURE OF IOT SECURITY

While IoT gadgets bring powerful correspondence between gadgets, robotize things, save time and cost and have various advantages, there is one thing actually concerning the clients IoT security. There have been explicit occurrences which have made the IoT gadgets testing to trust.

More Data Monitoring

A recent concern in IoT security concerns the entrance IoT needs to touchy information and the development of delicate information by and large. With sufficient opportunity, programmers could hypothetically utilize an associated pot to acquire your business' Wi-Fi secret phrase. The figure 4 shows the IoT Security Problems and issued by the variants.

Hence, IoT security relies upon intra-network information misfortune avoidance. This instrument guarantees that IoT gadgets can't just access information to which they aren't entitled. Further, it keeps pernicious entertainers from moving information through organization hubs or out of the organization; all things being equal, it keeps the entirety of the information put away safely until an approved client chooses to move it (Cai et al., 2016). This can apply to gadgets as much as individuals. Table 2 elaborates the Challenges, Threats and Security Requirements of IoT Security.

Joining with Backup

At the point when we observe IoT security, the discussion generally depends on endpoint security. All things considered, IoT gadgets speak to one more part of the equipment based computerized edge; every gadget opens another potential assault vector for outer danger entertainers. Without the perceivability into each gadget brought by endpoint security, programmers could locate a strong traction for contaminations. Even the most grounded cyber security can't forestall 100% of all malware. So we require hav-

Figure 4. IoT security problems

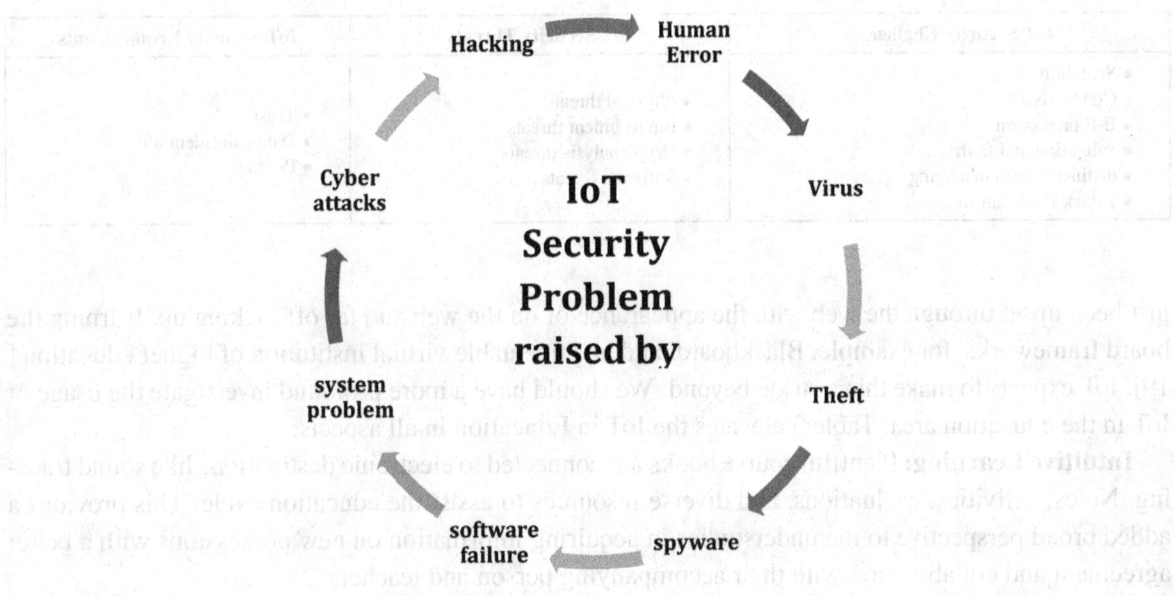

ing a support plan for your devices by methods for fortification and failure recovery courses of action. Those coordinate with endpoint security to relieve the harm done by ransom ware and different types of malware, all of which can taint IoT gadgets.

Pointless Capabilities

IoT security depends in huge part on your own obligation to cyber security .Numerous IoT gadgets accompany default head passwords which are effortlessly speculated or broken. So the security group needs to set aside the effort to reset these passwords at every possible opportunity. Further, to kill pointless capacities on every gadget this could hamper cyber security endeavors and assurances(Chahid et al., 2017). This is to restrict interruptions and alleviate the adequacy of interruptions which do happen.

Updates and Patches

IoT security relies upon ensuring that IoT gadgets get ordinary updates to their security firmware and software. Like all gadgets, updates these gadgets get contain imperative security patches and danger knowledge. Tragically, numerous IoT engineers neglect to make fixing these gadgets simple (Dhaya & Kanthavel, 2020b)

OUTLOOK OF IOT IN EDUCATION

The IoT is a progressive change occurring directly in front of us that vows to change a horde of areas including schooling. It not just tries to increase conventional human-to-human homeroom communications, yet additionally challenges training from a more extensive perspective. An instruction area has

Table 2. Challenges, threats; and security requirements of IoT security

IoT Security Challenges	IoT Security Threats	IoT Security Requirements
• Scalability • Connectivity • E-E protection • validation and faith • distinctiveness managing • Attack-Resistant safety	• Physical threats • Environment threats • Cryptanalysis threats • Software threats	• Trust • Data Confidentiality, • Privacy

just been upset through the web with the appearance of on the web and far off picking up, learning the board frameworks, for example, Blackboard, and an undeniable virtual institution of higher education [19]. IoT expects to make this a stride beyond. We should have a more profound investigate the usage of IoT in the education area. Table 3 elevates the IoT in Education in all aspects.

Intuitive Learning: Plentiful course books are connected to electronic destinations like sound tracking, Notes, activities, evaluations, and diverse resources to assist the education cycle. This provides a added broad perspective to the understudies in acquiring information on new possessions with a better agreement and collaboration with their accompanying person and teachers. .

Security: The students in an educational organization are obtainable to chances and need brilliant safety when differentiated and the general population at some other workplaces. IoT can add a huge motivation regarding improving the security of schools, college, campus and some other learning communities . For observing the understudy conduct, a savvy camera image can be used on the grounds. As of late, computer vision developments have improved a lot and can monitor at the surroundings.

Educational Applications: The educational applications uses IoT can be out looked as amazing inventive gadgets and are shifting the way by which instructing and learning is ended. They likewise empower teachers and students to make 3D illustrations syllabus volumes which highlight recordings and provide the capability to acquire the observations. These sorts of applications can be considered as distinct advantages as they give an enormous number of educational games. These games give various highlights that offer fascinating prospects with regards to educating and learning. This makes schooling more captivating than some other time in late memory.

Expanding Efficiency: In plentiful schools and universities, a ton of time is used up on workout that doesn't increase the value of the center point of their very incidence. With the assist of IoT devices, the information can be getting together and shipped off the office worker taking out the requirement for any human mediation (Dhaya & Kanthavel, 2020c).

FUTURE OF IOT IN AGRICULTURE

Use of IoT in agriculture could be a day to day existence transformer for humankind and the entire planet. Presently, we witness how extraordinary climate, disintegrating soil and drying lands, falling environments that assume a vital job in agriculture make food creation increasingly hard. Savvy agriculture is used for collecting the food creation rehearses fueled by IoT, enormous data and developmental survey improvement (Kassab et al., 2020). Table 5 enlightens the Benefits, Applications, Challenges and Solutions to Agricultural Problems using IoT. The most well-known IoT applications in savvy agriculture are:

Table 3. IoT in education

BENEFITS OF IOT IN EDUCATION
• Personalized Learning occurrence • Textbook enrichment • Smart Classrooms • assists Special-need Students • Robust Security for Learning Spaces • Task-based education
EDUCATION PROBLEMS SOLVED BY IOT
• Data Collection • Personalized Learning • More Human to-Machine Interaction • Security
POSSIBLE DRAWBACKS OF IOT IN EDUCATION
• Privacy • fuel the Global Digital-Divide • investment issues
REASON FOR EFFECTIVE EXECUTION OF IOT IN EDUCATION
• Security • Integration • Education Policies
CHALLENGES OF IOT IN EDUCATION
• More execution price. • In-class principles. • be short of of information processing infrastructure. • safety issues • Reliable Wi-Fi Connection
THE FUTURE OF IOT IN EDUCATION
• make IoT a part of mainstream education • technologies accessible and simple to use
EXAMPLES OF IOT IN THE EDUCATION SECTOR
• Promethean • Blackboard • Kaltura • Tynker • EdModo
IOT-HOW DOES HELP STUDENTS
- Helps students learn at their tempo With IoT, use your Smartphone to get further clarification. - IoT has open latest chances for people to study from anywhere at any time. - IoT permit students to follow their learning growth and assess their performance and results.
IOT- HOW IT HELPS EDUCATORS
o IoT provides you permit to the various huge number of materials with high feature. o IoT computerizes the learning series and permits you as a teacher to follow student attending. o IoT likewise gives you more opportunity as a teacher.

1. Sensor-based frameworks
2. Elegant agriculture automobiles, drones, self-ruling robots and actuators.
3. Linked agriculture places, for example, shrewd nurseries or aqua-farming.
4. Data investigation, representation and the board frameworks.

Wellbeing of Using IoT in Agriculture

Use of IoT in agriculture guarantees already inaccessible productivity, the decrease of assets and cost, robotization and information driven cycles. In agriculture, notwithstanding, these advantages don't go about as upgrades, yet rather the answers for the entire business going up against a scope of perilous issues.

Dominated Efficiency: IoT-enabled farming licenses to screen their item and conditions perpetually. They get pieces of information rapidly, can predict issues before they happen, and make taught decisions on the most capable technique to evade them. Additionally, IoT courses of action in agribusiness present computerization, for example, demand based water framework, planning and robot procuring.

Extension: IoT-based nurseries and water cultivating systems enable short food creation, organization and should have the alternative to deal with these people with new results of the dirt. Sharp shut cycle plant structures grant creating food basically all finished—in business sectors, on tall structures' dividers and rooftops, in steel trailers and so on (Namiot, 2016).

Diminished Resources: A great deal of IoT is based on propelling the use of resources like water, energy, land. Precision developing using IoT depends upon the data accumulated from arranged sensors in the field which helps farmers with dispensing resources inside one plant.

Cleaner Cycle: The comparison is appropriate to pesticides and composts. Not solely do IoT-based systems for precision developing assistance producers save water and energy and, thusly, make developing greener, yet moreover basically cut back on the usage of insect killers and compost..

Agility: One of the upsides of using IoT in horticulture is the extended preparation of the cycles. In view of steady checking and conjecture systems, farmers can quickly respond to any gigantic change in an atmosphere, dampness, air quality similarly as the adequacy of each reap or soil in the field.

Improved Item Quality: Data driven horticulture helps both with creating and better items. Using soil and gather sensors, raised robot noticing and farm arranging, farmers better understand itemized conditions among the circumstances and the idea of the yields via related systems, they can replicate the finest environment and addition; the dietary advantage of the items(Moreno-Cano et al., 2015).

IoT Challenges in Agriculture

Savvy agriculture framework utilizing IoT and large information innovation could be the guardian angel for the entire business. However, incorporating innovation in conventional farming cycles has not been without its own issues.

Set of the Connections: You need to give the network all through the farming climate—fields, storage facilities, horse shelters, nurseries, and so forth to make an IoT framework work. Preferably, it ought to likewise be a dependable continuous association which could withstand extreme climate occasions and open space conditions. Despondently, the availability actually represents an issue in the Internet of Things all in all, as assorted frameworks utilize various conventions and information transmission strategies.

Plan and Strength: Any IoT framework utilized in agriculture ought to have the option to deal with availability, however the states of outside spaces. Robots, compact sensors, IoT in savvy network and climate observing stations ought to have a straightforward yet practical plan and a specific degree of power to "work in the homestead." also the many-sided environment and strangeness of preparation an IoT item as a law (Zhiqiang & Junming, 2011).

Restricted Resources and Time: The part of IoT in agriculture is significant; however the coordination of savvy innovation here happens with regards to a continually changing climate and absence of time.

Table 4. Benefits, applications, challenges and solutions to agricultural problems using IoT

Benefits	Applications	Challenges	Solutions to Agricultural Problems
• Excelled efficiency • Remote control & Pest Control • Expansion • Reduced resources. • Cleaner process • Agility • Irrigation & animal tracking • Improved product quality	• Air Monitoring • Soil Monitoring • Water monitoring • Disease Monitoring • Environmental Condition Monitoring • Crop and Plant Growth Monitoring • Temperature Monitoring • Humidity Monitoring • Location Tracking	• Connectivity • Design and durability • Limited resources and time	• exactitude Farming • exactitude Livestock Farming

EDGE COMPUTING IN IOT

Edge computing is altering the method in which information is being dealt with, handled, and conveyed from a large number of gadgets around the world. It is as "a bit of an appropriated registering topography where information planning is found close to that. Edge figuring was made in light of the surprising advancement of IoT contraptions, which partner with the web for either accepting information from the cloud or conveying information back to the cloud. Furthermore, various IoT contraptions produce monstrous proportions of information all through their assignments (Mostafavi, 2019).

How Edge Computing Works?

Edge Computing authorizes information from IoT gadgets to be evaluated at the edge of the system prior to being shipped off server farm or cloud or data storage(Dhaya & Kanthavel, 2016). Figure 5 promotes the Working flow of Edge Computing.

Utilization of Edge Computing

Edge computing can be consolidated into an extensive assortment of utilizations, items, and administrations or networks. The Table 5 briefs the Pros and Cons of Edge Computing

A couple of conceivable outcomes include the

- IoT contraptions:
- Self-driving vehicles: Security system noticing such as
- More productive sharing
- Medical noticing devices:
- Video conferencing:

Key Merits of Edge Computing

Faster Response Time: Power of data accumulating and count is passed on and close by. No roundtrip to the cloud diminishes inaction and connects snappier responses. This will help forestall essential machine assignments from isolating or perilous scenes from happening.

Figure 5. Working flow of edge computing

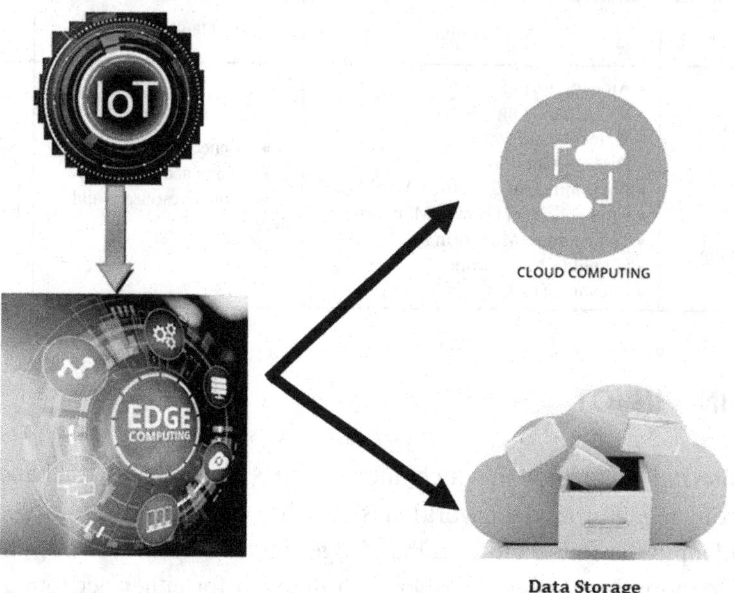

Table 5. Pros and cons of edge computing

EDGE COMPUTING	
PROS	**CONS**
✓ Minimum Latency ✓ Availability in Real time ✓ Real time data transmission ✓ Customer –Corporate Integration ✓ Fast response in customer part ✓ Increase productivity	✓ Limited or low redundancy ✓ Data corruption or data loss ✓ Takes longer time for producing output ✓ Lack of security in times ✓ High Risk

Reliable Undertakings When Irregular Accessibility: For most far off assets, checking or conflicting web network regions, for instance, oil wells, farm siphons, daylight based estates or windmills can be inconvenient. Edge devices' ability to locally store and cycle data ensures no data hardship or operational disillusionment if there should arise an occurrence of the limited web network (Khan et al., 2019).

Security and Consistence: Due to edge figuring's advancement, A huge load of data move among devices and the cloud is avoidable. It's possible to channel fragile information locally and simply convey critical data model construction information to the cloud. This grants customers to build an adequate security and consistence framework that is essential for huge business security and audits.

Monetarily Information Courses of Action: One of the judicious concerns around IoT determination is the candid cost on account of association move speed, data storing, and computational power. Edge processing can locally play out a huge load of data figuring's, which licenses associations to pick which organizations to run locally and which ones to transport off the cloud, which diminishes the last costs of an as a rule IoT game plan.

Interoperability among the Gadgets: Edge contraptions can go probably as a correspondence contact among the legacy and current machines. This grants legacy mechanical machines to connect with present day machines or IoT game plans and gives snappy points of interest of getting encounters from legacy or current machines (Chiang & Ha, 2017).

Advantages and Real-Life Use Cases For Edge Computing In IoT

The principle motivation behind edge computing is to decentralize information taking care of. This prompts various favorable circumstances over the conventional cloud. To be specific, there are five primary favorable circumstances of edge computing for IoT:

Expanded Data Security: While IoT arrangements speak to an ideal objective for digital assaults, edge computing can help you secure your organizations and improve generally information protection. Since the information is decentralized and conveyed among the gadgets where it is created, it's hard to bring down the entire organization or bargain the entirety of the information with a solitary assault(He et al., 2018).

Better App Performance: It takes some effort for information travel to and fro between the gadget and the server farm. By putting away and handling the information near its source, you decrease the slack time and improve the in general application execution. Subsequently, you can break down the information progressively, without delays.

Decreased Operational Costs: When you store and cycle the majority of the information "at the edge," you needn't bother with a wealth of distributed storage. Also, you can sift through the pointless data and reinforcement just the pertinent information (Shi et al., 2016).

Improved Business Efficiency and Reliability: Lower information traffic and diminished distributed storage, thus, prompts more effective business tasks. . This is because of the way that your gadgets can work self-governing, without an Internet association.

Limitless Scalability: In contrast to cloud, edge computing permits you to scale your IoT network varying, without reference to the accessible stockpiling.

CASE STUDIES IN THE FUTURE OF IOT

Here some case studies are elaborated in the domain wise.

IOT in Agriculture: Case Study: Precision Agriculture

Precision agriculture can help ranchers manage various difficulties, for example, water deficiencies, the restricted accessibility of reasonable grounds for crop plantings, the troubles ranchers have overseeing costs through the usage IoT frameworks and advancements to basically diminish likely stumbles and, thusly, amplify yields. Accuracy agribusiness uses IoT applications, which help farmers with extending the quality, sum, practicality and cost feasibility of cultivating creation. These instruments license the farmers to comprehend what seeds to plant, the proportion of fertilizer they need to use, the better an ideal chance to gather similarly as the ordinary yield yields(Porambage et al., 2018). Through the use of IoT, farmers can in like manner screen sensors that can be used to distinguish soil sogginess, crop advancement and animals feed levels, among other key limits. The sensors can in like manner indirectly supervise and control related authorities and water framework gear. Certain IoT stages used in the farming license to operate farmers to manage the colossal proportions of data assembled from sensors, cloud organizations, for instance, atmosphere or aides, related stuff and existing structures.

IOT in Education: Case Study: Smart Boards

The circumstances are different. The current day understudies appreciate keen sheets far more than boards. Smart boards are interactive white boards that undertakings subject pictures. It empowers the educators and understudies to interact with it. By essentially writing on it or moving it around the class. It is substantially more fun and exciting than it is appears right now. It isn't unexpected to think whether savvy sheets can supplant slates in all methods or not. The appropriate response is 'Yes'. Words and shown figures on a slate or course readings, miss the mark now and again to communicate the idea of an exercise in minute manners. Insight conflicts become normal and henceforth the study hall winds up in a pool of disarray. Here, utilizations of IoT in schooling have figured out how to make training and the trading of information basic, interesting and interactive. With savvy sheets, an instructor can take a murmur of alleviation. Info designs, instructional exercise recordings and complex formulae, be it for any subject and particularly of arithmetic, could be settled in more limited time periods.

IoT in Healthcare: Case Study: Medical IoT: 3D Imaging Technology

Medical imaging is an enormous market that continually advances with innovation advances, and there are numerous applications. One use case large numbers of us may not know about is the requirement for exact injury estimation. This is a worry with new injuries, regarding assessing seriousness, just as wounds that are progressing through the healing cycle. Eykona, a UK-based medical imaging organization, built up a Wound Measurement System to address this difficulty. The framework utilizes cameras and 3D imaging to photo, measure and guide twisted movement over the long run. By observing changes in volume and tissue structure, clinicians can assess wounds and the adequacy of treatment.

IoT in Retail: Smartphone Charging Solution for Retail Outlets

The Powermat organization utilized a custom Digi passage in an application that empowers clients to charge their telephones from Starbucks and other retail areas. The Powermat remote charging stations are implanted in tabletops and associated nearby with Zigbee network innovation. A Digi XBee Gateway interfaces Powermat safely to its cloud-based framework, and furthermore empowers information integration to catch information, for example, the areas of the "charging spot" stations.

IoT in Smart Cities: City Lighting Applications

Lighting is perhaps the most common instances of IoT applications for urban cities, and numerous districts nowadays are revolving to remote correspondences for price reserving and power decrease (Zhiqiang & Junming, 2011). The arrangement incorporates the ruggedized Digi WR44R venture class switch, which gives availability and information routing to different gadget hubs on the Smart Pole.

Case Study: IoT Transportation: Transit and Automotive IoT Solutions

TransData is an IoT framework integrator that creates applications for public travel, for example, installment and IDs frameworks, for the Slovak market. TransDatas leader item is a multi-faceted arrangement that underpins a wide scope of public vehicle capacities:

- Secure ticket exchanges
- Easy-to-utilize electronic card framework improves traveler encounters
- GPS-followed course direction limits delays
- Display neighborhood shops, cafés and focal points
- More dependable Internet access and rapid traveler Wi-Fi
- Monitor traffic movement with on-vehicle surveillance cameras
- Route interchanges through a focal terminal or dispatch

CONCLUSION

This chapter presented the futuristic research perspectives of IoT platforms elaborately that includes education, agriculture, industry, healthcare and security. The focus also has been given to advantages and real time manner for edge computing in IoT, in addition to the case study in Transportation for transit and Automotive IoT Solutions. From the investigations of these studies, it is induced that the future IoT seems splendid and empowering. With all the assumptions and thoughts in advancement, our lives will turn much more straightforward and gainful whether we are taking a gander at investigating around our metropolitan territories, collaborating at work or lodging in thc comfort of our own homes. In any case, there is one restriction of IoT contraptions face in all of these regions is that the issue of network and correspondence between all the devices. Hence this chapter concludes by saying that the future of IoT platform will be of no doubt as magnanimous as the users want to apply and utilize depending on the various needs in different platforms. The effectiveness of futuristic IoT will be playing a key role in globalization, privatization and industrialization towards the globe connectivity by means technological advancement and developments in terms of innovation.

REFERENCES

Ammar, M., Russello, G., & Crispo, B. (2018). *Internet of things: A survey on the security of iot frameworks* (Vol. 38). J Inf Secur Appl.

Anirudh, M., Thileeban, S. A., & Nallathambi, D. J. (2017). Use of honeypots for mitigating dos attacks targeted on IoT networks. In *2017 International conference on computer, communication and signal processing (ICCCSP)*. IEEE.

Arias, Wurm, Hoang, & Jin. (2015). Privacy and security in internet of things and wearable devices. IEEE Trans Multi Scale. *Comput Syst.*, *1*(2), 99–109.

Behrendt, F. (2019). Cycling the smart and sustainable city: Analyzing EC policy documents on internet of things, mobility and transport, and smart cities. *Sustainability*, *11*(3), 763. doi:10.3390u11030763

Bodeau, D. J., Graubart, R., & Fabius-Greene, J. (2010). Improving cyber security and mission assurance via cyber preparedness (cyber prep) levels. In *2010 IEEE Second international conference on social computing*. IEEE.

Cai, H., Xu, B., Jiang, L., & Vasilakos, A. V. (2016). IoT-Based Big Data Storage Systems in Cloud Computing: Perspectives and Challenges. *IEEE Internet of Things Journal*, *4*(1), 75–87. doi:10.1109/JIOT.2016.2619369

Chahid, Y., Benabdellah, M., & Azizi, A. (2017). Internet of things security. In *2017 International conference on wireless technologies, embedded and intelligent systems (WITS)*. IEEE.

Chen, J., Su, C., Yeh, K. H., & Yung, M. (2018). *Special issue on advanced persistent threat*. Elsevier. doi:10.1016/j.future.2017.11.005

Chiang, M., & Ha, S. (2017). Clarifying fog computing and networking: 10 questions and answers. *IEEE Communications Magazine*, *55*(4).

Dhaya, R., & Kanthavel, R. (2016). Smart Waste Management Using Internet of Things (IOT). *Middle East Journal of Scientific Research*, *24*(10), 3358–3361.

Dhaya, R., & Kanthavel, R. (2020a). A Wireless Collision Detection on Transmission Poles through IoT Technology. Journal of Trends in Computer Science and Smart Technology, 2(3), 165-172.

Dhaya, R., & Kanthavel, R. (2020b). *Reinforcement Learning Concepts Ministering Smart City Applications Using IoT*. EAI/Springer Innovations in Communication and Computing. doi:10.1007/978-3-030-34328-6_2

Dhaya, R., & Kanthavel, R. (2020c). Data Science for Internet of Things (IoT). Lecture Notes on Data Engineering and Communications Technologies, 44, 60-70.

Gaona-Garcia, Montenegro-Marin, Prieto, & Nieto. (2017). Analysis of security mechanisms based on clusters IoT environments. Int J Interact Multimed. *Artificial Intelligence*, *4*(3), 55–60.

He, D., Chan, S., & Guizani, M. (2018). Security in the Internet of Things Supported by Mobile Edge Computing. *IEEE Communications Magazine*, *56*(8), 56–61. doi:10.1109/MCOM.2018.1701132

Heer, T., Garcia-Morchon, O., Hummen, R., Keoh, S. L., Kumar, S. S., & Wehrle, K. (2011). Security challenges in the IP based internet of things. *Wireless Personal Communications*, *61*(3), 527–542. doi:10.100711277-011-0385-5

Kanthavel. (2018). Advanced LTE (5G) in Medical IOT-Research, Future and Scope. *Communications in Computer and Information Science, 876.*

Kassab, DeFranco, & Laplante. (2020). *A systematic literature review on Internet of things in education: Benefits and challenges*. doi:10.1111/jcal.12383

Khan, W. Z., Ahmed, E., Hakak, S., Yaqoob, I., & Ahmed, A. (2019). Edge computing: A survey. *Future Generation Computer Systems*, *97*, 219–235. doi:10.1016/j.future.2019.02.050

Kumar, S., Tiwari, P., & Zymbler, M. (2019). Internet of Things is a revolutionary approach for future technology enhancement: A review. *Journal of Big Data*, *6*(1), 111. doi:10.118640537-019-0268-2

Liu, J., Xiao, Y., & Philip-Chen, C. L. (2012). Authentication and access control in the internet of things. In *32nd international conference on distributed computing systems workshops*. IEEE Xplore. 10.1109/ICDCSW.2012.23

Moreno-Cano, V., Terroso-Saenz, F., & Skarmeta-Gómez, A. F. (2015). Big data for IoT services in smart cities. In *Internet of Things (WF-IoT) IEEE 2nd World Forum on*. IEEE. 10.1109/WF-IoT.2015.7389091

Mostafavi, S. A. (2019). Edge Computing for IoT: Challenges and Solutions. *Journal of Communications Technology, Electronics and Computer Science*, (26), 4–8.

Namiot. (2016). On Internet of Things and Smart Cities educational courses. *International Journal of Open Information Technologies*, *4* (5), 26-38.

Porambage, P., Okwuibe, J., Liyanage, M., Ylianttila, M., & Taleb, T. (2018). Survey on multi-access edge computing for internet of things realization. *IEEE Communications Surveys and Tutorials*, *20*(4), 2961–2991. doi:10.1109/COMST.2018.2849509

Shi, W., Cao, J., Zhang, Q., Li, Y., & Xu, L. (2016). Edge Computing: Vision and Challenges. *IEEE Internet of Things Journal*, *3*(no. 5), 637–646. doi:10.1109/JIOT.2016.2579198

Weber, R. H. (2010). Internet of things-new security and privacy challenges. *Computer Law & Security Review*, *26*(1), 23–30. doi:10.1016/j.clsr.2009.11.008

Zanella, A., Bui, N., Castellani, A., Vangelista, L., & Zorgi, M. (2014). Internet of things for smart cities. *IEEE IoT-Journal*, *1*(1), 22–32.

Zhiqiang, H., & Junming, Z. (2011). *The Application of Internet of Things in Education and Its Trend of Development*. Modern Distance Education Research.

Zhou, J., Cap, Z., Dong, X., & Vasilakos, A. V. (2017). Security and privacy for cloud-based IoT: Challenges. *IEEE Commun Mag. Vol*, *55*(1), 26–33. doi:10.1109/MCOM.2017.1600363CM

Compilation of References

Santucci, G. (2009, January). Internet of things–when your fridge orders your groceries. In *International Conference on Future Trends of the Internet (Vol. 28)*. Academic Press.

Atzori, L., Iera, A., & Morabito, G. (2010). The Internet of Things: A survey. *Computer Networks, 54*(15), 2787-2805. doi:10.1016/j.comnet.2010.05.010

Jia, X., Feng, Q., Fan, T., & Lei, Q. (2012). RFID technology and its applications in Internet of Things (IoT). *2012 2nd International Conference on Consumer Electronics, Communications and Networks (CECNet),* 1282-1285. 10.1109/CECNet.2012.6201508

De Caro, N., Colitti, W., Steenhaut, K., Mangino, G., & Reali, G. (2013). Comparison of two lightweight protocols for smartphone-based sensing. *2013 IEEE 20th Symposium on Communications and Vehicular Technology in the Benelux (SCVT),* 1-6. 10.1109/SCVT.2013.6735994

OData. (2015). *Libraries.* Retrieved January 14, 2016, from OData - the Best Way to REST: https://www.odata.org/libraries/

OData - the Best Way to REST. (n.d.). Retrieved January 14, 2016, from OData - the Best Way to REST: https://www.odata.org/

Vineetha, Misra, & Kishore. (2020). A real time IoT based patient health monitoring system using machine learning algorithms. *European Journal of Molecular & Clinical Medicine, 7*(4), 2912-2925.

Hiraguri, T., Aoyagi, M., Morino, Y., Akimoto, T., Nishimori, K., & Hiraguri, T. (2015). Proposal of ZigBee systems for the provision of location information and transmission of sensor data in medical welfare. *E-Health Telecommunication Systems and Networks, 4*(3), 45–55. doi:10.4236/etsn.2015.43005

Verma, N., Singh, S., & Prasad, D. (2021). A Review on existing IoT Architecture and Communication Protocols used in Healthcare Monitoring System. *J. Inst. Eng. India Ser. B.* doi:10.1007/s40031-021-00632-3

Pradhan, Bhattacharyya, & Pal. (2021). IoT-Based Applications in Healthcare Devices. *Journal of Healthcare Engineering*. doi:10.1155/2021/6632599

Buttyan, L., & Hubaux, J. P. (2007). *Security and cooperation in wireless networks: Thwarting malicious and selfish behavior in the age of ubiquitous computing.* Cambridge University Press. doi:10.1017/CBO9780511815102

Selvaraj, S., & Sundaravaradhan, S. (2020). Challenges and opportunities in IoT healthcare systems: A systematic review. *SN Appl. Sci., 2*(1), 139. doi:10.100742452-019-1925-y

Jaswal, K., Choudhury, T., Chhokar, R. L., & Singh, S. R. (2017). Securing the Internet of Things: A proposed framework. *2017 International Conference on Computing, Communication and Automation (ICCCA)*, 1277-1281. 10.1109/CCAA.2017.8230015

Wang, Y., Hu, M., Li, Q., Zhang, X., Zhai, G., & Yao, N. (2020). *Abnormal respiratory patterns classifier may contribute to large-scale screening of people infected with COVID-19 in an accurate and unobtrusive manner.* ArXiv, abs/2002.05534.

Chen, C., Jyan, H., Chien, S., Jen, H., Hsu, C., Lee, P., Lee, C.-F., Yang, Y.-T., Chen, M.-Y., Chen, L.-S., Chen, H.-H., & Chan, C.-C. (2020, May 5). Containing COVID-19 among 627,386 persons in contact with the Diamond Princess cruise ship passengers who disembarked in Taiwan: Big data analytics. *Journal of Medical Internet Research, 22*(5), e19540. doi:10.2196/19540 PMID:32353827

Materia, F. T., Faasse, K., & Smyth, J. M. (2020, May 25). Understanding and preventing health concerns about emerging mobile health technologies. *JMIR mHealth and uHealth, 8*(5), e14375. doi:10.2196/14375 PMID:32449688

Were, M. C., Sinha, C., & Catalani, C. (2019, August 1). A systematic approach to equity assessment for digital health interventions: Case example of mobile personal health records. *Journal of the American Medical Informatics Association, 26*(8-9), 884–890. doi:10.1093/jamia/ocz071 PMID:31188438

Hallur, S., Kulkarni, R., & Patavardhan, P. (2020). *Introduction, Security Challenges, and Threats in IoT, Internet of Things: Integration and Security Challenges*. CRC Press. doi:10.1201/9781003032441

Samaniego, M., & Deters, R. (2016). Management and Internet of Things. *The 13th International Conference on Mobile Systems and Pervasive Computing (MobiSPC 2016), 94*, 137 – 143. 10.1016/j.procs.2016.08.022

Al-Fuqaha, M., Guizani, M., Mohammadi, M., Aledhari, M., & Ayyash, M. (2015). Internet of Things: A Survey on Enabling Technologies, Protocols, and Applications. *IEEE Communications Surveys and Tutorials, 17*(4), 2347–2376. doi:10.1109/COMST.2015.2444095

Alaba, F. A., Othman, M., Hashem, I. A. T., & Alotaibi, F. (2017). Internet of things security: A survey. *Journal of Network and Computer Applications, 88*, 10–28. doi:10.1016/j.jnca.2017.04.002

Hallur, S. N., Torse, D. A., Aithal, V. K., & Santaji, S. S. (2018). Epilepsy Detection by Processing of EEG signals using LabVIEW Simulation. *2018 International Conference on Electrical, Electronics, Communication, Computer, and Optimization Techniques (ICEECCOT)*, 1101-1106. 10.1109/ICEECCOT43722.2018.9001570

Ammar, M., Russello, G., & Crispo, B. (2018). Internet of things: A survey on the security of IoT frameworks. *J. Inf. Security Appl., 38*, 8–27. doi:10.1016/j.jisa.2017.11.002

Khan, M. A., & Salah, K. (2018). IoT security: Review, blockchain solutions, and open challenges. *Future Generation Computer Systems, 82*, 395–411. doi:10.1016/j.future.2017.11.022

Sfar, R., Natalizio, E., Challal, Y., & Chtourou, Z. (2018). A roadmap for security challenges in the internet of things. *Digital Commun. Netw., 4*(2), 118–137. doi:10.1016/j.dcan.2017.04.003

Irshad, M. (2016). A Systematic Review of Information Security Frameworks in the Internet of Things (IoT). *2016 IEEE 18th International Conference on High Performance Computing and Communications*, 1270-1275. 10.1109/HPCC-SmartCity-DSS.2016.0180

Nguyen, K. T., Laurent, M., & Oualha, N. (2015). Survey on secure communication protocols for the internet of things. *Ad Hoc Networks, 32*, 17–31. doi:10.1016/j.adhoc.2015.01.006

Zhao, K., & Ge, L. (2013). A Survey on the Internet of Things Security. *2013 Ninth International Conference on Computational Intelligence and Security*, 663-667. 10.1109/CIS.2013.145

Shehab. (2018). Secure and Robust Fragile Watermarking Scheme for Medical Images. *IEEE Access, 6*, 10269-10278. . doi:10.1109/ACCESS.2018.2799240

Bairagi, Khondoker, & Islam. (2016). An efficient steganographic approach for protecting communication in the Internet of Things (IoT) critical infrastructures. *Information Security Journal: A Global Perspective, 25*(4-6), 197-212. doi:10.1080/19393555.2016.1206640

Anwar, Ghany, & El Mahdy. (2015). Improving the security of images transmission. *Int. J. Bio-Med. Inform. e-Health, 3*(4), 7-13.

Elhoseny, Salama, & Riad. (2018). A machine learning model for improving healthcare services on cloud computing environment. Measurement, 119, 117-128. doi:10.1016/j.measurement.2018.01.022

Decuir, J. (2015). The Story of the Internet of Things: Issues in utility, connectivity, and security. *IEEE Consumer Electronics Magazine, 4*(4), 54–61. doi:10.1109/MCE.2015.2463292

Yehia, L., Khedr, A., & Darwish, A. (2015). Hybrid security techniques for Internet of Things healthcare applications. *Adv. Internet Things, 5*, 21-25. https:// doi:10.4236/ait.2015.53004

Sreekutty, M. S., & Baiju, P. S. (2017). Security enhancement in image steganography for medical integrity verification system. *2017 International Conference on Circuit, Power and Computing Technologies (ICCPCT)*, 1-5. 10.1109/ICCPCT.2017.8074197

Khalil, M. I. (2017). Medical image steganography: Study of medical image quality degradation when embedding data in the frequency domain. *Int. J. Comput. Netw. Inf. Secur., 9*(2), 22–28. doi:10.5815/ijcnis.2017.02.03

Hallur & Bajantri. (2018). Myocardial Infraction Alert System using RFID Technology. *International Journal of Innovative Science and Research Technology, 3*(6), 45-49.

Thilakanathan, D., Calvo, R., Chen, S., & Nepal, S. (2013). Secure and Controlled Sharing of Data in Distributed Computing. *2013 IEEE 16th International Conference on Computational Science and Engineering*, 825-832. 10.1109/CSE.2013.125

Abomhara, M., & Køien, G. M. (2014). Security and privacy in the Internet of Things: Current status and open issues. *2014 International Conference on Privacy and Security in Mobile Systems (PRISMS)*, 1-8. 10.1109/PRISMS.2014.6970594

Bing, C., Yuebo, D., Bo, J., Xiang, Z., & Lijuan, Z. (2011). The RFID-based electronic identity security platform of the Internet of Things. *2011 International Conference on Mechatronic Science, Electric Engineering and Computer (MEC)*, 246-249. 10.1109/MEC.2011.6025447

Noura, M., Atiquzzaman, M., & Gaedke, M. (2019). Interoperability in Internet of Things: Taxonomies and Open Challenges. *Mobile Networks and Applications, 24*(3), 796–809. doi:10.100711036-018-1089-9

Djenna, D. & Saïdouni, E. (2018). Cyber Attacks Classification in IoT-Based-Healthcare Infrastructure. *2018 2nd Cyber Security in Networking Conference (CSNet)*, 1-4. 10.1109/CSNET.2018.8602974

Hussain, S., Schaffner, S., & Moseychuck, D. (2009). Applications of Wireless Sensor Networks and RFID in a Smart Home Environment. In *Proceedings of the 2009 Seventh Annual Communication Networks and Services Research Conference (CNSR '09)*. IEEE Computer Society. 10.1109/CNSR.2009.32

A performance-aware dynamic scheduling algorithm for cloud-based IoT applications. (2020). *Computer Communications, 160*, 512–520. doi:10.1016/j.comcom.2020.06.016

A, D., R, M.-O., M, D., D, H., & G, S. (2010). The Internet of Things for Ambient Assisted Living. *Seventh International Conference on Information Technology: New Generations*, 804-809.

Abdel-Basset, M., Manogaran, G., Gamal, A., & Chang, V. (2019). A Novel Intelligent Medical Decision Support Model Based on Soft Computing and IoT. *IEEE Internet of Things Journal*, 1–1. doi:10.1109/JIOT.2019.2931647

Abdul Minaam, D. S., & Abd-ELfattah, M. (2018). Smart drugs:Improving healthcare using Smart Pill Box for Medicine Reminder and Monitoring System. *Future Computing and Informatics Journal*, *3*(2), 443–456. doi:10.1016/j.fcij.2018.11.008

Ahad, A., Tahir, M., Aman Sheikh, M., Istiaque Ahmed, K., Mughees, A., & Numani, A. (2020). Technologies Trend towards 5G Network for Smart Health-Care Using IoT: A Review. *Sensors*.

Ahmed, E., Yaqoob, I., Hashem, I. A. T., Khan, I., Ahmed, A. I. A., Imran, M., & Vasilakos, A. V. (2017). The role of big data analytics in Internet of Things. *Computer Networks*, *129*(2), 459–471. doi:10.1016/j.comnet.2017.06.013

Akhtar, M. M., & Rizvi, D. R. (2021). Traceability and detection of counterfeit medicines in pharmaceutical supply chain using blockchain-based architectures. In *Sustainable and Energy Efficient Computing Paradigms For Society* (pp. 1–31). Springer. doi:10.1007/978-3-030-51070-1_1

Akmandor, A. O., & Jha, N. K. (2017). Smart health care: An edge-side computing perspective. *IEEE Consum. Electron. Mag.*, *7*(1), 29–37. doi:10.1109/MCE.2017.2746096

Al Bassam, N., Shaik Asif, H., Al Qaraghuli, A., Khan, J., Sumesh, E. P., & Lavanya, V. (2021). IoT Based Wearable Device to Monitor the Signs of Quarantined remote patients of COVID-19. *Informatics in Medicine Unlocked*, *100588*, 100588. Advance online publication. doi:10.1016/j.imu.2021.100588 PMID:33997262

Albahri, Alwan, Taha, Ismail, Hamid, Zaidan, Albahri, Zaidan, Alamoodi, & Alsalem. (2020). IoT-based telemedicine for disease prevention and health promotion: State-of-the-Art. *Journal of Network and Computer Applications*, (102873). Advance online publication. doi:10.1016/j.jnca.2020.102873

Alhussein, M., & Muhammad, G. (2018). Voice Pathology Detection Using Deep Learning on Mobile Healthcare Framework. *IEEE Access : Practical Innovations, Open Solutions*, *6*, 41034–44104. doi:10.1109/ACCESS.2018.2856238

Ali & Abu-Elkheir. (2015). *Internet of Nano-Things Healthcare Applications: requirements, opportunities, and challenges*. IEEE. doi:10.1109/WiMOB.2015.7347934

Ali, Z., & Alhamid, M. F. (2017). An Automatic Health Monitoring System for Patients Suffering from Voice Complications in Smart Cities. *IEEE Access : Practical Innovations, Open Solutions*, *5*(1), 3900–3908. doi:10.1109/ACCESS.2017.2680467

Al-khafajiy, M., Baker, T., Chalmers, C., Asim, M., Kolivand, H., Fahim, M., & Waraich, A. (2019). Remote health monitoring of elderly through wearable sensors. *Multimedia Tools and Applications*, *78*(17), 24681–24706. doi:10.100711042-018-7134-7

Alkhazaali, A. H. (2020). *International Congress on Human-Computer Interaction, Optimization and Robotic Applications (HORA)*. 10.1109/HORA49412.2020.9152923

Alloghani, M., Al-Jumeily, D., Hussain, A., Aljaaf, A. J., Mustafina, J., & Petrov, E. (2018). *Healthcare Services Innovations Based on the State of the Art Technology Trend Industry 4.0* [Paper Presentation]. *11th International Conference on Developments in e-Systems Engineering (DeSE)*, Cambridge, UK. 10.1109/DeSE.2018.00016

Aloi, G., Fortino, G., Gravina, R., Pace, P., & Savaglio, C. (2021). Simulation-Driven Platform for Edge-Based AAL Systems. *IEEE Journal on Selected Areas in Communications*, *39*(2), 446–462. doi:10.1109/JSAC.2020.3021544

Alonsa, G. S., Arambarri, J., Lopez Coronado, M., & de la Toree Diez, I. (2019). Proposing new blockchain challenges in e-health. *Journal of Medical Systems*, *43*(64).

Altexsoft. (2020). *Comparing Machine Learning as a Service: Amazon, Microsoft Azure, Google Cloud AI, IBM Watson.* https://www.altexsoft.com/blog/datascience/comparing-machine-learning-as-a-service-amazon-microsoft-azure-google-cloud-ai-ibm-watson/

Ambrosini, G. L., Hurworth, M., Giglia, R., Trapp, G., & Strauss, P. (2018). Feasibility of a commercial smartphone application for dietary assessment in epidemiological research and comparison with 24-h dietary recalls. *Nutrition Journal, 17*(1), 5. Advance online publication. doi:10.118612937-018-0315-4 PMID:29316930

Amin, S. U., Alsulaiman, M., Muhammad, G., Mekhtiche, M. A., & Shamim Hossain, M. (2019). Deep Learning for EEG motor imagery classification based on multi-layer CNNs feature fusion. *Future Generation Computer Systems, 101*, 542–554. doi:10.1016/j.future.2019.06.027

Ammar, M., Russello, G., & Crispo, B. (2018). *Internet of things: A survey on the security of iot frameworks* (Vol. 38). J Inf Secur Appl.

Anirudh, M., Thileeban, S. A., & Nallathambi, D. J. (2017). Use of honeypots for mitigating dos attacks targeted on IoT networks. In *2017 International conference on computer, communication and signal processing (ICCCSP)*. IEEE.

Ara, A., & Ara, A. (2017). Case study: Integrating IoT, streaming analytics and machine learning to improve intelligent diabetes management system. *2017 International Conference on Energy, Communication, Data Analytics and Soft Computing (ICECDS)*. 10.1109/ICECDS.2017.8390043

Archundia Herrera, M., & Chan, C. (2018). Narrative Review of New Methods for Assessing Food and Energy Intake. *Nutrients, 10*(8), 1064. doi:10.3390/nu10081064 PMID:30103401

Arias, Wurm, Hoang, & Jin. (2015). Privacy and security in internet of things and wearable devices. IEEE Trans Multi Scale. *Comput Syst., 1*(2), 99–109.

Arsene, C. (2021). *Artificial Intelligence in Healthcare: The Future Is Amazing.* https://healthcareweekly.com/artificial-intelligence-in-healthcare/

Ashman, A., Collins, C., Brown, L., Rae, K., & Rollo, M. (2017). Validation of a Smartphone Image-Based Dietary Assessment Method for Pregnant Women. *Nutrients, 9*(1), 73. doi:10.3390/nu9010073 PMID:28106758

Atitallah, S. B., Driss, M., Boulila, W., & Ghézala, H. B. (2020). Leveraging Deep Learning and IoT big data analytics to support the smart cities development: Review and future directions. *Computer Science Review, 38*, 100303. doi:10.1016/j.cosrev.2020.100303

Atlam, H. F., Alenezi, A., Alharthi, A., Walters, R. J., & Wills, G. B. (2017). Integration of Cloud Computing with Internet of Things: Challenges and Open Issues. *2017 IEEE International Conference on Internet of Things (IThings) and IEEE Green Computing and Communications (GreenCom) and IEEE Cyber, Physical and Social Computing (CPSCom) and IEEE Smart Data (SmartData)*. 10.1109/iThings-GreenCom-CPSCom-SmartData.2017.105

Attaia, O. (2019). An IoT-blockchain architecture based on hyperledger framework for healthcare monitoring application. In *Proceedings: 10th IFIP International Conference on New Technologies, Mobility And Security (NTMS)*. IEEE Publications. 10.1109/NTMS.2019.8763849

Atul, K., Ken, A., David, S., & Fera, B. (2019). *The future of artificial intelligence in health care.* https://www.modernhealthcare.com/technology/future-artificial-intelligence-health-care

Ayaz, M., Ammad-uddin, M., Sharif, Z., Mansour, A., & Aggoune, E.-H. M. (2019). Internet-of-Things (IoT) based Smart Agriculture: Towards Making the Fields Talk. *IEEE Access: Practical Innovations, Open Solutions, 7*, 1–1. doi:10.1109/ACCESS.2019.2932609

Azana, Hassan, Sameen, Bash, Alizadeh, & Latiff. (2020). IoMT amid COVID-19 pandemic: Application, architecture, technology, and security. *Journal of Network and Computer Applications*. Advance online publication. doi:10.1016/j.jnca.2020.102886

Azbeg, K., Ouchetto, O., Andaloussi, S. J., & Fetjah, L. (2011). A Taxonomic Review of the Use of IoT and Blockchain in Healthcare Applications. *IRBM*. Advance online publication. doi:10.1016/j.irbm.2021.05.003

Babaei & Schiele. (2019). *Physical Unclonable Functions in the Internet of Things: State of the Art and Open Challenges*. doi:10.3390/s19143208

Bai, H. X., Hsieh, B., Xiong, Z., Halsey, K., Choi, J. W., Tran, T. M. L., & Liao, W. H. (2020). Performance of radiologists in differentiating COVID-19 from non-COVID-19 viral pneumonia at chest CT. *Radiology*, *296*(2), E46–E54. doi:10.1148/radiol.2020200823 PMID:32155105

Bakar, Ab Hamid, Yunus, Zawani, Halim, & Zainuddin. (2020). Descriptive Analysis of Type 2 Diabetes Mellitus Patients Using Data From Hospital. *Information Systems*, *16*, 94.

Bally, L., Dehais, J., Nakas, C. T., Anthimopoulos, M., Laimer, M., Rhyner, D., Rosenberg, G., Zueger, T., Diem, P., Mougiakakou, S., & Stettler, C. (2016). Carbohydrate Estimation Supported by the GoCARB System in Individuals with Type 1 Diabetes: A Randomized Prospective Pilot Study. *Diabetes Care*, *40*(2), e6–e7. doi:10.2337/dc16-2173 PMID:27899490

Barabde, M. & Danve, S. (2015). Real Time Water Quality Monitoring System. *International Journal of Innovative Research in Computer and Communication Engineering*.

Barcelo, M., Correa, A., Llorca, J., Tulino, A. M., Vicario, J. L., & Morell, A. (2016). IoT-Cloud Service Optimization in Next Generation Smart Environments. *IEEE Journal on Selected Areas in Communications*, *34*(12), 4077–4090. doi:10.1109/JSAC.2016.2621398

Barla, N. (2021). *Data Science and Machine Learning in the Medical Industry*. https://neptune.ai/blog/data-science-and-machine-learning-in-the-medical-industry

Bassoli, M., Bianchi, V., De Munari, I., & Ciampolini, P. (2017). An IoT Approach for an AAL Wi-Fi-Based Monitoring System. *IEEE Transactions on Instrumentation and Measurement*, *66*(12), 3200–3209. doi:10.1109/TIM.2017.2753458

Beck, R. (2018). Beyond bitcoin: The rise of blockchain world. *Computer*, *51*(2), 54–58. doi:10.1109/MC.2018.1451660

Behrendt, F. (2019). Cycling the smart and sustainable city: Analyzing EC policy documents on internet of things, mobility and transport, and smart cities. *Sustainability*, *11*(3), 763. doi:10.3390u11030763

Ben Fekih, R., & Lahami, M. (2020). *The Impact of Digital Technologies on Public Health in Developed and Developing Countries. International Conference on Smart Homes and Health Telematics*, 268-276.

Berry, S. E., Valdes, A. M., Drew, D. A., Asnicar, F., Mazidi, M., Wolf, J., Capdevila, J., Hadjigeorgiou, G., Davies, R., Al Khatib, H., Bonnett, C., Ganesh, S., Bakker, E., Hart, D., Mangino, M., Merino, J., Linenberg, I., Wyatt, P., Ordovas, J. M., ... Spector, T. D. (2020). Human postprandial responses to food and potential for precision nutrition. *Nature Medicine*, *26*(6), 964–973. doi:10.103841591-020-0934-0 PMID:32528151

Bertsimas, D., Kallus, N., Weinstein, A. M., & Zhuo, Y. D. (2016). Personalized Diabetes Management Using Electronic Medical Records. *Diabetes Care*, *40*(2), 210–217. doi:10.2337/dc16-0826 PMID:27920019

Bharati, Podder, Mondal, & Paul. (2021). *Applications and Challenges of Cloud Integrated IoMT*. doi:10.1007/978-3-030-55833-8_4

Bhatia, K., Arora, S., & Tomar, R. (2016, October). Diagnosis of diabetic retinopathy using machine learning classification algorithm. In *2016 2nd International Conference on Next Generation Computing Technologies (NGCT)* (pp. 347-351). IEEE. 10.1109/NGCT.2016.7877439

Bianchi, V., Bassoli, M., Lombardo, G., Fornacciari, P., Mordonini, M., & De Munari, I. (2019). IoT Wearable Sensor and Deep Learning: An Integrated Approach for Personalized Human Activity Recognition in a Smart Home Environment. *IEEE Internet of Things Journal, 6*(5), 8553–8562. doi:10.1109/JIOT.2019.2920283

Bin Zikria, Ali, Afzal, & Kim. (2021). *Next Generation Internet of Things (IoT): Opportunities, Challenges, and Solutions Sensors.* . doi:10.3390/s21041174

Boakye, A., & Olumide, O. B. (2020). The role of internet of things (IoT) to support health services in rural communities. A case study of Ghana and Sierra Leone. *Transnational Corporations Review.*

Bodeau, D. J., Graubart, R., & Fabius-Greene, J. (2010). Improving cyber security and mission assurance via cyber preparedness (cyber prep) levels. In *2010 IEEE Second international conference on social computing*. IEEE.

Brandt, B., Rashidiani, S., Bán, Á., & Rauch, T. A. (2019). DNA Methylation-Governed Gene Expression in Autoimmune Arthritis. *International Journal of Molecular Sciences, 20*(22), 5646. Advance online publication. doi:10.3390/ijms20225646 PMID:31718084

Bronze-da-Rocha, E. (2014). MicroRNAs Expression Profiles in Cardiovascular Diseases. *BioMed Research International, 2014*, 1–23. doi:10.1155/2014/985408 PMID:25013816

Bucher Della Torre, S., Carrard, I., Farina, E., Danuser, B., & Kruseman, M. (2017). Development and Evaluation of e-CA, an Electronic Mobile-Based Food Record. *Nutrients, 9*(1), 76. doi:10.3390/nu9010076 PMID:28106767

Buterin, V. (2014). *A next generation smart contract decentralized application platform.* Academic Press.

Cai, H., Xu, B., Jiang, L., & Vasilakos, A. V. (2016). IoT-Based Big Data Storage Systems in Cloud Computing: Perspectives and Challenges. *IEEE Internet of Things Journal, 4*(1), 75–87. doi:10.1109/JIOT.2016.2619369

Castelo, M. (2020). *The Future of Artificial Intelligence in Healthcare.* https://healthtechmagazine.net/article/2020/02/future-artificial-intelligence-healthcare

Catrin, S., Zaid, A., Niamh, O. N., Mehdi, K., & Ahmed, K. (2020). World Health Organization declares global emergency: A review of the 2019 novel corona virus (COVID-19). *International Journal of Surgery, 76*, 71–76. doi:10.1016/j.ijsu.2020.02.034 PMID:32112977

Chahid, Y., Benabdellah, M., & Azizi, A. (2017). Internet of things security. In *2017 International conference on wireless technologies, embedded and intelligent systems (WITS).* IEEE.

Chakraborty, S., Aich, S., & Kim, H. C. (2019). A secure healthcare system design framework using blockchain technology. In *Proceedings: 21st International Conference on Advanced Communication Technology (ICACT).* IEEE Publications. 10.23919/ICACT.2019.8701983

Chelvachandran, N., Trifuljesko, S., Drobotowicz, K., Kendzierskyj, S., Jahankhani, H., & Shah, Y. (2020). Considerations for the Governance of AI and Government Legislative Frameworks. In H. Jahankhani, S. Kendzierskyj, N. Chelvachandran, & J. Ibarra (Eds.), *Cyber Defence in the Age of AI, Smart Societies and Augmented Humanity. Advanced Sciences and Technologies for Security Applications.* Springer. doi:10.1007/978-3-030-35746-7_4

Chen, G., Ding, C., Li, Y., Hu, X., Li, X., Ren, L., Ding, X., Tian, P., & Xue, W. (2020). Prediction of Chronic Kidney Disease Using Adaptive Hybridized Deep Convolutional Neural Network on the Internet of Medical Things Platform. *IEEE Access: Practical Innovations, Open Solutions, 8*, 100497–100508. doi:10.1109/ACCESS.2020.2995310

Chen, J., Su, C., Yeh, K. H., & Yung, M. (2018). *Special issue on advanced persistent threat.* Elsevier. doi:10.1016/j.future.2017.11.005

Chen, S., Yang, J., Yang, W., Wang, C., & Barnighausen, T. (2020). COVID-19 Control in China during Mass Population Movements at New Year. *Lancet, 395*(10226), 764–766. Advance online publication. doi:10.1016/S0140-6736(20)30421-9 PMID:32105609

Chiang, M., & Ha, S. (2017). Clarifying fog computing and networking: 10 questions and answers. *IEEE Communications Magazine, 55*(4).

Cohen, G., & Mello, M. (2018). HIPAA and protecting health information in the 21st century. *Journal of the American Medical Association, 320*(3), 231–232. doi:10.1001/jama.2018.5630 PMID:29800120

Corella, D., & Ordovás, J. M. (2012). Interactions between dietary n-3 fatty acids and genetic variants and risk of disease. *British Journal of Nutrition, 107*(S2), S271–S283. doi:10.1017/S0007114512001651 PMID:22591901

Craft, L. (2017). *Emerging Applications of Ai for Health care Providers.* Gartner. https://www.gartner.com/document/3753763?ref=solrAll&refval=224860044&qid=d68fd7aaf33dc5ae74c5e8

Cui, X. R., Abbod, M. F., Liu, Q., Shieh, J.-S., Chao, T. Y., Hsieh, C. Y., & Yang, Y. C. (2010). Ensembled artificial neural networks to predict the fitness score for body composition analysis. *The Journal of Nutrition, Health & Aging, 15*(5), 341–348. doi:10.100712603-010-0260-1 PMID:21528159

D, H., & S, K. (2021). Patch-SIFT: Enhanced feature descriptor to learn human facial emotions using an Ensemble approach. *Indian Journal of Science and Technology*, 1740-1747.

Danneskiold-Samsøe, N. B., Dias de Freitas Queiroz Barros, H., Santos, R., Bicas, J. L., Cazarin, C. B. B., Madsen, L., Kristiansen, K., Pastore, G. M., Brix, S., & Maróstica Júnior, M. R. (2019). Interplay between food and gut microbiota in health and disease. *Food Research International, 115*, 23–31. doi:10.1016/j.foodres.2018.07.043 PMID:30599936

Data Flair. (2019a). *IoT Tutorial for Beginners | What is Internet of Things?* Dataflair Team. https://data-flair.training/blogs/iot-tutorial

Data Flair. (2019b). *IoT Analytics – 3 Major Uses Cases of Internet of Things Analytics.* https://data-flair.training/blogs/iot-analytics

Data Flair. (2019c). *IoT Analytics at the Edge Vertica Brings Analytics to Where the "Things" are.* https://www.microfocus.com/media/white-paper/iot_analytics_at_the_edge_wp.pdf

de Moraes Lopes, M. H. B., Ferreira, D. D., Ferreira, A. C. B. H., da Silva, G. R., Caetano, A. S., & Braz, V. N. (2020). Use of artificial intelligence in precision nutrition and fitness. *Artificial Intelligence in Precision Health*, 465–496. doi:10.1016/B978-0-12-817133-2.00020-3

de Vries, J., Antoine, J.-M., Burzykowski, T., Chiodini, A., Gibney, M., Kuhnle, G., Méheust, A., Pijls, L., & Rowland, I. (2013). Markers for nutrition studies: Review of criteria for the evaluation of markers. *European Journal of Nutrition, 52*(7), 1685–1699. doi:10.100700394-013-0553-3 PMID:23955424

DeBusk, R. (2010). The Role of Nutritional Genomics in Developing an Optimal Diet for Humans. *Nutrition in Clinical Practice, 25*(6), 627–633. doi:10.1177/0884533610385700 PMID:21139127

Deebak, B. D., Al-Turjman, F., Aloqaily, M., & Alfandi, O. (2020). IoT-BSFCAN: A smart context-aware system in IoT-Cloud using mobile-fogging. *Future Generation Computer Systems, 109*, 368–381. doi:10.1016/j.future.2020.03.050

Dehais, J., Anthimopoulos, M., Shevchik, S., & Mougiakakou, S. (2017). Two-View 3D Reconstruction for Food Volume Estimation. *IEEE Transactions on Multimedia, 19*(5), 1090–1099. doi:10.1109/TMM.2016.2642792

DelPrete. (2016). *Self Service Kiosks: Improving Collections, Efficiency and Patient Experience.* American Association of Orthopedic Executives. https://www.aaoe.net/news/315967/self-service-kiosks-improving-collections-efficiency-and-patient-experience.html

Demirci, F., Akan, P., Kume, T., Sisman, A. R., Erbayraktar, Z., & Sevinc, S. (2016). Artificial Neural Network Approach in Laboratory Test Reporting. *American Journal of Clinical Pathology, 146*(2), 227–237. doi:10.1093/ajcp/aqw104 PMID:27473741

Deng, Z., Ren, Y., Liu, Y., Yin, X., Shen, Z., & Kim, H.-J. (2019). Blockchain-based trusted electronic records preservation in cloud storage. *Computers, Materials & Continua, 58*(1), 135–151. doi:10.32604/cmc.2019.02967

Deo, R. C. (2020). Machine Learning in Medicine. *Circulation, 142*(16), 1521–1523. doi:10.1161/CIRCULATIONAHA.120.050583 PMID:33074761

Devika, N. T., & Raman, K. (2019). Deciphering the metabolic capabilities of Bifidobacteria using genome-scale metabolic models. *Scientific Reports, 9*(1), 18222. Advance online publication. doi:10.103841598-019-54696-9 PMID:31796826

Dey, Ashour, & Bhatt. (2017). *Internet of Things Driven Connected Healthcare: Internet of Things and Big Data Technologies for Next Generation Healthcare.* Springer International Publishing. doi.. doi:10.1007/978-3-319-49736-5_1

Dhaya, R., & Kanthavel, R. (2020a). A Wireless Collision Detection on Transmission Poles through IoT Technology. Journal of Trends in Computer Science and Smart Technology, 2(3), 165-172.

Dhaya, R., & Kanthavel, R. (2020c). Data Science for Internet of Things (IoT). Lecture Notes on Data Engineering and Communications Technologies, 44, 60-70.

Dhaya, R., & Kanthavel, R. (2016). Smart Waste Management Using Internet of Things (IOT). *Middle East Journal of Scientific Research, 24*(10), 3358–3361.

Dhaya, R., & Kanthavel, R. (2020b). *Reinforcement Learning Concepts Ministering Smart City Applications Using IoT.* EAI/Springer Innovations in Communication and Computing. doi:10.1007/978-3-030-34328-6_2

Dhillon & Singh. (2019). Machine Learning in Healthcare Data Analysis: A Survey. *Journal of Biology and Today's World, 8*(6), 1-10.

Diabetes statistics: Read the facts. (2020, September 29). Retrieved from The Checkup website: https://www.singlecare.com/blog/news/diabetes-statistics/

Dialani, P. (2021). *How Virtual Reality Is Helping to Deal with Covid-19.* https://www.analyticsinsight.net/virtualreality-helping-deal-covid-19/

Dietary assessment a resource guiDe to method selection and application in low resource settings. (n.d.). https://www.fao.org/3/i9940en/I9940EN.pdf

Difference-data-analytics-data-analysis. (2020). *What's the Difference Between Data Analytics and Data Analysis? | FAQs.* https://www.getsmarter.com/blog/career-advice/difference-data-analytics-data-analysis/

Dobrescu, R., Merezeanu, D., & Mocanu, S. (2019). Context-Aware Control and Monitoring System with IoT and Cloud Support. *Computers and Electronics in Agriculture, 160*(May), 91–99. doi:10.1016/j.compag.2019.03.005

Dong, Y., Hoover, A., Scisco, J., & Muth, E. (2012). A New Method for Measuring Meal Intake in Humans via Automated Wrist Motion Tracking. *Applied Psychophysiology and Biofeedback*, *37*(3), 205–215. doi:10.100710484-012-9194-1 PMID:22488204

Doni, A., & Chidananda, M. M. (2018). Water Quality Monitoring System using IoT. *International Journal of Engineering Research & Technology*.

Dubovitskaya, A., Xu, Z., Ryn, S., Schumacher, M., & Wang, F. (2017). Secure and trustable electronic medical records sgaring using blockchain. *AMIA Annual Symposium Proceedings*, 650-659.

Durairaj, M., & Ranjani, V. (2013). Data Mining Applications In Healthcare Sector: A Study. *International Journal of Scientific & Technology Research*, *2*(10).

Edison & Somasundaram. (2013). Monitoring Water Quality Using RF Module. *International Journal of Engineering and Innovative Technology, 3*(1).

Education, K. is passionate to write about A. driving technological change. (2020, June 11). *The Rise of Data: Data Science, Big Data and Data Analytics for Seamless Business Operations*. Retrieved from https://www.analyticsinsight.net/the-rise-of-data-data-science-big-data-and-data-analytics-for-seamless-business-operations/

Edwards, J. (2019). *How Mobility Solutions are Increasing Patient Satisfaction in Health care.* https://healthtechmagazine.net/article/2018/05/thoughtful-healthcare-mobility-deployments-improve-patient-satisfaction

Elezabeth, L., Mishra, V. P., & Dsouza, J. (2018). *The Role of Big Data Mining in Healthcare Applications*. IEEE. doi:10.1109/ICRITO.2018.8748434

El-Latif, A., Abd-El-Atty, B., Hossain, M. S., Elmougy, S., & Ghoneim, A. (2018). Secure Quantum Steganography Protocol for Fog Cloud Internet of Things. *IEEE Access : Practical Innovations, Open Solutions*, *6*, 10332–10340. doi:10.1109/ACCESS.2018.2799879

Elmadfa, I., & Meyer, A. L. (2010). Importance of food composition data to nutrition and public health. *European Journal of Clinical Nutrition*, *64*(S3), S4–S7. doi:10.1038/ejcn.2010.202 PMID:21045848

Fang, S., & Kerr, B. (2019). An End-to-End Image-Based Automatic Food Energy Estimation Technique Based on Learned Energy Distribution Images: Protocol and Methodology. *Nutrients*, *11*(4), 877. doi:10.3390/nu11040877 PMID:31003547

Fernández-Caramés, T. M., & Fraga-Lamas, P. (2018). A review on the use of blockchain for the internet of things. *IEEE Access: Practical Innovations, Open Solutions*, *6*, 32979–33001. doi:10.1109/ACCESS.2018.2842685

Fernández-Caramés, T., & Fraga-Lamas, P. (2018). Design of a Fog Computing, Blockchain and IoT-Based Continuous Glucose Monitoring System for Crowdsourcing mHealth. *Proceedings.*, *4*(1), 5757. doi:10.3390/ecsa-5-05757

Fong, D. S., Aiello, L., Gardner, T. W., King, G. L., Blankenship, G., Cavallerano, J. D., Ferris, F. L., & Klein, R. (2004). Retinopathy in diabetes. *Diabetes Care*, *27*(suppl1), s84–s87. doi:10.2337/diacare.27.2007.S84 PMID:14693935

Forooghifar, F., Aminifar, A., & Atienza, D. (2019). Resource-Aware Distributed Epilepsy Monitoring Using Self-Awareness From Edge to Cloud. *IEEE Transactions on Biomedical Circuits and Systems*, *13*(6), 1338–1350. doi:10.1109/TBCAS.2019.2951222 PMID:31689205

Forsee. (2020). *AI in Healthcare*. https://www.foreseemed.com/artificial-intelligence-in-healthcare

Forster, H., Walsh, M. C., Gibney, M. J., Brennan, L., & Gibney, E. R. (2015). Personalised nutrition: The role of new dietary assessment methods. *The Proceedings of the Nutrition Society*, *75*(1), 96–105. doi:10.1017/S0029665115002086 PMID:26032731

Fountaine, T., McCarthy, B., & Saleh, T. (2019). *Building the AI-Powered Organization.* Academic Press.

Fremantle, P. (2016). *White paper, A Reference Architecture for the Internet of Things*. https://wso2.com/whitepapers/a-reference-architecture-for-the-internet-of- things/

Friedewald, M., Önen, M., Lievens, E., Krenn, S., & Fricker, S. (2020). Distributed ledger for provenance tracking of artificial intelligence assets. *IFIP Advances in Information and Communication Technology*. Advance online publication. doi:10.1007/978-3-030-42504-3

Fuellen, G., Schofield, P., Flatt, T., Schulz, R.-J., Boege, F., Kraft, K., Rimbach, G., Ibrahim, S., Tietz, A., Schmidt, C., Köhling, R., & Simm, A. (2015). Living Long and Well: Prospects for a Personalized Approach to the Medicine of Ageing. *Gerontology, 62*(4), 409–416. doi:10.1159/000442746 PMID:26675034

G7. (2018). *Charlevoix: Common Vision for the Future of Artificial Intelligence*. https://g7.gc.ca/wp-content/uploads/2018/06/FutureArtificialIntelligence.pdf

Gahan, B. G. (2019). A Portable Color Sensor Based Urine Analysis System to Detect Chronic Kidney Disease. *11th International Conference on Communication Systems & Networks (COMSNETS)*, 876-881. 10.1109/COMSNETS.2019.8711466

Gallucci, M., Pallucca, C., Di Battista, M. E., Fougère, B., & Grossi, E. (2019). Artificial Neural Networks Help to Better Understand the Interplay Between Cognition, Mediterranean Diet, and Physical Performance: Clues from TRELONG Study. *Journal of Alzheimer's Disease, 71*(4), 1321–1330. doi:10.3233/JAD-190609 PMID:31524170

Gaona-Garcia, Montenegro-Marin, Prieto, & Nieto. (2017). Analysis of security mechanisms based on clusters IoT environments. Int J Interact Multimed. *Artificial Intelligence, 4*(3), 55–60.

García-Magariño, I., Lacuesta, R., & Lloret, J. (2018). Agent-Based Simulation of Smart Beds With Internet-of-Things for Exploring Big Data Analytics. *IEEE Access: Practical Innovations, Open Solutions, 6*, 366–379. doi:10.1109/ACCESS.2017.2764467

Gatteschi, V., Lamberti, F., Demartini, C., Pranteda, C., & Santamaria, V. (2018). Blockchain and smart contracts for insurance: Is the technology mature enough? *Future Internet, 10*(2), 20. doi:10.3390/fi10020020

Geng, D., & Rishi, V. (2018). *Tricking Neural Networks: Create Your Own Adversarial Examples.* https://ml.berkeley.edu/blog/2018/01/10/adversarial-examples/

Georgescu, L. (2018). *What Artificial Intelligence Is and How It Can Be Used.* Academic Press.

GGVS. (2019). *Importance of AI in healthcare*. https://www.gavstech.com/importance-of-ai-in-healthcare/

Gharagyozyan, H. (2019). *A Practical Application of Machine Learning in Medicine.* https://www.macadamian.com/learn/a-practical-application-of-machine-learning-in-medicine/

Ghassemi, Naumann, Schulam, Beam, Chen, & Ranganath. (2019). *A Review of Challenges and Opportunities in Machine Learning for Health.* Academic Press.

Ghoneim, A., Muhammad, G., Amin, S. U., & Gupta, B. (2018). Medical image forgery detection for smart healthcare. *IEEE Communications Magazine, 56*(4), 33–37. doi:10.1109/MCOM.2018.1700817

Giacconi, R., Malavolta, M., Bürkle, A., Moreno-Villanueva, M., Franceschi, C., Capri, M., Slagboom, P. E., Jansen, E. H. J. M., Dollé, M. E. T., Grune, T., Weber, D., Hervonen, A., Stuetz, W., Breusing, N., Ciccarone, F., Zampieri, M., Aversano, V., Caiafa, P., Formentini, L., ... Cardelli, M. (2019). Nutritional Factors Modulating Alu Methylation in an Italian Sample from The Mark-Age Study Including Offspring of Healthy Nonagenarians. *Nutrients, 11*(12), 2986. doi:10.3390/nu11122986 PMID:31817660

Gil Press. (2021). *The Future of AI in Healthcare.* https://www.forbes.com/sites/gilpress/2021/04/29/the-future-of-ai-in-healthcare/?sh=31809939163b

Gill, S. S., Tuli, S., Xu, M., Singh, I., Singh, K. V., Lindsay, D., Tuli, S., Smirnova, D., Singh, M., Jain, U., Pervaiz, H., Sehgal, B., Kaila, S. S., Misra, S., Aslanpour, M. S., Mehta, H., Stankovski, V., & Garraghan, P. (2019). Transformative effects of IoT, Blockchain and Artificial Intelligence on cloud computing: Evolution, vision, trends and open challenges. *Internet of Things*, *8*, 100118. doi:10.1016/j.iot.2019.100118

Gkouskou, K., Vlastos, I., Karkalousos, P., Chaniotis, D., Sanoudou, D., & Eliopoulos, A. G. (2020). The "Virtual Digital Twins" Concept in Precision Nutrition. *Advances in Nutrition*, *11*(6), 1405–1413. doi:10.1093/advances/nmaa089 PMID:32770212

Goel, P., Jain, P., Pasman, H. J., Pistikopoulos, E. N., & Datta, A. (2020). Integration of data analytics with cloud services for safer process systems, application examples and implementation challenges. *Journal of Loss Prevention in the Process Industries*, *68*, 104316. doi:10.1016/j.jlp.2020.104316

Gokhale, Bhat, & Bhat. (2018). Introduction to IOT. IARJSET, 5(1).

Gokhale, P., Bhat, O., & Bhat, S. (2018). Introduction to IOT. *International Advanced Research Journal in Science, Engineering and Technology*, *5*(1), 41–44.

Gomez-Delgado, F., Alcala-Diaz, J. F., Garcia-Rios, A., Delgado-Lista, J., Ortiz-Morales, A., Rangel-Zuñiga, O., Tinahones, F. J., Gonzalez-Guardia, L., Malagon, M. M., Bellido-Muñoz, E., Ordovas, J. M., Perez-Jimenez, F., Lopez-Miranda, J., & Perez-Martinez, P. (2014). Polymorphism at the TNF-alpha gene interacts with Mediterranean diet to influence triglyceride metabolism and inflammation status in metabolic syndrome patients: From the CORDIOPREV clinical trial. *Molecular Nutrition & Food Research*, *58*(7), 1519–1527. doi:10.1002/mnfr.201300723 PMID:24753491

Gong, L., Wong, C.-H., Idol, J., Ngan, C. Y., & Wei, C.-L. (2019). Ultra-long Read Sequencing for Whole Genomic DNA Analysis. *Journal of Visualized Experiments*, *145*(145). Advance online publication. doi:10.3791/58954 PMID:30933081

Guanjing, Z. (2012a). *Patent No. CN202821362U-Internet-of-things human body data blood pressure collecting and transmitting device.* China.

Guanjing, Z. (2012b). *Patent No. CN202838653U-Somatic data blood glucose collection transmission device for internet of things.* China.

Gupta, R., Ghosh, A., Singh, A. K., & Misra, A. (2020, May). Clinical considerations for patients with diabetes in times of COVID-19 epidemic. *Diabetes & Metabolic Syndrome*, *14*(3), 211–212. doi:10.1016/j.dsx.2020.03.002 PMID:32172175

Gurudath, N., Celenk, M., & Riley, H. B. (2014, December). Machine learning identification of diabetic retinopathy from fundus images. In *2014 IEEE Signal Processing in Medicine and Biology Symposium (SPMB)* (pp. 1-7). IEEE. 10.1109/SPMB.2014.7002949

Han, J., Rodriguez, J. C., & Beheshti, M. (2008, December 1). *Diabetes Data Analysis and Prediction Model Discovery Using RapidMiner.* doi:10.1109/FGCN.2008.226

Handelman, G. S., Kok, H. K., Chandra, R. V., Razavi, A. H., Lee, M. J., & Asadi, H. (2018). eDoctor: Machine learning and the future of medicine. *Journal of Internal Medicine*, *284*(6), 603–619. doi:10.1111/joim.12822 PMID:30102808

Han, Y., Han, Z., Wu, J., Yu, Y., Gao, S., Hua, D., & Yang, A. (2020). Artificial Intelligence Recommendation System of Cancer Rehabilitation Scheme Based on IoT Technology. *IEEE Access: Practical Innovations, Open Solutions*, *8*, 44924–44935. doi:10.1109/ACCESS.2020.2978078

Haq, I., & Esuka, O. M. (2018). Blockchain technology in pharmaceutical industry to prevent counterfeit drugs. *International Journal of Computers and Applications*, *975*, 8887.

Hatzivasilis, Soultatos, Ioannidis, Verikoukis, Demetriou, & Tsatsoulis. (n.d.). *Review of Security and Privacy for the Internet of Medical Things (IoMT)*. IEEE. doi:. doi:10.1109/DCOSS.2019.00091

He, D., Chan, S., & Guizani, M. (2018). Security in the Internet of Things Supported by Mobile Edge Computing. *IEEE Communications Magazine*, *56*(8), 56–61. doi:10.1109/MCOM.2018.1701132

Heer, T., Garcia-Morchon, O., Hummen, R., Keoh, S. L., Kumar, S. S., & Wehrle, K. (2011). Security challenges in the IP based internet of things. *Wireless Personal Communications*, *61*(3), 527–542. doi:10.100711277-011-0385-5

Hemalatha, P. (2021). Monitoring and securing the healthcare data harnessing IOT and blockchain technology. *Turkish Journal of Computer and Mathematics Education*, *12*(2), 2554–2561.

Hernandez, D. (2017). *How AI Is Transforming Drug Creation*. https://www.wsj.com/articles/how-ai-is-transforming-drug-creation-1498442760

Heydarian, H., Adam, M., Burrows, T., Collins, C., & Rollo, M. E. (2019). Assessing Eating Behaviour Using Upper Limb Mounted Motion Sensors: A Systematic Review. *Nutrients*, *11*(5), 1168. doi:10.3390/nu11051168 PMID:31137677

Hossain, M. S. (2019). Applying Deep Learning for Epilepsy Seizure Detection and Brain Mapping Visualization. ACM Trans. Multimedia Comput. Commun. Appl., 15(1S). doi:10.1145/3241056

Hossain, M., & Muhammad, G. (2014). Cloud-Based Collaborative Media Service Framework for HealthCare. International Journal of Distributed Sensor Networks. doi:10.1155/2014/858712

Hossain, M. S., & Muhammad, G. (2020). Deep Learning Based Pathology Detection for Smart Connected Healthcare. *IEEE Network*, *34*(6), 120–125. doi:10.1109/MNET.011.2000064

Hoy, M. B. (2017). An introduction to the blockchain and its implications for libraries and medicine. *Medical Reference Services Quarterly*, *36*(3), 273–279. doi:10.1080/02763869.2017.1332261 PMID:28714815

Hsu, C.-Y., Huang, L.-C., Chen, T. M., Chen, L.-F., & Chao, J. C.-J. (2011). A Web-Based Decision Support System for Dietary Analysis and Recommendations. *Telemedicine Journal and e-Health*, *17*(2), 68–75. doi:10.1089/tmj.2010.0104 PMID:21385024

Hu, Z., Ge, Q., Jin, L., & Xiong, M. (2020). *Artificial intelligence forecasting of COVID-19 in China* [Unpublished Manuscript].

Huzooree, G., Khedo, K. K., & Joonas, N. (2017, July 1). *Glucose prediction data analytics for diabetic patients monitoring*. doi:10.1109/NEXTCOMP.2017.8016197

Iansiti, M., & Lakhani, K. R. (2017). The truth about blockchain. *Harvard Business Review*, *95*(1), 118–127.

Imaging Technology News. (2020). *Integrating Artificial Intelligence in Treatment Planning*. https://www.itnonline.com/article/integrating-artificial-intelligence-treatment-planning

Imran, I., Iqbal, N., Ahmad, S., & Kim, D. H. (2021). Health Monitoring System for Elderly Patients Using Intelligent Task Mapping Mechanism in Closed Loop Healthcare Environment. *Symmetry*, *13*(2), 357. doi:10.3390ym13020357

Irfan & Naim Ahmad. (2018). *Internet of Medical Things: Architectural Model, Motivational Factors and Impediments*. Dept. of Computer Science, King Khaild University.

Islam, M., Rahaman, A., & Islam, R. (2020). *Development of Smart Healthcare Monitoring System in IoT Environment*. SN Computer Science. doi:10.100742979-020-00195-y

Jabbar, Samreen, & Aluvalu. (2018). The Future of Health care: Machine Learning. *International Journal of Engineering & Technology*, *7*(4.6), 23-25.

Jæger, B., & Mishra, A. (2020). IoT Platform for Seafood Farmers and Consumers. *Sensors (Basel)*, *20*(15), 4230. doi:10.339020154230 PMID:32751365

Jamali, M. A. J. (2020). *IoT architecture towards the internet of things*. Springer. doi:10.1007/978-3-030-18468-1

Jamil, F., Ahmad, S., Iqbal, N., & Kim, D.-H. (2020). Towards a remote monitoring of patient vital signs based on IoT-based blockchain integrity management platforms in smart hospitals. *Sensors (Basel)*, *20*(8), 2195. doi:10.339020082195 PMID:32294989

Jamil, F., Hang, L., Kim, K., & Kim, D. (2019). A novel medical blockchain model for drug supply chain integrity management in a smart hospital. *Electronics (Basel)*, *8*(5), 505. doi:10.3390/electronics8050505

Javaid, M., Haleem, A., Vaishya, R., Bahl, S., Suman, R., & Vaish, A. (2018). Industry 4.0 technologies and their applications in fighting COVID-19 pandemic. *Diabetes & Metabolic Syndrome*, *14*(4), 419–422. doi:10.1016/j.dsx.2020.04.032 PMID:32344370

Jeon, M., Sethi, I. K., & Xu, B. (2017). Machine Learning Theory and Applications for Healthcare. *Journal of Healthcare Engineering*. PMID:29090076

Jiang, S., Cao, J., Wu, H., Yang, Y., Ma, M., & He, J. (2018). A blockchain-based platform for healthcare information exchange. *IEEE International Conference on Smart Computing*, 49-56. 10.1109/SMARTCOMP.2018.00073

Jianxin, T., Min, B., & Mingjie, J. (2012). Patent No. CN202875315U-Carry-on blood pressure/pulse rate/blood oxygen monitoring location intelligent terminal based on internet of things. China.

Jin, H., Luo, Y., Li, P., & Mathew, J. (2019). A review of secure and privacy-preserving medical data sharing. *IEEE Access: Practical Innovations, Open Solutions*, *7*, 61656–61669. doi:10.1109/ACCESS.2019.2916503

Joel, J. P. C. (2021). *Internet of Medical Things in the Context of COVID-19*. Academic Press.

Jones, S., & Edwards, R. T. (2010). Diabetic retinopathy screening: A systematic review of the economic evidence. *Diabetic Medicine*, *27*(3), 249–256. doi:10.1111/j.1464-5491.2009.02870.x PMID:20536486

Junjian, Z., Zhanli, K., & Zhuang, M. (2012). *Patent No. CN102811185A-Temperature measurement system and method based on home gateway*. China.

Junnila, A. (n.d.). *Trackinno*. Retrieved 2021, from Trackinno: https://trackinno.com/2018/07/06/how-iot-works-part-3-data-processing/

Kaggle. (n.d.). https://www.kaggle.com/c/diabetic-retinopathy-detection

Kamruzzaman, M. M. (2020). *Architecture of Smart Health Care System Using Artificial Intelligence*. doi:10.1109/ICMEW46912.2020.9106026

Kanthavel. (2018). Advanced LTE (5G) in Medical IOT-Research, Future and Scope. *Communications in Computer and Information Science, 876*.

Kaput, J., & Rodriguez, R. L. (2004). Nutritional genomics: The next frontier in the postgenomic era. *Physiological Genomics*, *16*(2), 166–177. doi:10.1152/physiolgenomics.00107.2003 PMID:14726599

Karthikeyan, S., & Pandian, M. S. (2021). Science and Technology in the Modern Agricultural Sector: An Overview. *Science and Technology, 7*(2).

Kassab, DeFranco, & Laplante. (2020). *A systematic literature review on Internet of things in education: Benefits and challenges*. doi:10.1111/jcal.12383

Kathleen. (2020). *The Increasing Use Of AI In The Pharmaceutical Industry*. https://www.forbes.com/sites/cognitiveworld/2020/12/26/the-increasing-use-of-ai-in-the-pharmaceutical-industry/?sh=74a4b0cb4c01

Kawano, Y., & Yanai, K. (2014). FoodCam: A real-time food recognition system on a smartphone. *Multimedia Tools and Applications*, *74*(14), 5263–5287. doi:10.100711042-014-2000-8

Kechit, G. (2021). *Artificial Intelligence in Pharmaceutical Industry: 8 Exciting Applications in 2021*. https://www.upgrad.com/blog/artificial-intelligence-in-pharmaceutical-industry/

Kelly, Campbell, Gong, & Ham. (2020). The Internet of Things: Impact and Implications for Health Care Delivery. *Journal of Medical Internet Research*. Advance online publication. doi:10.2196/20135

Khanam, J. J., & Foo, S. Y. (2021). *A comparison of machine learning algorithms for diabetes prediction*. ICT Express. doi:10.1016/j.icte.2021.02.004

Khan, W. Z., Ahmed, E., Hakak, S., Yaqoob, I., & Ahmed, A. (2019). Edge computing: A survey. *Future Generation Computer Systems*, *97*, 219–235. doi:10.1016/j.future.2019.02.050

Kirk, D., Catal, C., & Tekinerdogan, B. (2021). Precision nutrition: A systematic literature review. *Computers in Biology and Medicine*, *133*, 104365. doi:10.1016/j.compbiomed.2021.104365 PMID:33866251

Kizza, J. M. (2017). Internet of things (IoT): Growth, challenges, and security. In *Guide to Computer Network Security* (pp. 517–531). Springer. doi:10.1007/978-3-319-55606-2_24

Kraft, F., & Kurth, I. (2019). Long-read sequencing in human genetics. *Medizinische Genetik*, *31*(2), 198–204. doi:10.100711825-019-0249-z

Kritzinger, W., Karner, M., Traar, G., Henjes, J., & Sihn, W. (2018). Digital Twin in manufacturing: A categorical literature review and classification. *IFAC-PapersOnLine*, *51*(11), 1016–1022. doi:10.1016/j.ifacol.2018.08.474

Kulkarni, P., Mahabaleshwarkar, A., Kulkarni, M., Sirsikar, N., & Gadgil, K. (2019). Conversational AI: An Overview of Methodologies, Applications & Future Scope. *2019 5th International Conference on Computing, Communication, Control and Automation (ICCUBEA)*. 10.1109/ICCUBEA47591.2019.9129347

Kumar, N. M. S., Eswari, T., Sampath, P., & Lavanya, S. (2015). Predictive Methodology for Diabetic Data Analysis in Big Data. *Procedia Computer Science, 50*, 203–208. doi:10.1016/j.procs.2015.04.069

Kumar, T. (2018). Blockchain utilization in healthcare: Key requirements and challenges. In *Proceedings: IEEE 20th International Conference on E-Health Networking, Applications and Services (Healthcom)*. IEEE Publications. 10.1109/HealthCom.2018.8531136

Kumar, Thiwari, & Zymbler. (2019). Internet of Things is a revolutionary approach for future technology enhancement: a review. *Journal of Big Data*. doi:10.1186/s40537-019-0268-2

Kumari, A., & Kumar, N. (2018). Fog computing for healthcare 4.0 environment: Opportunities and challenges. *Computers & Electrical Engineering*, *72*, 1–13. doi:10.1016/j.compeleceng.2018.08.015

Kumar, N. M., & Mallick, P. K. (2018). Blockchain technology for security issues and challenges in IoT. *Procedia Computer Science*, *132*, 1815–1823. doi:10.1016/j.procs.2018.05.140

Kura, B., Parikh, M., Slezak, J., & Pierce, G. N. (2019). The Influence of Diet on MicroRNAs that Impact Cardiovascular Disease. *Molecules (Basel, Switzerland)*, *24*(8), 1509. doi:10.3390/molecules24081509 PMID:30999630

Lam, C., Yi, D., Guo, M., & Lindsey, T. (2018). Automated detection of diabetic retinopathy using deep learning. *AMIA Joint Summits on Translational Science Proceedings AMIA Summit on Translational Science*, *2018*, 147. PMID:29888061

Larson, E. C., Goel, M., Boriello, G., Heltshe, S., Rosenfeld, M., & Patel, S. N. (2012). *SpiroSmart: Using a Microphone to Measure Lung Function on a Mobile Phone*. Ubicomp. doi:10.1145/2370216.2370261

Lashari, S. A., Ibrahim, R., & Senan, N. N. S. A. M. (2018). Application of Data Mining Techniques for Medical Data Classification: A Review. *MATEC Web of Conferences.*

Latha, R., & Vetrivelan, P. (2020). *Wireless Body Area Network (WBAN)-Based Telemedicine for Emergency Care.* School of Electronics Engineering. *Vellore Institute of Technology, Chennai.* Advance online publication. doi:10.339020072153

Latif, G., Shankar, A., Alghazo, J., Kalyanasundaram, V., Boopathi, C. S., & Arfan Jaffar, M. (2020). I-CARES: Advancing health diagnosis and medication through IoT. *Wireless Networks*, *26*(4), 2375–2389. Advance online publication. doi:10.100711276-019-02165-6

Li, Y.H., Yeh, N.N., Chen, S.J., & Chung, Y.C. (2019). Computer-assisted diagnosis for diabetic retinopathy based on fundus images using deep convolutional neural network. *Mobile Information Systems.*

Li, H., Zhu, L., Shen, M., Gao, F., Tao, X., & Liu, S. (2018). Blockchain Based Data Preservation System for Medical Data. *Journal of Medical Systems*, *42*(8), 141. doi:10.100710916-018-0997-3 PMID:29956058

Li, L., Qin, L., Xu, Z., Yin, Y., Wang, X., Kong, B., & Xia, J. (2020). Artificial intelligence distinguishes COVID-19 from community acquired pneumonia on chest CT. *Radiology*. Advance online publication. doi:10.1148/radiol.2020200905

Lin, K., Li, C., Tian, D., Ghoneim, A., Hossain, M. S., & Amin, S. U. (2019). Artificial-Intelligence-Based Data Analytics for Cognitive Communication in Heterogeneous Wireless Networks. *IEEE Wireless Communications*, *26*(3), 83–89. doi:10.1109/MWC.2019.1800351

Linn, L. A., & Koo, M. B. (2016). Blockchain for health data and its potential use in health IT and health care related research. Proceedings of the ONC/NIST use of Blockchain for Healthcare and Research Workshop.

Linthicum, D. S. (2017). Making Sense of AI in Public Clouds. *IEEE Cloud Computing*, *4*(6), 70–72. doi:10.1109/MCC.2018.1081067

Liu, J., Xiao, Y., & Philip-Chen, C. L. (2012). Authentication and access control in the internet of things. In *32nd international conference on distributed computing systems workshops.* IEEE Xplore. 10.1109/ICDCSW.2012.23

Liu, B., & Qian, S.-B. (2011). Translational Regulation in Nutrigenomics. *Advances in Nutrition*, *2*(6), 511–519. doi:10.3945/an.111.001057 PMID:22332093

Liu, D., Yan, Z., & Wenxiu, D. M. A. (2019). *A Survey on Secure Data Analytics in Edge Computing*. *IEEE Internet of Things Journal*. doi:10.1109/JIOT.2019.2897619

Liu, Y., Wang, Y., Ni, Y., Cheung, C. K. Y., Lam, K. S. L., Wang, Y., Xia, Z., Ye, D., Guo, J., Tse, M. A., Panagiotou, G., & Xu, A. (2020). Gut Microbiome Fermentation Determines the Efficacy of Exercise for Diabetes Prevention. *Cell Metabolism*, *31*(1), 77–91.e5. doi:10.1016/j.cmet.2019.11.001 PMID:31786155

Lloyd-Price, J., Abu-Ali, G., & Huttenhower, C. (2016). The healthy human microbiome. *Genome Medicine*, *8*(1), 51. Advance online publication. doi:10.118613073-016-0307-y PMID:27122046

Lo, F., Sun, Y., Qiu, J., & Lo, B. (2018). Food Volume Estimation Based on Deep Learning View Synthesis from a Single Depth Map. *Nutrients*, *10*(12), 2005. doi:10.3390/nu10122005 PMID:30567362

Loucks, J., Davenport, T., & Schatsky, D. (2018). *State of AI in the Enterprise.* https://www2.deloitte.com/content/dam/insights/us/articles/4780_State-of-AI-in-the-enterprise/AICognitiveSurvey2018_Infographic.pdf

Lu, Y., Stathopoulou, T., Vasiloglou, M. F., Pinault, L. F., Kiley, C., Spanakis, E. K., & Mougiakakou, S. (2020). goFOODTM: An Artificial Intelligence System for Dietary Assessment. *Sensors (Basel)*, *20*(15), 4283. Advance online publication. doi:10.339020154283 PMID:32752007

Maghdid, Ghafoor, Sadiq, Curran, & Rabie. (2020). *A Novel AI-Enabled Framework to Diagnose Corona virus Covid 19 Using Smartphone Embedded Sensors: Design study* [Unpublished Manuscript].

Maghdid, H. S., Asaad, A. T., Ghafoor, K. Z., Sadiq, A. S., Mirjalili, S., & Khan, M. K. (2021). Diagnosing COVID-19 pneumonia from X-ray and CT images using deep learning and transfer learning algorithms. Multimodal Image Exploitation and Learning, 11734. doi:10.1117/12.2588672

Mahdavinejad, M. S., Rezvan, M., Barekatain, M., Adibi, P., Barnaghi, P., & Sheth, A. P. (2018). Machine learning for internet of things data analysis: A survey. *Digital Communications and Networks*, *4*(3), 161–175. doi:10.1016/j.dcan.2017.10.002

Mahdi, Miraz, Ali, & Picking. (2018). *Internet of Nano-Things, Things and Everything: Future Growth Trends.* doi:10.3390/fi10080068

Maheshwari, R., Moudgil, K., Parekh, H., & Sawant, R. (2018). A Machine Learning Based Medical Data Analytics and Visualization Research Platform. *2018 International Conference on Current Trends towards Converging Technologies (ICCTCT)*, 1-5. 10.1109/ICCTCT.2018.8550953

Mahmud, S., Iqbal, R., & Doctor, F. (2016). Cloud enabled data analytics and visualization framework for health-shocks prediction. *Future Generation Computer Systems*, *65*, 169–181. doi:10.1016/j.future.2015.10.014

Mallardi, G., & Bellifemine, F. (2017). Telemedicine solutions and services: a new challenge that supports active participation of patients. *i-CiTies 2017 (3rd CINI Annual Conference on ICT for Smart Cities & Communities).*

Manghnani, D. (2021). *Robotics: A Layman's Guide.* https://blogs.systweak.com/robotics-a-laymans-guide/

Marshall, S. (2021). *How AI is Transforming the Future of Healthcare.* https://www.internationalsos.com/client-magazines/in-this-issue-3/how-ai-is-transforming-the-future-of-healthcare

Masud, M., Hossain, M. S., & Alamri, A. (2012). Data Interoperability and Multimedia Content Management in e-Health Systems. *IEEE Transactions on Information Technology in Biomedicine*, *16*(6), 1015–1023. doi:10.1109/TITB.2012.2202244 PMID:22677322

Mathur, N., & Glesk, I. (2016). A practical design and implementation of a low cost platform for remote monitoring of lower limb health of amputees in the developing world. *IEEE Access : Practical Innovations, Open Solutions*, *4*, 7440–7451. doi:10.1109/ACCESS.2016.2622163

Mazlan, A. A., Mohd Daud, S., Mohd Sam, S., Abas, H., Rasid, S. Z. A., & Yusof, M. F. (2020). Scalability challenges in healthcare blockchain system-a systematic review. *IEEE Access: Practical Innovations, Open Solutions*, *8*, 23663–23673. doi:10.1109/ACCESS.2020.2969230

McGee, E. E., Kiblawi, R., Playdon, M. C., & Eliassen, A. H. (2019). Nutritional Metabolomics in Cancer Epidemiology: Current Trends, Challenges, and Future Directions. *Current Nutrition Reports*, *8*(3), 187–201. doi:10.100713668-019-00279-z PMID:31129888

Mckinsey.com. (2020). *Transforming healthcare with AI: The impact on the workforce and organizations.* https://www.mckinsey.com/industries/healthcare-systems-and-services/our-insights/transforming-healthcare-with-ai

Meloni, A., Pegoraro, P. A., Atzori, L., Benigni, A., & Sulis, S. (2018). Cloud-based IoT solution for state estimation in smart grids: Exploiting virtualization and edge-intelligence technologies. *Computer Networks*, *130*, 156–165. doi:10.1016/j.comnet.2017.10.008

Midha, M. K., Wu, M., & Chiu, K.-P. (2019). Long-read sequencing in deciphering human genetics to a greater depth. *Human Genetics*, *138*(11-12), 1201–1215. doi:10.100700439-019-02064-y PMID:31538236

Miller, W. L., & Jaffe, A. S. (2015). Biomarkers in heart failure: The importance of inconvenient details. *ESC Heart Failure*, *3*(1), 3–10. doi:10.1002/ehf2.12071 PMID:27774262

Minihane, A. M., Armah, C. K., Miles, E. A., Madden, J. M., Clark, A. B., Caslake, M. J., Packard, C. J., Kofler, B. M., Lietz, G., Curtis, P. J., Mathers, J. C., Williams, C. M., & Calder, P. C. (2016). Consumption of Fish Oil Providing Amounts of Eicosapentaenoic Acid and Docosahexaenoic Acid That Can Be Obtained from the Diet Reduces Blood Pressure in Adults with Systolic Hypertension: A Retrospective Analysis. *The Journal of Nutrition*, *146*(3), 516–523. doi:10.3945/jn.115.220475 PMID:26817716

Minnie, A. (2019). *AI can reduce mammography screening's workload.* https://www.auntminnie.com/index.aspx?sec=sup&sub=aic&pag=dis&ItemID=124880

Miraz, M. H., & Picking, R. (2015). *A review on internet of things (IoT), internet of everything (IoE) and internet of nano things (IoNT). In 2015 Internet Technologies and Applications.* ITA. doi:10.1109/ITechA.2015.7317398

Modgil, S. (2009). Reasoning about preferences in argumentation frameworks. *Artificial Intelligence*, *173*(9), 901–934. doi:10.1016/j.artint.2009.02.001

Moghadas, E., Rezazadeh, J., & Farahbakhsh, R. (2020). An IoT patient monitoring based on fog computing and data mining: Cardiac arrhythmia usecase. *Internet of Things*, *11*, 100251. doi:10.1016/j.iot.2020.100251

Moreno-Cano, V., Terroso-Saenz, F., & Skarmeta-Gómez, A. F. (2015). Big data for IoT services in smart cities. In *Internet of Things (WF-IoT) IEEE 2nd World Forum on.* IEEE. 10.1109/WF-IoT.2015.7389091

Morgan, P. (2020). Blockchain technology: Principles and applications in medical imaging. *Journal of Digital Imaging*, *33*(3), 726–734. doi:10.100710278-019-00310-3 PMID:31898037

Mostafavi, S. A. (2019). Edge Computing for IoT: Challenges and Solutions. *Journal of Communications Technology, Electronics and Computer Science*, (26), 4–8.

Motilal, Tayade, & Karandikar. (2013). Role of Data Mining Techniques in Healthcare sector in India. *Scholars Journal of Applied Medical Sciences.*

Mufareh, A. (2021). *Artificial Intelligence Technology Benefits.* https://yourstory.com/mystory/artificial-intelligence-technology-benefits

Muhammad, G., Hossain, M. S., & Kumar, N. (2021, February). EEG-Based Pathology Detection for Home Health Monitoring. *IEEE Journal on Selected Areas in Communications*, *39*(2), 603–610. Advance online publication. doi:10.1109/JSAC.2020.3020654

Muhammad, M. (2011). Formant analysis in dysphonic patients and automatic Arabic digit speech recognition. *Biomedical Engineering.* PMID:21624137

Mujawar, S., & Joshi, A. (2015). Data Analytics Types, Tools and their Comparison. *International Journal of Advanced Research in Computer and Communication Engineering, 4*(2). Advance online publication. doi:10.17148/IJARCCE.2015.42110

Munna, Islam, Hoque, & Bhattacharya. (2015). *A Study on Water Quality Parameters of Water Supply in Sylhet City Corporation Area.* Science Publishing Group.

Munoz, R., Vilalta, R., Yoshikane, N., Casellas, R., Martinez, R., Tsuritani, T., & Morita, I. (2018). Integration of IoT, Transport SDN, and Edge/Cloud Computing for Dynamic Distribution of IoT Analytics and Efficient Use of Network Resources. *Journal of Lightwave Technology, 36*(7), 1420–1428. doi:10.1109/JLT.2018.2800660

Musacchio, N., Giancaterini, A., Guaita, G., Ozzello, A., Pellegrini, M. A., Ponzani, P., Russo, G. T., Zilich, R., & de Micheli, A. (2020). Artificial Intelligence and Big Data in Diabetes Care: A Position Statement of the Italian Association of Medical Diabetologists. *Journal of Medical Internet Research, 22*(6), e16922. doi:10.2196/16922 PMID:32568088

Myint, C. Z., Gopal, L., & Aung, Y. L. (2017), Reconfigurable Smart Water Quality Monitoring System in IoT Environment. *IEEE International Conference on Information Systems (ICIS).*

Myung, S.-K. (2012). Efficacy of Omega-3 Fatty Acid Supplements (Eicosapentaenoic Acid and Docosahexaenoic Acid) in the Secondary Prevention of Cardiovascular Disease. *Archives of Internal Medicine, 172*(9), 686. doi:10.1001/archinternmed.2012.262 PMID:22493407

Nakamoto, S. (2008). *Bitcoin: A peer to peer electronic cash system.* Academic Press.

Namiot. (2016). On Internet of Things and Smart Cities educational courses. *International Journal of Open Information Technologies, 4* (5), 26-38.

Nandyala, C. S., & Kim, H. K. (2016). From cloud to fog and iot-based real-time u-healthcare monitoring for smart homes and hospitals. *International Journal of Smart Home, 10*(2), 187–196. doi:10.14257/ijsh.2016.10.2.18

Narvekar, Menezes, Angle, Lotlekar, Naik, & Purohit. (n.d.). *Students Performance Prediction using Data Mining Techniques.* Academic Press.

Nasrullah, P. (n.d.). *Peerbits.* Retrieved from https://www.peerbits.com/blog/internet-of-things-healthcare-applications-benefits-and-challenges.html

Nasser, N., Ali, A., Karim, L., & Belhaouari, S. (2013), An Efficient Wireless Sensor Network-based Water Quality Monitoring System. *Proceedings of the 2013 ACS International Conference on Computer Systems and Applications (AICCSA'13).*

Naz, H., & Ahuja, S. (2020). Deep learning approach for diabetes prediction using PIMA Indian dataset. *Journal of Diabetes and Metabolic Disorders, 19*(1), 391–403. doi:10.100740200-020-00520-5 PMID:32550190

Neelima, A., Amit, K. B., & Mangamoori, L. N. (2020). The role of artificial intelligence in tackling COVID-19. *Future Virology, 15*(11), 717–724. Advance online publication. doi:10.2217/fvl-2020-0130

Nguyen, T. T., Waurn, G., & Campus, P. (2021). *Artificial intelligence in the battle against corona virus (COVID-19): A survey and future research directions.* https://www.thepeninsula.org.in/2020/04/28/artificial-intelligence-in-the-battle-against-coronavirus-covid-19-a-survey-and-future-research-directions/

Nguyen, Q. H., Muthuraman, R., Singh, L., Sen, G., Tran, A. C., Nguyen, B. P., & Chua, M. (2020). Diabetic retinopathy detection using deep learning. *Proceedings of the 4th International Conference on Machine Learning and Soft Computing*, 103-107. 10.1145/3380688.3380709

Nicolae, A., Morton, G., Chung, H., Loblaw, A., Jain, S., Mitchell, D., Lu, L., Helou, J., Al-Hanaqta, M., Heath, E., & Ravi, A. (2017). Evaluation of a Machine-Learning Algorithm for Treatment Planning in Prostate Low-Dose-Rate Brachytherapy. *International Journal of Radiation Oncology, Biology, Physics*, *97*(4), 822–829. doi:10.1016/j.ijrobp.2016.11.036 PMID:28244419

Nigam & Bhatia. (2016). Impact of Cloud Computing on Health Care. *International Research Journal of Engineering and Technology, 3*(5).

Noecker, C., & Borenstein, E. (2016). Getting Personal About Nutrition. *Trends in Molecular Medicine*, *22*(2), 83–85. doi:10.1016/j.molmed.2015.12.010 PMID:26776092

O'herrin, J. K., Fost, N., & Kudsk, K. A. (2004). Health Insurance Portability Accountability Act (HIPAA) regulations: Effect on medical record research. *Annals of Surgery*, *239*(6), 772–778. doi:10.1097/01.sla.0000128307.98274.dc PMID:15166956

Ogundele, I.O., Popoola, O.L., Oyesola, O.O., & Orija, K.T. (2018). A Review on Data Mining in Healthcare. *International Journal of Advanced Research in Computer Engineering & Technology, 7*(9).

Ohlhorst, S. D., Russell, R., Bier, D., Klurfeld, D. M., Li, Z., Mein, J. R., Milner, J., Ross, A. C., Stover, P., & Konopka, E. (2013). Nutrition research to affect food and a healthy lifespan. *Advances in Nutrition*, *4*(5), 579–584. doi:10.3945/an.113.004176 PMID:24038264

Oikonomopoulos, S., Bayega, A., Fahiminiya, S., Djambazian, H., Berube, P., & Ragoussis, J. (2020). Methodologies for Transcript Profiling Using Long-Read Technologies. *Frontiers in Genetics*, *11*, 606. Advance online publication. doi:10.3389/fgene.2020.00606 PMID:32733532

Olivia Li, J.-P., Liu, H., Ting, D. S. J., Jeon, S., & Chan, R. V. P., Kim, J. E., Sim, D. A., Thomas, P. B. M., Lin, H., Chen, Y., Sakomoto, T., Loewenstein, A., Lam, D. S. C., Pasquale, L. R., Wong, T. Y., Lam, L. A., & Ting, D. S. W. (2020). Digital technology, tele-medicine and artificial intelligence in ophthalmology: A global perspective. *Progress in Retinal and Eye Research, 100900*. Advance online publication. doi:10.1016/j.preteyeres.2020.100900

Ordovas, J. M., Ferguson, L. R., Tai, E. S., & Mathers, J. C. (2018). Personalised nutrition and health. *BMJ*, k2173. doi:10.1136/bmj.k2173

Özdemir, V., & Kolker, E. (2016). Precision Nutrition 4.0: A Big Data and Ethics Foresight Analysis—Convergence of Agrigenomics, Nutrigenomics, Nutriproteomics, and Nutrimetabolomics. *OMICS: A Journal of Integrative Biology*, *20*(2), 69–75. doi:10.1089/omi.2015.0193 PMID:26785082

Paganelli, A. I., Velmovitsky, P. E., Miranda, P., Branco, A., Alencar, P., Cowan, D., Endler, M., & Morita, P. P. (2021). A conceptual IoT-based early-warning architecture for remote monitoring of COVID-19 patients in wards and at home. *Internet of Things*, *100399*, 100399. Advance online publication. doi:10.1016/j.iot.2021.100399

Palou, M., Torrens, J. M., Castillo, P., Sánchez, J., Palou, A., & Picó, C. (2019). Metabolomic approach in milk from calorie-restricted rats during lactation: A potential link to the programming of a healthy phenotype in offspring. *European Journal of Nutrition*, *59*(3), 1191–1204. doi:10.100700394-019-01979-6 PMID:31069458

Panarello, A., & Puliafito, A. (2018). Blockchain and IoT integration: A systematic survey. *Sensors (Basel)*, *18*(8), 2575. doi:10.339018082575 PMID:30082633

Pandey, P. (2018). *Building a Simple Chatbot from Scratch in Python (Using NLTK)*. https://medium.com/analytics-vidhya/building-a-simple-chatbot-in-python-using-nltk-7c8c8215ac6e

Pandian, M. S. (2020). Impact of new agriculture technology in prediction of modern robotic system. *Dogo Rangsang Research Journal, 10*(06), 85–94.

Patel & Patel. (2016). Survey Of Data Mining Techniques Used In Healthcare Domain. *International Journal of Information Sciences and Techniques, 6.*

Patil. (2015). Survey Of Data Mining Techniques In Healthcare. *International Research Journal of Innovative Engineering, 1*(9).

Patra, R., & khuntia, B. (2021). Analysis and Prediction Of Pima Indian Diabetes Dataset Using SDKNN Classifier Technique. *IOP Conference Series. Materials Science and Engineering, 1070*(1), 012059. doi:10.1088/1757-899X/1070/1/012059

Peng, W., Gao, W., & Liu, J. (2019). AI-enabled Massive Devices Multiple Access for Smart City. *IEEE Internet of Things Journal, 6*(5), 1–1. doi:10.1109/JIOT.2019.2902448

Picó, C., Serra, F., Rodríguez, A. M., Keiper, J., & Palou, A. (2019). Biomarkers of Nutrition and Health: New Tools for New Approaches. *Nutrients, 11*(5), 1092. doi:10.3390/nu11051092 PMID:31100942

Pirouz, B., Shaffiee Haghshenas, S., & Piro, P. (2020). Investigating a Serious Challenge in the Sustainable Development Process: Analysis of Confirmed Cases of COVID-19 (New Type of Corona Virus) through a Binary Classification Using Artificial Intelligence and Regression Analysis. *Sustainability, 12*(6), 24–27. doi:10.3390u12062427

Ponnusamy, V., Coumaran, A., Shunmugam, A. S., Rajaram, K., & Senthilvelavan, S. (2020, July). Smart Glass: Real-Time Leaf Disease Detection using YOLO Transfer Learning. In *2020 International Conference on Communication and Signal Processing (ICCSP)* (pp. 1150-1154). IEEE. 10.1109/ICCSP48568.2020.9182146

Ponnusamy, V., & Malarvihi, S. (2017). Hardware impairment detection and prewhitening on MIMO precoder for spectrum sharing. *Wireless Personal Communications, 96*(1), 1557–1576. doi:10.100711277-017-4256-6

Porambage, P., Okwuibe, J., Liyanage, M., Ylianttila, M., & Taleb, T. (2018). Survey on multi-access edge computing for internet of things realization. *IEEE Communications Surveys and Tutorials, 20*(4), 2961–2991. doi:10.1109/COMST.2018.2849509

Porwal, P., Pachade, S., Kamble, R., Kokare, M., Deshmukh, G., Sahasrabuddhe, V., & Meriaudeau, F. (2018). Indian diabetic retinopathy image dataset (IDRiD): A database for diabetic retinopathy screening research. *Data, 3*(3), 25. doi:10.3390/data3030025

Potischman, N. (2003). Biologic and Methodologic Issues for Nutritional Biomarkers. *The Journal of Nutrition, 133*(3). doi:10.1093/jn/133.3.875S

Prabhu, P., & Selvabharathi, S. (2019, July 1). *Deep Belief Neural Network Model for Prediction of Diabetes Mellitus.* doi:10.1109/ICISPC.2019.8935838

Pranto, B., Mehnaz, S. M., Momen, S., & Huq, S. M. (2020). Prediction of diabetes using cost sensitive learning and oversampling techniques on Bangladeshi and Indian female patients. In *2020 5th International Conference on Information Technology Research (ICITR)* (pp. 1-6). IEEE. 10.1109/ICITR51448.2020.9310892

Price, N. (2019). *Risks and Remedies For Artificial Intelligence In Health Care.* https://www.brookings.edu/research/risks-and-remedies-for-artificial-intelligence-in-health-care/

Pundir, M., Sharma, M., & Singh, Y. (2016). IJARCCE Internet of Things (IoT): Challenges and Future Directions. *International Journal of Advanced Research in Computer and Communication Engineering, 5.* Advance online publication. doi:10.17148/IJARCCE.2016.53226

Queralta, J. P., & Westerlund, T. (2019). Edge-AI in lorabased health monitoring: Fall detection system with fog computing and LSTM recurrent neural networks. In *2019 42nd International Conference on Telecommunications and Signal Processing (TSP)*. IEEE.

R. S. H., I., S, H., N. Y., P., & A, S. (2011). The potential of Internet of m-health Things "m-IoT" for non-invasive glucose level sensing. *Annu Int Conf IEEE Eng Med Biol Soc.*

Raden, N. (2020). *Digital twins for personalized medicine - a critical assessment.* Diginomica. Retrieved from https://diginomica.com/digital-twins-personalized-medicine-critical-assessment

Rahmani, A. M., & Liljeberg, P. (2018). Exploiting smart e-health gateways at the edge of healthcare internetof-things: A fog computing approach. *Future Generation Computer Systems, 78*, 641–658. doi:10.1016/j.future.2017.02.014

Raiten, D. J., Namasté, S., Brabin, B., Combs, G., L'Abbe, M. R., Wasantwisut, E., & Darnton-Hill, I. (2011). Executive summary—Biomarkers of Nutrition for Development: Building a Consensus. *The American Journal of Clinical Nutrition, 94*(2). doi:10.3945/ajcn.110.008227

Raja Singh, R., Yash, S. M., Shubham, S. C., Indragandhi, V., Vijayakumar, V., Saravanan, P., & Subhramaniya, S. (2020). IoT embedded cloud-based intelligent power quality monitoring system for industrial drive application. *Future Generation Computer Systems, 112*, 884–898. doi:10.1016/j.future.2020.06.032

Rajeswari, S. V. K. R., & Vijayakumar, P. (2021). Prediction of Diabetes Mellitus Using Machine Learning Algorithm. *Annals of the Romanian Society for Cell Biology*, 5655–5662. https://www.annalsofrscb.ro/index.php/journal/article/view/6653

Rajkamal. (2017). *Internet of Things: Architecture and Design Principles.* Chennai: McGraw-Hill Education.

Rajkomar, A., Dean, J., & Kohane, I. (2019). Machine Learning in Medicine. *The New England Journal of Medicine, 380*(14), 1347–1358. doi:10.1056/NEJMra1814259 PMID:30943338

Ram, S. S., & Shiratori. (2019). A machine learning framework for edge computing to improve prediction accuracy in mobile health monitoring. In *International Conference on Computational Science and Its Applications.* Springer. 10.1007/978-3-030-24302-9_30

Ramesh, S., & Perros, H. G. (2000). A multilayer client-server queueing network model with synchronous and asynchronous messages. *IEEE Transactions on Software Engineering, 26*(11), 1086–1100. doi:10.1109/32.881719

Ramos-Lopez, O., Milagro, F. I., Allayee, H., Chmurzynska, A., Choi, M. S., Curi, R., De Caterina, R., Ferguson, L. R., Goni, L., Kang, J. X., Kohlmeier, M., Marti, A., Moreno, L. A., Pérusse, L., Prasad, C., Qi, L., Reifen, R., Riezu-Boj, J. I., San-Cristobal, R., ... Martínez, J. A. (2017). Guide for Current Nutrigenetic, Nutrigenomic, and Nutriepigenetic Approaches for Precision Nutrition Involving the Prevention and Management of Chronic Diseases Associated with Obesity. *Journal of Nutrigenetics and Nutrigenomics, 10*(1-2), 43–62. doi:10.1159/000477729 PMID:28689206

Rathee, P. (2020). Introduction to blockchain and IoT. *Studies in Big Data*, 1–14.

Raval, S. (2016). *Decentralized applications: Harnessing Bitcoin's Blockchain technology.* O'Reilly Media, Inc.

Ray, R. (2018). Advances in Data Mining: Healthcare Applications. *International Research Journal of Engineering and Technology, 5*(3).

Ray, P. P., Dash, D., Salah, K., & Kumar, N. (2020). Blockchain for IoT-based healthcare: Background, consensus, platforms, and use cases. *IEEE Systems Journal.*

Reale, A. (2017). *A guide to Edge IoT analytics.* White paper. https://www.ibm.com/blogs/internet-of-things/edge-iot-analytics/

Recio-Rodriguez, J. I., Rodriguez-Martin, C., Gonzalez-Sanchez, J., Rodriguez-Sanchez, E., Martin-Borras, C., Martínez-Vizcaino, V., Arietaleanizbeaskoa, M. S., Magdalena-Gonzalez, O., Fernandez-Alonso, C., Maderuelo-Fernandez, J. A., Gomez-Marcos, M. A., Garcia-Ortiz, L., & Investigators, E. (2019). EVIDENT Smartphone App, a New Method for the Dietary Record: Comparison with a Food Frequency Questionnaire. *JMIR mHealth and uHealth, 7*(2), e11463. doi:10.2196/11463 PMID:30735141

Reddy, S. (2018). *Use of Artificial Intelligence in Healthcare Delivery, eHealth - Making Health Care Smarter.* https://www.intechopen.com/chapters/60562

Reddy, S., Fox, J., & Purohit, M. P. (2019). Artificial Intelligence-Enabled Healthcare Delivery. *Journal of the Royal Society of Medicine, 112*(1), 22–28. doi:10.1177/0141076818815510 PMID:30507284

Reports, V. (n.d.). *Streaming Analytics Market is Projected to Reach USD 52,190.0 Million by 2027 at CAGR 26.8% | Valuates Reports.* Retrieved October 14, 2021, from www.prnewswire.com website: https://www.prnewswire.com/news-releases/streaming-analytics-market-is-projected-to-reach-usd-52-190-0-million-by-2027-at-cagr-26-8--valuates-reports-301287553.html

Reyna, A., Martín, C., Chen, J., Soler, E., & Diaz, M. (2018). On blockchain and its integration with IoT. Challenges and opportunities. *Future Generation Computer Systems, 88*, 173–190. doi:10.1016/j.future.2018.05.046

Rhyner, D., Loher, H., Dehais, J., Anthimopoulos, M., Shevchik, S., Botwey, R. H., Duke, D., Stettler, C., Diem, P., & Mougiakakou, S. (2016). Carbohydrate Estimation by a Mobile Phone-Based System Versus Self-Estimations of Individuals with Type 1 Diabetes Mellitus: A Comparative Study. *Journal of Medical Internet Research, 18*(5), e101. doi:10.2196/jmir.5567 PMID:27170498

Ridhawi, I., Aloqaily, M., & Jararweh, Y. (2020). *An incentive-based mechanism for volunteer computing using blockchain.* Academic Press.

Roehrs, A., Da Costa, C. A., & Da Rosa Righi, R. (2017). OmniPHR: A distributed architecture model to integrate personal health records. *Journal of Biomedical Informatics, 71*, 70–81. doi:10.1016/j.jbi.2017.05.012 PMID:28545835

Rojas-Fernandez, C. H., & Tyber, K. (2016). Benefits, Potential Harms, and Optimal Use of Nutritional Supplementation for Preventing Progression of Age-Related Macular Degeneration. *The Annals of Pharmacotherapy, 51*(3), 264–270. doi:10.1177/1060028016680643 PMID:27866147

Rong, G., Mendez, A., Bou Assi, E., Zhao, B., & Sawan, M. (2020). Artificial Intelligence in Healthcare: Review and Prediction Case Studies. Engineering, 6(3), 291-301.

Ruchi. (2021). https://www.kaggle.com/ruchi798/siim-covid-19-detection-eda-data-augmentation

Rupasinghe, T., Burstein, F., Rudolph, C., & Strange, S. (2019). Towards a blockchain based fall prediction model for aged care. *Proceedings of the Australasian Computer Science Week Multiconference*, 1–10, 10.1145/3290688.3290736

S, S., P, S., & M, S. (2018). IoT based measurement of body temperature using MAX30205. *International Research Journal of Engineering and Technology*, 3913-3915.

Sadiku, Kelechi, Sarhan, & Musa Roy. (2018). Wireless Sensor Networks for Healthcare. *Perry College of Engineering, Prairie View A&M University, Journal of Scientific and Engineering Research, 5*(7), 210-213.

Sadoughi, F., Behmanesh, A., & Sayfouri, N. (2020). Internet of things in medicine: A systematic mapping study. *Journal of Biomedical Informatics, 103*, 103383. doi:10.1016/j.jbi.2020.103383 PMID:32044417

Sak, J., & Suchodolska, M. (2021). Artificial Intelligence in Nutrients Science Research: A Review. *Nutrients, 13*(2), 322. doi:10.3390/nu13020322 PMID:33499405

Salam, H., & Moussa, A. (2020). Edge-Computing Architectures for Internet of Things Applications: A Survey. *Sensors (Basel), 1*(20), 1–52.

Santhoshkumar. (2021). https://www.kaggle.com/santhoshkumarv/covid19indiadata

Sarda, S., & Hannenhalli, S. (2014). Next-Generation Sequencing and Epigenomics Research: A Hammer in Search of Nails. *Genomics & Informatics, 12*(1), 2. doi:10.5808/GI.2014.12.1.2 PMID:24748856

Sarkar, T. (2020). *AI and machine learning for healthcare article.* https://towardsdatascience.com/ai-and-machine-learning-for-healthcare-7a70fb3acb67

Satija, U., & Manikandan, M. S. (2017). Real-time signal qualityaware ECG telemetry system for IoT-based health care monitoring. *IEEE Internet of Things Journal, 4*(3), 815–823. doi:10.1109/JIOT.2017.2670022

Scholes, S. (2016). Politics, Business, Technology, and the Arts. *Slate Magazine.* http://www.slate.com

Sciarrone, A., Bisio, I., Garibotto, C., Lavagetto, F., Staude, G. H., & Knopp, A. (2021). Leveraging IoT Wearable Technology Towards Early Diagnosis of Neurological Diseases. *IEEE Journal on Selected Areas in Communications, 39*(2), 582–592. doi:10.1109/JSAC.2020.3021573

Sengupta, R. (2021). *PM Modi to Address the Nation Again Tonight amid the Corona Virus Crisis.* https://yourstory.com/2020/03/pm-modi-address-tonight-coronavirus-crisis?utm_pageloadtype=scroll

Shailaja, K., Seetharamulu, B., & Jabbar, M. A. (2018). Machine Learning in Healthcare: A Review. *2018 Second International Conference on Electronics, Communication and Aerospace Technology (ICECA),* 910-914. 10.1109/ICECA.2018.8474918

Sha, K., Yang, T. A., Wei, W., & Davari, S. (2020). A survey of edge computing-based designs for IoT security. *Digital Communications and Networks, 6*(2), 195–202. doi:10.1016/j.dcan.2019.08.006

Shaown, T., Hasan, I., Mim, M. R., & Hossain, S. (2019). *1st International Conference on Advances in Science, Engineering and Robotics Technology (ICASERT).* Academic Press.

Sharma, Pawbake, Patel, & Potdar. (2018). Water Quality Monitoring System Using IOT. *International Journal of Advance Research and Innovative Ideas in Education, 4*(5). doi:10.1109/ICCPCT.2015.7159459

Shima, H., Masuda, S., Date, Y., Shino, A., Tsuboi, Y., Kajikawa, M., Inoue, Y., Kanamoto, T., & Kikuchi, J. (2017). Exploring the Impact of Food on the Gut Ecosystem Based on the Combination of Machine Learning and Network Visualization. *Nutrients, 9*(12), 1307. doi:10.3390/nu9121307 PMID:29194366

Shi, W., Cao, J., Zhang, Q., Li, Y., & Xu, L. (2016). Edge Computing: Vision and Challenges. *IEEE Internet of Things Journal, 3*(no. 5), 637–646. doi:10.1109/JIOT.2016.2579198

Shugalo, I. (2019, April 29). *Digital Twin Technology: Should Healthcare Jump on the Bandwagon?* https://hitconsultant.net/2019/04/29/digital-twin-technology-should-healthcare-jump-on-the-bandwagon/#.Xsy9OGj7RPZ

Singh, H. (2021). *The Impact of Artificial Intelligence in Healthcare 2020.* https://blogs.systweak.com/the-impact-of-artificial-intelligence-in-healthcare/

Singh, A. (2020). Tools for metabolomics. *Nature Methods, 17*(1), 24–24. doi:10.103841592-019-0710-6 PMID:31907484

Slatko, B. E., Gardner, A. F., & Ausubel, F. M. (2018). Overview of Next-Generation Sequencing Technologies. *Current Protocols in Molecular Biology, 122*(1), e59. doi:10.1002/cpmb.59 PMID:29851291

Somasundaram, S. K., & Alli, P. (2017). A machine learning ensemble classifier for early prediction of diabetic retinopathy. *Journal of Medical Systems, 41*(12), 201. doi:10.100710916-017-0853-x PMID:29124453

Sperandei, S. (2014). Understanding logistic regression analysis. *Biochemia Medica, 24*(1), 12–18. doi:10.11613/BM.2014.003 PMID:24627710

Stagnaro, C. (2017). *White paper: Innovative blockchain uses in health care*. Freed Associates.

Stefanini. (2020). *The Usage of AI in Pharma Has Been Relatively Slow; However, Unknown to Many, It Offers Immense Benefits*. https://stefanini.com/en/trends/news/a-guide-to-ai-in-the-pharmaceutical-industry

Steinhubl, S. R., Muse, E. D., Barrett, P. M., & Topol, E. J. (2016). Off the cuff: Rebooting blood pressure treatment. *Lancet, 388*(10046), 749. doi:10.1016/S0140-6736(16)31348-4 PMID:27560266

Sudalairajkumar. (2021). https://www.kaggle.com/sudalairajkumar/covid19-in-india?select=covid_19_india.csv

Sun, M., Fernstrom, J. D., Jia, W., Hackworth, S. A., Yao, N., Li, Y., Li, C., Fernstrom, M. H., & Sclabassi, R. J. (2010). A Wearable Electronic System for Objective Dietary Assessment. *Journal of the American Dietetic Association, 110*(1), 45–47. doi:10.1016/j.jada.2009.10.013 PMID:20102825

Swayam Siddha, S., & Mohanty, C. (2020). Application of cognitive Internet of Medical Things for COVID-19 pandemic. *Diabetes & Metabolic Syndrome, 8*. Advance online publication. doi:10.1016/j.dsx.2020.06.014.8

Szablewski, L., & Sulima, A. (2017). The structural and functional changes of blood cells and molecular components in diabetes mellitus. *Biological Chemistry, 398*(4), 411–423. doi:10.1515/hsz-2016-0196 PMID:27768581

Tachibana, C. (2015). Transcriptomics today: Microarrays, RNA-seq, and more. *Science, 349*(6247), 544–546. doi:10.1126cience.349.6247.544

Tang, W., & Shen, X. S. (2019). Fogenabled smart health: Toward cooperative and secure healthcare service provision. *IEEE Communications Magazine, 57*(5), 42–48. doi:10.1109/MCOM.2019.1800234

Tawalbeh, L. A., Mehmood, R., Benkhlifa, E., & Song, H. (2016). Mobile Cloud Computing Model and Big Data Analysis for Healthcare Applications. *IEEE Access: Practical Innovations, Open Solutions, 4*, 6171–6180. doi:10.1109/ACCESS.2016.2613278

Telenti, A., Pierce, L. C. T., Biggs, W. H., di Iulio, J., Wong, E. H. M., Fabani, M. M., Kirkness, E. F., Moustafa, A., Shah, N., Xie, C., Brewerton, S. C., Bulsara, N., Garner, C., Metzker, G., Sandoval, E., Perkins, B. A., Och, F. J., Turpaz, Y., & Venter, J. C. (2016). Deep sequencing of 10,000 human genomes. *Proceedings of the National Academy of Sciences of the United States of America, 113*(42), 11901–11906. doi:10.1073/pnas.1613365113 PMID:27702888

The Economic Times. (2021). *Can your Fitbit or Apple Watch detect corona virus infection early?* https://economictimes.indiatimes.com/tech/can-your-fitbit-or-apple-watch-detect-coronavirus-infection-early/tech-wearables-in-the-fight/slideshow/76319430.cms

Thinxtream's White Paper. (2018). *IoT Edge Analytics & Machine Learning for Real-time Device Control*. https://www.thinxtream.com/whitepapers/thinxtream-iot-edge-analytics-machine-learning-real-time-device-control-wp-003.pdf

Thompson, F. E., Subar, A. F., Loria, C. M., Reedy, J. L., & Baranowski, T. (2010). Need for Technological Innovation in Dietary Assessment. *Journal of the American Dietetic Association, 110*(1), 48–51. doi:10.1016/j.jada.2009.10.008 PMID:20102826

TI. (n.d.). https://www.ti.com/tool/CC3200-LAUNCHXL

Townsend & Term. (2001). Article. *Medical Electronics*, 48-54.

Truong, H-L. (2018). *Enabling Edge Analytics of IoT Data: The Case of LoRaWAN*. doi:10.1109/GIOTS.2018.8534429

Udgata, S. K., & Suryadevara, N. K. (2021). *COVID-19, Sensors, and Internet of Medical Things (IoMT), Internet of Things and Sensor Network for COVID-19*. Springer Nature Singapore Pte Ltd. doi:10.1007/978-981-15-7654-6

Upendra. (2020). *Artificial Intelligence in Healthcare: Top Benefits, Risks and Challenges*. https://www.tristatetechnology.com/blog/artificial-intelligence-in-healthcare-top-benefits-risks-and-challenges/

Vaishya, R., Javaid, M., Khan, I. H., & Haleemb, A. (2020). Artificial Intelligence (AI) applications for COVID-19 pandemic. *Diabetes & Metabolic Syndrome, 14*(4), 337–339. doi:10.1016/j.dsx.2020.04.012 PMID:32305024

van Dijk, E. L., Jaszczyszyn, Y., Naquin, D., & Thermes, C. (2018). The Third Revolution in Sequencing Technology. *Trends in Genetics, 34*(9), 666–681. doi:10.1016/j.tig.2018.05.008 PMID:29941292

Varshney, R. (2021). *Coronavirus: This IIT-Delhi alumni startup develops camera to detect face masks, social distancing in crowded places*. https://yourstory.com/2020/05/coronavirus-iit-delhi-alumni-camera-face-masks-social-distancing

Vasiloglou, M., Mougiakakou, S., Aubry, E., Bokelmann, A., Fricker, R., Gomes, F., Guntermann, C., Meyer, A., Studerus, D., & Stanga, Z. (2018). A Comparative Study on Carbohydrate Estimation: GoCARB vs. Dietitians. *Nutrients, 10*(6), 741. doi:10.3390/nu10060741 PMID:29880772

Verma, S., & Kato, N. (2017). A survey on network methodologies for real-time analytics of massive IoT data and open research issues. *IEEE Commun. Surveys Tuts., 19*(3), 1457–1477. doi:10.1109/COMST.2017.2694469

Vijayakumar, N., & Ramya, R. (2015). The real time monitoring of water quality in IoT environment. *International Conference on Circuits, Power and Computing Technologies.*

Vishnu, S., Jino Ramson, S. R., & Jegan, R. (2020). Internet of medical things (IoMT)- Overview. *5th International Conference on Devices, Circuits and Systems (ICDCS).*

Vollmer & Bohner. (2020). *Machine learning and artificial intelligence research for patient benefit: 20 critical questions on transparency, replicability, ethics, and effectiveness*. doi:10.1136/bmj.l6927

Walter, M. (2019). *6 Serious Risks Associated With AI in Healthcare*. https://www.aiin.healthcare/topics/diagnostics/6-risks-ai-healthcare-artificial-intelligence

Wang, D. D., & Hu, F. B. (2018). Precision nutrition for prevention and management of type 2 diabetes. *The Lancet. Diabetes & Endocrinology, 6*(5), 416–426. doi:10.1016/S2213-8587(18)30037-8 PMID:29433995

Wang, J., Chen, W., Wang, L., Ren, Y., & Simon Sherratt, R. (2020). Blockchain-based data storage mechanism for industrial internet of things. *Intelligent Automation & Soft Computing, 26*(5), 1157–1172. doi:10.32604/iasc.2020.012174

Wang, Q., Zhu, F., Ji, S., & Ren, Y. (2020). Secure provenance of electronic records based on blockchain. *Computers, Materials & Continua, 65*(2), 1753–1769. doi:10.32604/cmc.2020.07366

Weber, R. H. (2010). Internet of things-new security and privacy challenges. *Computer Law & Security Review, 26*(1), 23–30. doi:10.1016/j.clsr.2009.11.008

Wei, J., & Xu, C.-Z. (2006). eQoS: Provisioning of Client-Perceived End-to-End QoS Guarantees in Web Servers. *IEEE Transactions on Computers, 55*(12), 1543–1556. doi:10.1109/TC.2006.197

Wilson, T. (2020). *No longer Science Fiction, AI and Robotics Are Transforming Healthcare*. https://www.pwc.com/gx/en/industries/healthcare/publications/ai-robotics-new-health/transforming-healthcare.html

Woldaregay, A. Z., Årsand, E., Botsis, T., Albers, D., Mamykina, L., & Hartvigsen, G. (2019). Data-Driven Blood Glucose Pattern Classification and Anomalies Detection: Machine-Learning Applications in Type 1 Diabetes. *Journal of Medical Internet Research, 21*(5), e11030. doi:10.2196/11030 PMID:31042157

Woldaregay, A. Z., Årsand, E., Walderhaug, S., Albers, D., Mamykina, L., Botsis, T., & Hartvigsen, G. (2019). Data-driven modelling and prediction of blood glucose dynamics: Machine learning applications in type 1 diabetes. *Artificial Intelligence in Medicine, 98*, 109–134. doi:10.1016/j.artmed.2019.07.007 PMID:31383477

Wolever, T. M. S. (2016). Personalized nutrition by prediction of glycaemic responses: Fact or fantasy? *European Journal of Clinical Nutrition, 70*(4), 411–413. doi:10.1038/ejcn.2016.31 PMID:27050901

Wood, G. (2014). *Ethereum: A secure decentralized generalized transaction ledger*. Academic Press.

Wu, C., Buyya, R., & Ramamohanarao, K. (2016). *Big Data Analytics = Machine Learning + Cloud Computing*. doi:10.1016/B978-0-12-805394-2.00001-5

Wu, T., Wu, F., Qiu, C., Redoute, J.-M., & Yuce, M. R. (2020). A Rigid-Flex Wearable Health Monitoring Sensor Patch for IoT-Connected Healthcare Applications. *IEEE Internet of Things Journal, 7*(8), 1–1. doi:10.1109/JIOT.2020.2977164

Xavier Olleros, F. (2016). Blockchain technology: Principles and applications. *Research Handbook on Digital Transformations*, 225.

Xia, Q., Sifah, E. B., Asamoah, K. O., Gao, J., Du, X., & Guizani, M. (2017). MeDShare: Trust-less medical data sharing among cloud service providers via blockchain. *IEEE Access: Practical Innovations, Open Solutions, 5*, 14757–14767. doi:10.1109/ACCESS.2017.2730843

Xie, J. (2019). A survey of blockchain technology applied to smart cities: Research issues and challenges. *IEEE Commun. Surveys Tuts., 21*(3), 2794–2830.

Xu, X., Huang, S., Feagan, L., Chen, Y., Qiu, Y., & Wa, Y. (2017). EAaaS: Edge Analytics as a Service. *IEEE International Conference on Web Services (ICWS)*. 10.1109/ICWS.2017.130

Yang, C., Ambayo, H., De Baets, B., Kolsteren, P., Thanintorn, N., Hawwash, D., Bouwman, J., Bronselaer, A., Pattyn, F., & Lachat, C. (2019). An Ontology to Standardize Research Output of Nutritional Epidemiology: From Paper-Based Standards to Linked Content. *Nutrients, 11*(6), 1300. doi:10.3390/nu11061300 PMID:31181762

Yang, X., Wang, X., Li, X., Gu, D., Li, C., & Li, K. (2020). Exploring emerging IoT technologies in smart health research: A knowledge graph analysis. *BMC Medical Informatics and Decision Making, 20*(1), 260. doi:10.118612911-020-01278-9 PMID:33032598

Youbi, A. (2020). *Diabetic retinopathy detection through deep learning techniques: A review*. Informatics in Medicine Unlocked.

Yu, D.-J., Hu, J., Yan, H., Yang, X.-B., Yang, J.-Y., & Shen, H.-B. (2014). Enhancing protein-vitamin binding residues prediction by multiple heterogeneous subspace SVMs ensemble. *BMC Bioinformatics, 15*(1), 297. Advance online publication. doi:10.1186/1471-2105-15-297 PMID:25189131

Yue, X., Wing, H., Jin, D., Li, M., & Jiang, W. (2016). Healthcare data gateways: Found healthcare intelligence on blockchain with novel privacy risk control. *Journal of Medical Systems, 40*(10), 218. doi:10.100710916-016-0574-6 PMID:27565509

Zanella, A., Bui, N., Castellani, A., Vangelista, L., & Zorgi, M. (2014). Internet of things for smart cities. *IEEE IoT-Journal*, *1*(1), 22–32.

Zeevi, D., Korem, T., Zmora, N., Israeli, D., Rothschild, D., Weinberger, A., Ben-Yacov, O., Lador, D., Avnit-Sagi, T., Lotan-Pompan, M., Suez, J., Mahdi, J. A., Matot, E., Malka, G., Kosower, N., Rein, M., Zilberman-Schapira, G., Dohnalová, L., Pevsner-Fischer, M., ... Segal, E. (2015). Personalized Nutrition by Prediction of Glycemic Responses. *Cell*, *163*(5), 1079–1094. doi:10.1016/j.cell.2015.11.001 PMID:26590418

Zhang, V. (2017). *The pros and cons of IoT edge analytics, White paper*. https://internetofthingsagenda.techtarget.com/blog/IoT-Agenda/The-pros-and-cons-of-IoT-edge-analytics

Zhang, A., & Lin, X. (2018). Towards secure and privacy-preserving data sharing in e-health systems via consortium blockchain. *Journal of Medical Systems*, *42*(8), 140. doi:10.100710916-018-0995-5 PMID:29956061

Zhang, P., White, J., Schmidt, D. C., Lenz, G., & Rosenbloom, S. T. (2018). FHIRChain: Applying blockchain to securely and scalably share clinical data. *Computational and Structural Biotechnology Journal*, *16*, 267–278. doi:10.1016/j.csbj.2018.07.004 PMID:30108685

Zhanyang, X. & Wentao, L. (2020). Artificial Intelligence for Securing IoT Services in Edge Computing: A Survey. *Security and Communication Networks*, 1–13.

Zhao, S., Fung-Leung, W.-P., Bittner, A., Ngo, K., & Liu, X. (2014). Comparison of RNA-Seq and Microarray in Transcriptome Profiling of Activated T Cells. *PLoS One*, *9*(1), e78644. doi:10.1371/journal.pone.0078644 PMID:24454679

Z. Zheng, S. Xie, H. Dai, X. Chen, & H. Wang (Eds.). (2017). Big data (bigdata congress) *IEEE International Congress on 2017*. IEEE Publications.

Zhiqiang, H., & Junming, Z. (2011). *The Application of Internet of Things in Education and Its Trend of Development*. Modern Distance Education Research.

Zhou, J., Cap, Z., Dong, X., & Vasilakos, A. V. (2017). Security and privacy for cloud-based IoT: Challenges. *IEEE Commun Mag. Vol*, *55*(1), 26–33. doi:10.1109/MCOM.2017.1600363CM

Zhou, L., Wang, L., & Sun, Y. (2018). MIStore: A blockchain-based medical insurance storage system. *Journal of Medical Systems*, *42*(8), 149. doi:10.100710916-018-0996-4 PMID:29968202

Zou, Xu, Wang, Li, Chen, & Hu. (2017). A Survey on Secure Wireless Body Area Networks. *Hindawi Security and Communication Networks*. . doi:10.1155/2017/3721234

Zymr. (n.d.). Retrieved from https://www.zymr.com/5-key-benefits-of-cloud-computing-in-healthcare-industry/

About the Contributors

D. Jeya Mala has a Ph.D. in Software Engineering with Specialization on Software Testing and is Associate Professor in Thiagarajar College of Engineering, –a leading educational and philanthropic institution in Tamil Nadu, India. She had been in the industry for about 4 years. She has a profound teaching and research experience of more than 12 years. She has published a book on "Object Oriented Analysis and Design using UML" for Tata McGraw Hill Publishers. She has published more than forty (40) papers about her research works at leading international journals and conferences such as IET, ACM, Springer, World Scientific, Computing and Informatics etc. As a researcher, Dr. Jeya Mala had investigated practical aspects of software engineering and object oriented paradigms for effective software development. Her work on Software Testing has fetched grants from UGC under Major Research Project scheme. Her dissertation has been listed as one of the best Ph.D. thesis in the CSIR – Indian Science Abstracts. She has successfully guided numerous Software Development based projects for the IBM- The Great Mind Challenge (TGMC) contest. The project she has mentored during 2007, has received national level Best Top 10 Project Award – 2007, from IBM. Currently she is guiding Ph.D. and M.Phil research scholars under the areas of Software Engineering and optimization techniques. She is a life member of Computer Society of India and an invited member of ACEEE. She forms the reviewer board in Journals like IEEE Transactions on Software Engineering, Elsevier – Information Sciences, Springer, World Scientific, International Journal of Metaheuristics etc. She has organized several sponsored national level conferences and workshops, notably she is one of the organizers of "Research Ideas in Software Engineering and Security (RISES'13) – A run-up event of ICSE 2014 sponsored by Computer Society of India". She has been listed in Marquis Who's Who list in 2011. She has completed certification on Software Testing Fundamentals, Brain bench certification on Java 1.1 programming, IBM certification as Associate Developer Websphere Application Studio. She is a proud recipient of several laurels from industries like Honeywell, IBM and Microsoft for her remarkable contributions in the field of Software Development and Object Orientation.

* * *

Vishweshkumar Aithal has been working as Assistant Professor in the Department of Electronics and Communication Engineering of KLS Gogte Institute of Technology, Belagavi, an autonomous institute affiliated to Visvesvaraya Technological University, Belagavi since 3+ years. He has completed his Masters in Signal Processing. His research interests include the domain of Signal and Image Processing, Computer Vision. He has his papers published in reputed international conferences and journals. He intends to continue to do great contribution to his field of research interests mentioned above.

Anto Cordelia Tanislaus Antony Dhanapal received her Ph. D in Food Science and Nutrition from Avinashilingam Institute for Home Science and Higher Education for Women, Coimbatore, TN, India and is currently attached to the Center for Biomedical and Nutrition Research (CBNR), Faculty of Science, Universiti Tunku Abdul Rahman, Kampar, Malaysia. She is actively involved in teaching and research for the past two decades. She has published in various peer reviewed indexed journals and book chapters. She is the recipient of many national and international grants in the field of Food Science and Nutrition. She is also the member of Nutrition Society of Malaysia (NSM), Nutrition Society of India, Malaysian Association for then study of obesity (MASO) and Malaysian Body Composition Society. She is Editorial Board Member for numerous journals and is now serving as Assistant Professor in the Department of Chemical Science, UTAR, Malaysia.

Anil B. Malali is Head of the Department of Commerce and Management, Àcharya Institute of Graduate Studies. He has received his Ph.D., in Commerce from Alagappa University, Tamilnadu. He is known for his proficiency in Accounts and Finance. He is having 20 years of teaching experience in the field of Commerce and Management. He has published several research articles in the leading National as well as International Journals. His current research interests are Accounts and Finance.

G. Vinoth Chakkaravarthy received Ph.D in Computer Science and Engineering from Anna University Chennai, M.E degree in Computer Science and Engineering in Anna University Chennai and B.E degree in Computer Science and Engineering from Madurai Kamaraj University. He is an Associate Professor of Computer Science and Engineering in Velammal College of Engineering & Technology. He has authored more than 15 publications in journals and conferences. He is the Co-PI of the funded project from DST, India, MNRE India by MNRE and IEDC, DST. His research interests include Cryptography, Network Security, data security and privacy, Internet of Things and VANET security.

Hema D. is a passionate professor of Computer Science and an active researcher. Her subject interests include Computer architecture, Microcontroller, Machine learning algorithms, and Image Processing. She is the coordinator of the Centre for Communication and Multimedia at Lady Doak College. She received a letter of appreciation from IIT Bombay for conducting training and certification of MOOCs for the Lady Doak College community. Her research focuses on machine learning and deep learning techniques for Computer Vision. She has published over 6 research articles in national and international peer-reviewed journals indexed by Scopus, Web of Science, etc. She has also been a reviewer for the International Journal of Computer Applications. She was funded by the National Science Foundation (NSF) to attend a Semester Workshop at ICERM, USA. She got selected under CSIR Summer Research Training Program and worked in an interdisciplinary project on computational chemistry to contribute to the building of knowledge society. She has written a chapter in the book "A learner-centered instruction manual for Environmental education".

Sofia G. has been working as an Associate Professor in the Department of Computer Science, Lady Doak College, Madurai with more than 19 years of teaching experience. She has completed M.C.A, M.Phil., and Ph.D in Computer Science. She has also involved herself in various academic activities, attended many national and international seminars, conferences and presented numerous research papers and served as resource persons. She has presented many papers in National and International conferences and receive best paper award. As a contribution to her research 8 papers are published well reputed International journals. Her areas of specialization are Image Processing and Data Science.

Sudhakar Hallur has been working as Assistant Professor in the Department of Electronics and Communication Engineering of KLS Gogte Institute of Technology, Belagavi, an autonomous institute, affiliated to Visvesvaraya Technological University, Belagavi since 4+ years. He has completed his Masters in Digital Communication and Networking with a Gold Medal. He also has a strong working experience on Software Development and Testing in Industry. His research interests include the domain of Biomedical Signal Processing, Computer Networking, Cryptography, Automobiles and Electrical Vehicles. He has his papers and book chapters published in reputed international conferences and journals. He intends to continue to do great contribution to his field of research interests mentioned above.

Roopa Kulkarni has been working as Associate Professor with Dayanand Sagar Academy of Technology and Management, Bengaluru, affiliated to Visvesvaraya Technological University, Belagavi, Karnataka for more than 1+ years. She has previously worked as Associate Professor, KLS Gogte Institute of Technology, Belagavi for more than 16 years. She has significantly contributed to the domain of Embedded Systems, Low Power VLSI, HDL and others with a huge number of papers and book chapters published in national and International conferences and journals. She has guided with more than 40 projects at various levels and have secured various funds and awards.

Sudha M. is currently working as Assistant Professor and Head of the Department of Management, Acharya Institute of Graduate Studies. She has received her Ph.D., in the Management domain from Alagappa University, Tamilnadu. She is known for his proficiency in Marketing and Finance and has 14 years of teaching experience in the field of Commerce and Management, and three years of Industrial Experience. She has also received an Award from the GSN Publications for her Academic Excellence in the year 2021. She has published several research articles in the leading National as well as International Jou1nals. Her current research interest is in marketing management.

Subramaniam Meenakshi Sundaram is currently working as Professor and Head in the Department of Computer Science and Engineering at GSSS Institute of Engineering and Technology for Women, Mysuru. He obtained his Bachelor Degree in Computer Science & Engineering from Bharathidasan University, Tiruchirappalli in 1989, M.Tech from National Institute of Technology, Tiruchirappalli in 2006 and Ph.D. in Computer Science & Engineering from Anna University Chennai in 2014. He has published 53 papers in refereed International Journals, presented 3 papers in International Conferences and has delivered more than 40 seminars. He is a reviewer of Springer – Soft Computing Journal, International Journal of Ah Hoc Network Systems, Journal of Engineering Science and Technology, Taylor's University, Malaysia and International Journal of Computational Science & Engineering, Inderscience Publishers, UK. He has organized more than 40 seminars / Workshops / FDPs.He has attended more than 45 Workshops / Seminars. His area of interest includes Computer Networks, Wireless Communication, Software Engineering, Optical Networks and Data Mining. He is a Life Member of Indian Society for Technical Education (ISTE) and a member of Computer Society of India (CSI). He has 30 Years of teaching experience and 10 years of research experience. Currently 7 research scholars are pursuing Ph.D. in VTU Belagavi, India under his guidance.

Sumathy Mohan, M.Com., M.B.A., (M) M.B.A., (F)., PGDCA., M.A(WS)., M.Phil., PhD, D.Litt., completed her Schooling in St.Theresa,s Girls Higher Secondary School, Karur, Graduated and Post Graduated in Seethalakshmi Ramasamy College, Tiruchirapalli and did her M.Phil in H.H.The Raja's College, Pudukottai, She pursued her Doctoral Degree from Jamal Mohamed College and degree been awarded by Bharathidasan University, Tiruchirapalli. She served as Dean, School of Commerce, Professor, Associate Professor, Reader in Bharathiar University, Coimbatore and currently working as Professor & Head, Department of Commerce Bharathiar University, Coimbatore, TamilNadu, has put in three decades of teaching in the field of Commerce and Management Subjects. Previously she served as Faculty, HOD and Principal in Srisarada Niketan College of Science for Women, Karur and Head of the Department of Commerce and Corporate Secretaryship in Vivekanandha College of Arts and Science for women, Tiruchengode and as Lecturer and Assistant Professor of Commerce in Periyar University, Salem. She guided 70 Post Graduate Commerce and Management Students, 51 M.Phil and 18 PhD Scholars have been awarded. She authored 15 Books including edited Volumes and textbooks and to name a few "Banking Industry in India", "Globalization and Consumerism-issues and Challenges", "Consumer Awareness, Welfare and Protection Problems", Research Paradigms in Social Sciences Research, Teaching of Commerce etc., A Handbook of e-governance in India. Her 188 research papers have been published in various National, International, Refereed, Peer-Reviewed, Scopus, and Web of Science Journals with impact factor also contributed 17 chapters for the edited book. She has participated and chaired International and National Seminars/conferences and presented 163 research papers in India and Abroad. During COVID 19 pandemic she participated 44 Online workshops/Training /Faculty Development Programmes and 15 Certificate Programmes including Leadership Programmes. She organized 27 Programmes like National Seminars, Research methodology workshops, Anveshan: Research Convention for faculty and Scholars including funded programmes with a tune of Rs. 15,73,000/- from various National funding Agencies including the Ministry of Consumer Affairs and MHRD.GoI, Association of Indian Universities, New Delhi. She has completed Six Major Research Projects and Five Minor Research Projects with funding of Rs.45,58,610 sponsored by UGC, ICSSR,IIPA, RUSA New Delhi and worked as the Project Director for the research projects sponsored by the Ministry of Consumer Affairs, New Delhi, NCDEX Mumbai and Tamilnadu Rural Development Projects including Malcolm Elizabeth Adishesiah Trust Chennai. She is the Co-ordinator of the UGC SAP DRS-I project on the Topic," Environmental Accounting and Audit for Sustainable Development" with funding of Rs.41,00,000/- She has been registered three copyrights on the topics Perception of Women on New Economic Policy, Evaluative Model on Perception of Users towards E-Governance Practices, A Hand-Book of e-Governance Practices in India, SWOT Analysis Model on e-Governance Practices. During her period she signed Three MoU with ICSI, New Delhi and NSE Academy, Mumbai and AIC-NIFTEA, Tirupur . She is a member of the editorial board and Review Board for 15 National and International journals and the Life Member of various Academic Associations such as All India Commerce Association (ICA) TN 029 Association of Economist of Tamil Nadu (AET) All India Accounting Association Indian Institute of Public Administration, New Delhi (IIPA) Regional Association for women Studies (RAWS) Indian Academic Researchers Association (IARA). She acted as a Resource Person and delivered 129 lectures. She has Participated and Presented 163 research Papers in the National and International Conference including Malaysia, Sri Lanka, Sharjah, UAE, Singapore, Thailand and Vietnam. She is the recipient of four awards for various academic purposes Travel Award for The Ninth IIMS International Conference, Honai, Vietnam and chaired a Session and ICSSR New Delhi granted Rs. 40,756/- She got. Certificate of Appreciation Appreciation Towards the Spread of Digital Financial Literacy in Effecting to Excel and Achieve Second Rank Among top Best 20 Institutions out of

4896 Institutions and also towards meritorious service and valuable contribution as coordinator National Anveshan (SRC)2017-18. She served as NSS Programme officer, Deputy Warden, Warden in Periyar and Bharathiar Universities, Karur District Railway consultative committee Member, Coordinator for Academic Activities, Vice-Chancellor Nominee and also as Chairman, Member Board of Studies. She also served as Presiding Officer in the Lok Sabha Elections. Now she is the recipient of The Esteemed TANSA Award in Social Sciences Category from the government of Tamilnadu. Her current research interests include Banking Marketing, Finance, Rural Development, She.

Tejaswini R. Murgod received B.E. Degree in Computer Science and Engineering from Visvesvarya Technological University, Belagavi, India in June 2008. She acquired her Master's Degree in from Visvesvarya Technological University, Belagavi, India in Jan 2015. At present she is working as Assistant Professor at GSSS Institute of Technology for women, Mysuru. Currently she is pursuing Ph. D at Visvesvaraya Technological University, Belagavi and completed comprehensive viva. Her research focus includes underwater communication, Optical networks and wireless networks.

Jin Yong Park is a Professor of Marketing in School of Business, Konkuk University, Seoul, Korea. He holds a Ph.D. from Yonsei University, Seoul, Korea. His research interests include channels of distribution, retailing management, online consumer behaviors, information quality in marketing channels, and e-business research. His papers appear in marketing, information technology, and management-related journals and proceedings of international conferences.

Prashant Patavardhan has been serving as Professor and Head of the Department of Electronics and Communication Engineering in RVITM, Bengaluru, affiliated to Visveswaraya Technological University, Belagavi, Karnataka for more than 1+ years. He has previously worked as Professor in Dayanand Sagar University and KLS Gogte Institute of Technology, Belagavi for more than 22 years. He has significantly contributed to the domain of Image Processing, Embedded Systems, Biometrics, Networks, Video Analytics and others with a huge number of papers and book chapters published in national and International conferences and journals. He has guided with more than 40 projects at various levels and have secured various funds and awards.

Kanthavel R. has 22 years of experience in teaching and research in the field of information and Communication Engineering. He has the credit of more than 100 research articles in peer reviewed international Journals. His areas of interests are computer networking, Machine Learning and AI, Cooperative communication, computing and mobile networks.

Lavanya Raja received B.E and M.E degree in Computer Science and Engineering in Anna University .She is an Assistant Professor of Computer Science and Engineering in Thiagarajar College of Engineering, Madurai. She has authored more than 10 publications in journals and conferences. Her research interests include Cryptography, Network Security, data security and privacy, Internet of Things security.

S. V. K. R. Rajeswari is a Research Scholar in SRMIST, Kattankulathur, Chennai-Tamil Nadu, India. She is pursuing her Ph.D. from the faculty of Electronics and Communication Engineering department. She completed her M.Tech in 2013 with Embedded Systems Technology as her specialization. She received her Bachelor's of Technology from J.N.T.U.H, India. She is driven with her research in the Embedded Systems. Her current area of research is IoT, Machine Learning & Deep Learning.

Dhaya Ramakrishnan has 16 years of experience in teaching and research in the field of Computer Science and Engineering. She published more than 80 research papers in peer reviewed international Journals. She was the recipient of IEI Young women Engineer award. Her areas of interests are wireless sensor networks, embedded systems, Machine Learning, Communication Systems.

Gopalakrishnan Subramaniyan is presently working as Head-Research and Development Dept. and Associate Professor, Department of Commerce & Management, Acharya Institute of Graduate Studies, Bangalore. He has 25 years of experience including 12 years of industry and 12 years of management teaching experience. He was holding responsibilities of vice principal in his previous assignment and he has got an International experience of 1 year worked in Nigeria as Lecturer-Coordinator at University of UYO. His Industry experience includes holding positions like Senior Manager - Education & Training at Pentagon Global Solutions-Chennai, Academics Head at Aptech Limited-Chennai, HOD for Department of Management. He authored more than 30 Publications in National Level and International Journals and presented papers in conferences. He authored a book titled "Strategic Management & Corporate Governance" by Thakur Publications for III semester MBA students, Bangalore University. He was awarded with a Research Project for 8 Lakhs on "Solid Waste Management" by Central Government department ICSSR (Indian Council for Social Sciences Research, New Delhi). His professional association includes, ISTE & IAAC.

Dhanabalan Thangam is presently working as an Assistant Professor in Commerce and Management at Acharya Institute of Graduate Studies, Banglore, India. Earlier he was worked as Post - Doctoral researcher at Konkuk School of Business, Konkuk University, Seoul, Korea South. He received his Ph.D. degree in Management from Alagappa University, Tamilnadu, India. His current research interests are marketing, small business management, and artificial intelligence in management fields. He has authored several books, research articles, and proceedings presented at many professional conferences and venues.

Ponnusamy Vijayakumat has completed his Ph.D. from SRM IST (2018), Master in applied Electronics from the college of engineering Guindy(2005), B.E in Electronics and Communication Engineering, Madras University (2000). He is a Certified "IoT specialist" and "Data scientist. His current research interests are in machine learning, Deep learning and applications, data analytics, IoT-based intelligent system design, cognitive radio networks, and smart systems. He is a senior member of IEEE. He is currently working as Professor in the ECE Department, SRM IST, Chennai, Tamil Nadu, and India.

Index

R

S

T

Z

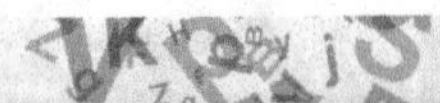

Recommended Reference Books

IGI Global's reference books are available in three unique pricing formats: Print Only, E-Book Only, or Print + E-Book.

Shipping fees may apply.

www.igi-global.com

ISBN: 978-1-5225-9687-5
EISBN: 978-1-5225-9689-9
© 2020; 405 pp.
List Price: US$ **225**

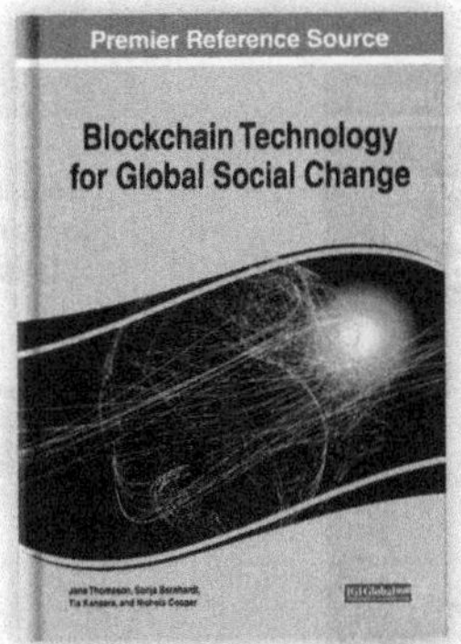

ISBN: 978-1-5225-9578-6
EISBN: 978-1-5225-9580-9
© 2019; 243 pp.
List Price: US$ **195**

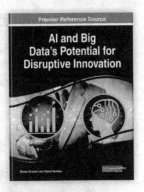

ISBN: 978-1-5225-5912-2
EISBN: 978-1-5225-5913-9
© 2019; 349 pp.
List Price: US$ **215**

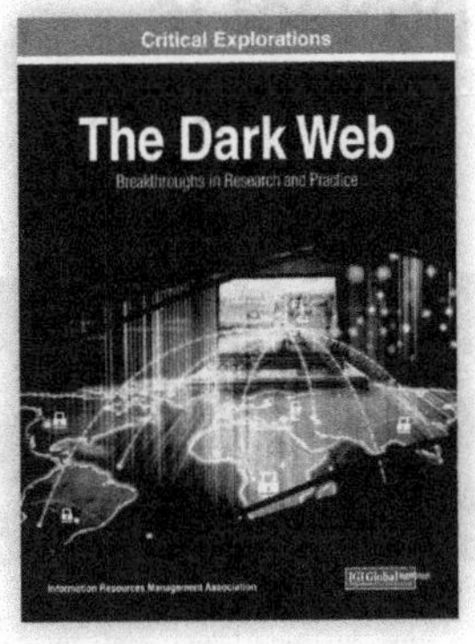

ISBN: 978-1-5225-3163-0
EISBN: 978-1-5225-3164-7
© 2018; 377 pp.
List Price: US$ **395**

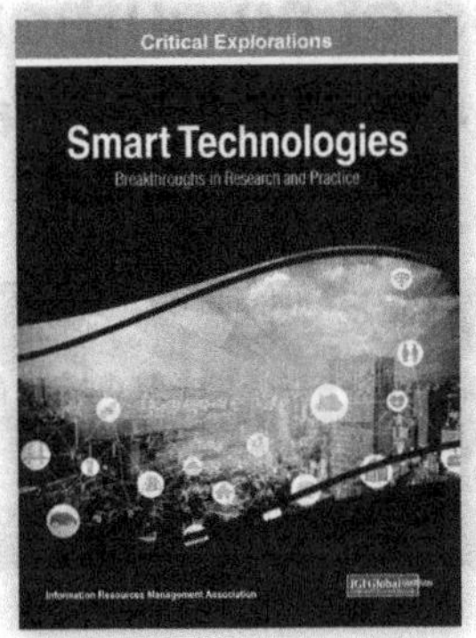

ISBN: 978-1-5225-2589-9
EISBN: 978-1-5225-2590-5
© 2018; 602 pp.
List Price: US$ **345**

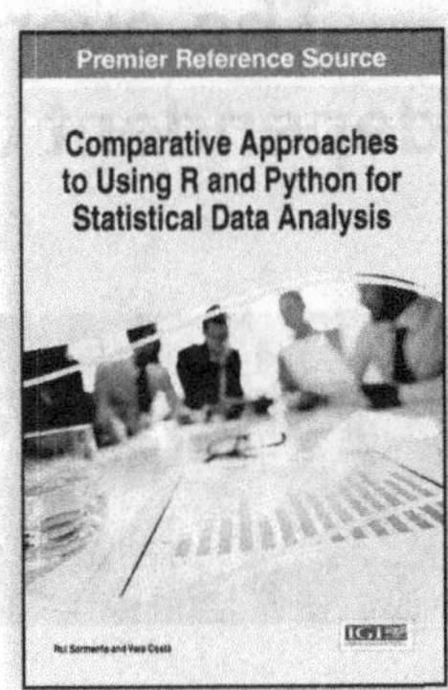

ISBN: 978-1-68318-016-6
EISBN: 978-1-5225-1989-8
© 2017; 197 pp.
List Price: US$ **180**

Do you want to stay current on the latest research trends, product announcements, news, and special offers?

Join IGI Global's mailing list to receive customized recommendations, exclusive discounts, and more.
Sign up at: **www.igi-global.com/newsletters.**

Publisher of Peer-Reviewed, Timely, and Innovative Academic Research

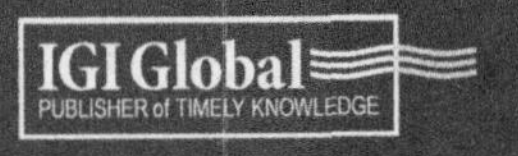

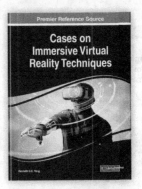

www.igi-global.com Sign up at www.igi-global.com/newsletters facebook.com/igiglobal twitter.com/igiglobal linkedin.com/igiglobal

Ensure Quality Research is Introduced to the Academic Community

Become an Evaluator for IGI Global Authored Book Projects

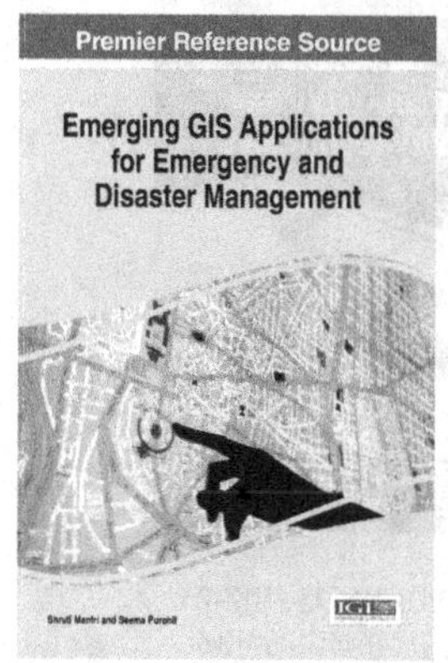

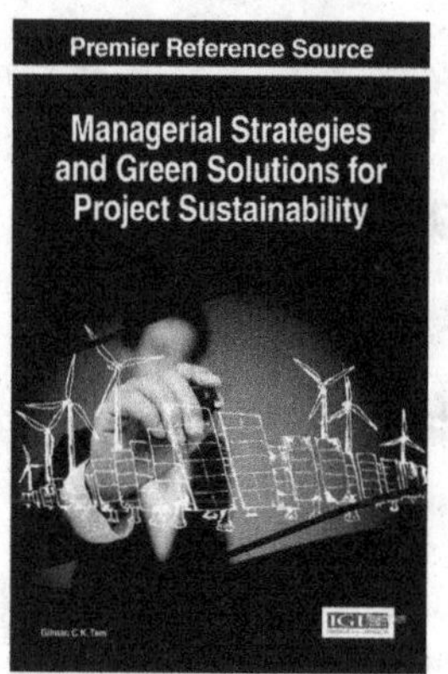

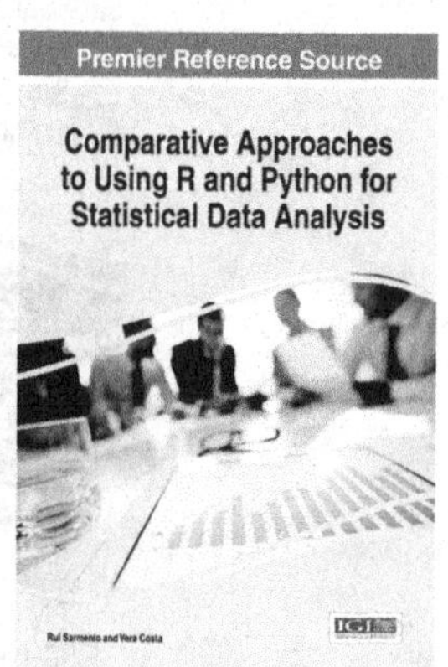

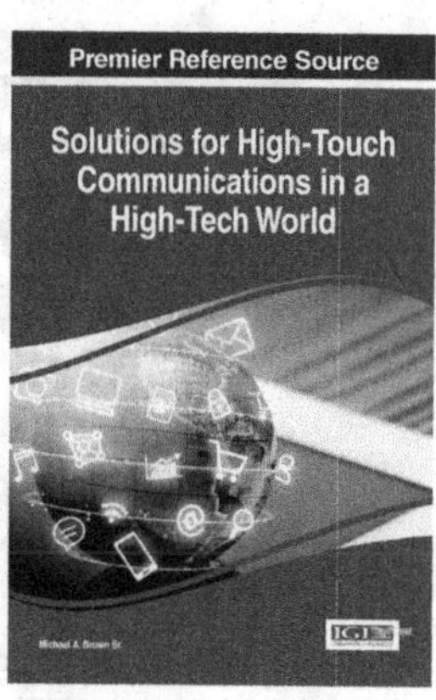

The overall success of an authored book project is dependent on quality and timely manuscript evaluations.

Applications and Inquiries may be sent to:
development@igi-global.com

Applicants must have a doctorate (or equivalent degree) as well as publishing, research, and reviewing experience. Authored Book Evaluators are appointed for one-year terms and are expected to complete at least three evaluations per term. Upon successful completion of this term, evaluators can be considered for an additional term.

If you have a colleague that may be interested in this opportunity, we encourage you to share this information with them.

IGI Global Author Services

Providing a high-quality, affordable, and expeditious service, IGI Global's Author Services enable authors to streamline their publishing process, increase chance of acceptance, and adhere to IGI Global's publication standards.

Benefits of Author Services:

- **Professional Service:** All our editors, designers, and translators are experts in their field with years of experience and professional certifications.
- **Quality Guarantee & Certificate:** Each order is returned with a quality guarantee and certificate of professional completion.
- **Timeliness:** All editorial orders have a guaranteed return timeframe of 3-5 business days and translation orders are guaranteed in 7-10 business days.
- **Affordable Pricing:** IGI Global Author Services are competitively priced compared to other industry service providers.
- **APC Reimbursement:** IGI Global authors publishing Open Access (OA) will be able to deduct the cost of editing and other IGI Global author services from their OA APC publishing fee.

Author Services Offered:

English Language Copy Editing
Professional, native English language copy editors improve your manuscript's grammar, spelling, punctuation, terminology, semantics, consistency, flow, formatting, and more.

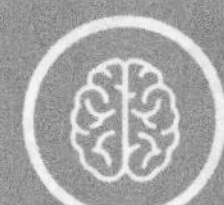

Scientific & Scholarly Editing
A Ph.D. level review for qualities such as originality and significance, interest to researchers, level of methodology and analysis, coverage of literature, organization, quality of writing, and strengths and weaknesses.

Figure, Table, Chart & Equation Conversions
Work with IGI Global's graphic designers before submission to enhance and design all figures and charts to IGI Global's specific standards for clarity.

Translation
Providing 70 language options, including Simplified and Traditional Chinese, Spanish, Arabic, German, French, and more.

Hear What the Experts Are Saying About IGI Global's Author Services

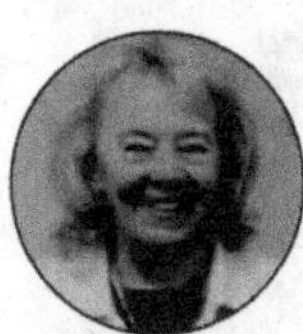

"Publishing with IGI Global has been ***an amazing experience*** *for me for sharing my research. The* ***strong academic production*** *support ensures quality and timely completion."* – **Prof. Margaret Niess, Oregon State University, USA**

"The service was ***very fast, very thorough, and very helpful*** *in ensuring our chapter meets the criteria and requirements of the book's editors. I was* ***quite impressed and happy*** *with your service."* – **Prof. Tom Brinthaupt, Middle Tennessee State University, USA**

Learn More or Get Started Here:

For Questions, Contact IGI Global's Customer Service Team at cust@igi-global.com or 717-533-8845

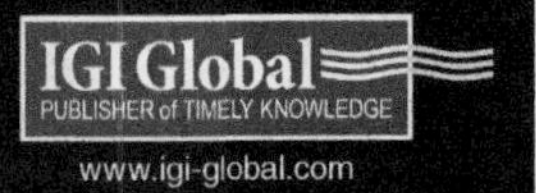

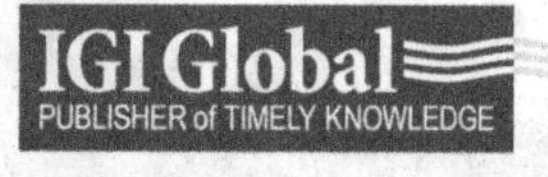

www.igi-global.com

Celebrating Over 30 Years of Scholarly Knowledge Creation & Dissemination

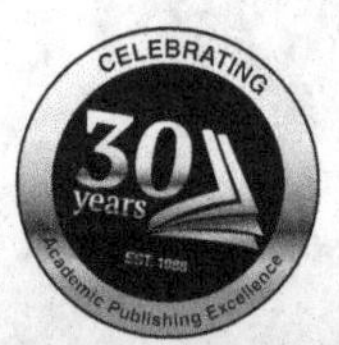

InfoSci®-Books

A Database of Nearly 6,000 Reference Books Containing Over 105,000+ Chapters Focusing on Emerging Research

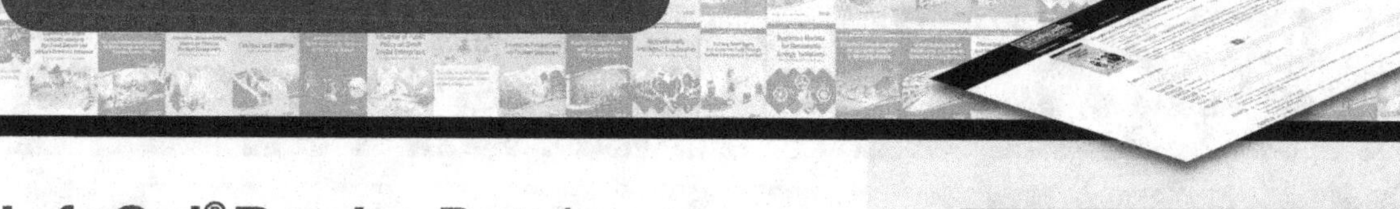

GAIN ACCESS TO **THOUSANDS** OF REFERENCE BOOKS AT **A FRACTION** OF THEIR INDIVIDUAL LIST **PRICE**.

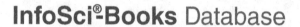

InfoSci®-Books Database

The **InfoSci®-Books** is a database of nearly 6,000 IGI Global single and multi-volume reference books, handbooks of research, and encyclopedias, encompassing groundbreaking research from prominent experts worldwide that spans over 350+ topics in 11 core subject areas including business, computer science, education, science and engineering, social sciences, and more.

Open Access Fee Waiver (Read & Publish) Initiative

For any library that invests in IGI Global's InfoSci-Books and/or InfoSci-Journals (175+ scholarly journals) databases, IGI Global will match the library's investment with a fund of equal value to go toward **subsidizing the OA article processing charges (APCs) for their students, faculty, and staff** at that institution when their work is submitted and accepted under OA into an IGI Global journal.*

INFOSCI® PLATFORM FEATURES

- Unlimited Simultaneous Access
- No DRM
- No Set-Up or Maintenance Fees
- A Guarantee of No More Than a 5% Annual Increase for Subscriptions
- Full-Text HTML and PDF Viewing Options
- Downloadable MARC Records
- COUNTER 5 Compliant Reports
- Formatted Citations With Ability to Export to RefWorks and EasyBib
- No Embargo of Content (Research is Available Months in Advance of the Print Release)

**The fund will be offered on an annual basis and expire at the end of the subscription period. The fund would renew as the subscription is renewed for each year thereafter. The open access fees will be waived after the student, faculty, or staff's paper has been vetted and accepted into an IGI Global journal and the fund can only be used toward publishing OA in an IGI Global journal. Libraries in developing countries will have the match on their investment doubled.*

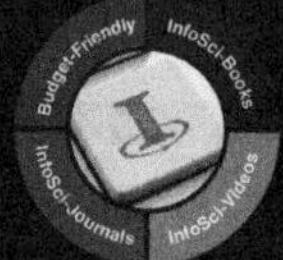

To Recommend or Request a Free Trial:
www.igi-global.com/infosci-books
eresources@igi-global.com • Toll Free: 1-866-342-6657 ext. 100 • Phone: 717-533-8845 x100

IGI Global
PUBLISHER of TIMELY KNOWLEDGE
www.igi-global.com

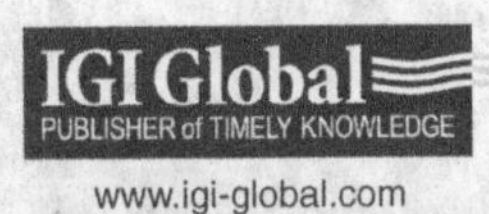

www.igi-global.com

Publisher of Peer-Reviewed, Timely, and Innovative Academic Research Since 1988

IGI Global's Transformative Open Access (OA) Model: How to Turn Your University Library's Database Acquisitions Into a Source of OA Funding

Well in advance of Plan S, IGI Global unveiled their OA Fee Waiver (Read & Publish) Initiative. Under this initiative, librarians who invest in IGI Global's InfoSci-Books and/or InfoSci-Journals databases will be able to subsidize their patrons' OA article processing charges (APCs) when their work is submitted and accepted (after the peer review process) into an IGI Global journal.

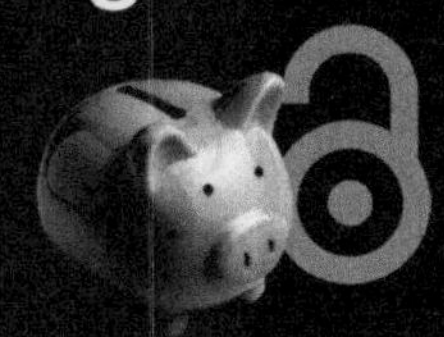

How Does it Work?

Step 1: **Library Invests in the InfoSci-Databases:** A library perpetually purchases or subscribes to the InfoSci-Books, InfoSci-Journals, or discipline/subject databases.

Step 2: **IGI Global Matches the Library Investment with OA Subsidies Fund:** IGI Global provides a fund to go towards subsidizing the OA APCs for the library's patrons.

Step 3: **Patron of the Library is Accepted into IGI Global Journal (After Peer Review):** When a patron's paper is accepted into an IGI Global journal, they option to have their paper published under a traditional publishing model or as OA.

Step 4: **IGI Global Will Deduct APC Cost from OA Subsidies Fund:** If the author decides to publish under OA, the OA APC fee will be deducted from the OA subsidies fund.

Step 5: **Author's Work Becomes Freely Available:** The patron's work will be freely available under CC BY copyright license, enabling them to share it freely with the academic community.

Note: *This fund will be offered on an annual basis and will renew as the subscription is renewed for each year thereafter. IGI Global will manage the fund and award the APC waivers unless the librarian has a preference as to how the funds should be managed.*

Hear From the Experts on This Initiative:

"I'm very happy to have been able to make one of my recent research contributions ***freely available*** along with having access to the ***valuable resources*** found within IGI Global's InfoSci-Journals database."

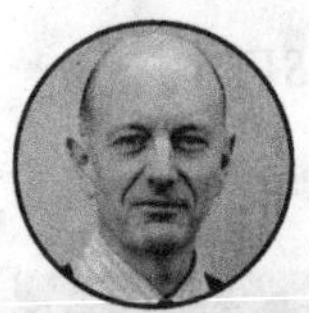

– **Prof. Stuart Palmer,** Deakin University, Australia

"Receiving the support from IGI Global's OA Fee Waiver Initiative ***encourages me to continue my research work without any hesitation.***"

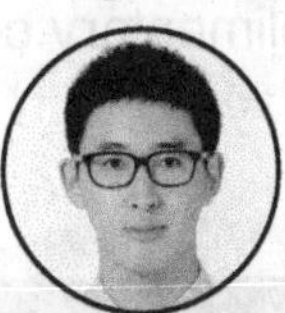

– **Prof. Wenlong Liu,** College of Economics and Management at Nanjing University of Aeronautics & Astronautics, China

For More Information, Scan the QR Code or Contact:
IGI Global's Digital Resources Team at eresources@igi-global.com.

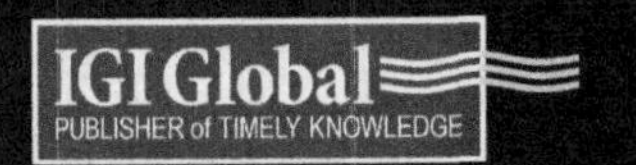

Are You Ready to **Publish Your Research?**

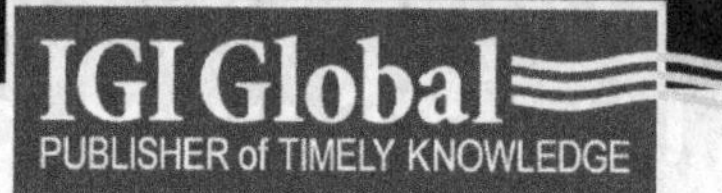

IGI Global offers book authorship and editorship opportunities across 11 subject areas, including business, computer science, education, science and engineering, social sciences, and more!

Benefits of Publishing with IGI Global:

- Free one-on-one editorial and promotional support.
- Expedited publishing timelines that can take your book from start to finish in less than one (1) year.
- Choose from a variety of formats, including: Edited and Authored References, Handbooks of Research, Encyclopedias, and Research Insights.
- Utilize IGI Global's eEditorial Discovery® submission system in support of conducting the submission and double-blind peer review process.
- IGI Global maintains a strict adherence to ethical practices due in part to our full membership with the Committee on Publication Ethics (COPE).
- Indexing potential in prestigious indices such as Scopus®, Web of Science™, PsycINFO®, and ERIC – Education Resources Information Center.
- Ability to connect your ORCID iD to your IGI Global publications.
- Earn honorariums and royalties on your full book publications as well as complimentary copies and exclusive discounts.

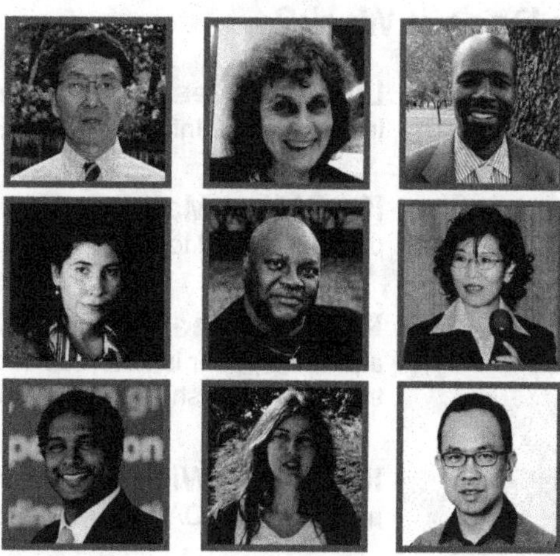

Join Your Colleagues from Prestigious Institutions, Including:

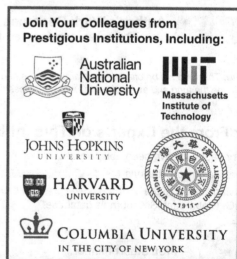

Learn More at: www.igi-global.com/publish

or Contact IGI Global's Aquisitions Team at: acquisition@igi-global.com

Purchase Individual IGI Global InfoSci-OnDemand Book Chapters and Journal Articles

InfoSci®-OnDemand

Pay-Per-View Articles and Chapters from IGI Global

For More Information, Visit: www.igi-global.com/e-resources/infosci-ondemand

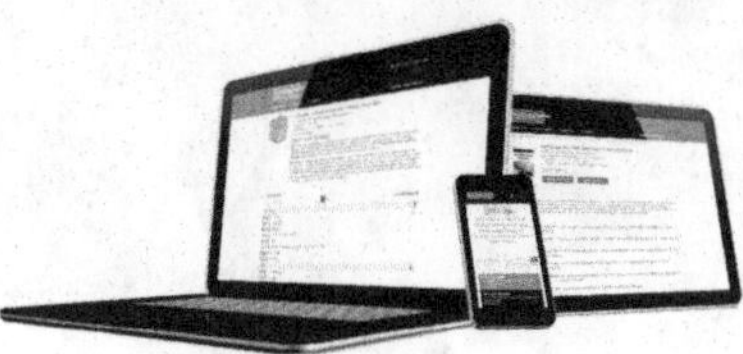

Browse through nearly 150,000+ articles/chapters to find specific research related to their current studies and projects that have been contributed by international researchers from prestigious institutions, including MIT, Harvard University, Columbia University, and many more.

Easily Identify, Acquire, and Utilize Published Peer-Reviewed Findings in Support of Your Current Research:

Accurate and Advanced Search:	Utilize the advanced InfoSci-OnDemand search engine to identify research in your area of interest.
Affordably Acquire Research:	Provide an affordable alternative to purchasing an entire reference book or scholarly journal.
Fast and Easy One-Click Shopping:	Simply utilize the OnDemand "Buy Now" button on the webpage.
Instantly Download/Access Your Content:	Receive an immediate link to download your InfoSci-OnDemand content to your personal computer and device.
Access Anywhere, Anytime, and on Any Device:	Additionally, receive access to your OnDemand articles and chapters through a personal electronic library.
Benefit from the InfoSci Platform Features:	Providing formatted citations, full-text PDF and HTML format, no embargo of content, no DRM, and more.

"It really provides **an excellent entry into the research literature of the field**. It presents a manageable number of **highly relevant sources** on topics of interest to a wide range of researchers. The sources are **scholarly, but also accessible** to 'practitioners'."

- Ms. Lisa Stimatz, MLS, University of North Carolina at Chapel Hill, USA

Interested in Additional Savings and Acquiring Multiple Articles and Chapters Through InfoSci-OnDemand?

Subscribe to InfoSci-OnDemand Plus

Learn More

Printed in the United States
by Baker & Taylor Publisher Services

Printed in the United States
by Baker & Taylor Publisher Services